Gastrointestinal Transplantation

Editors

ENRICO BENEDETTI
IVO G. TZVETANOV

GASTROENTEROLOGY CLINICS OF NORTH AMERICA

www.gastro.theclinics.com

Consulting Editor
ALAN L. BUCHMAN

June 2018 • Volume 47 • Number 2

ELSEVIER

1600 John F. Kennedy Boulevard ● Suite 1800 ● Philadelphia, Pennsylvania, 19103-2899
http://www.theclinics.com

GASTROENTEROLOGY CLINICS OF NORTH AMERICA Volume 47, Number 2
June 2018 ISSN 0889-8553, ISBN-13: 978-0-323-58401-2

Editor: Kerry Holland
Developmental Editor: Sara Watkins

Gastroenterology Clinics of North America (ISSN 0889-8553) is published quarterly by Elsevier Inc., 360 Park Avenue South, New York, NY 10010-1710. Months of issue are March, June, September, and December. Business and Editorial Offices: 1600 John F. Kennedy Blvd., Suite 1800, Philadelphia, PA 19103-2899. Customer Service Office: 6277 Sea Harbor Drive, Orlando, FL 32887-4800. Periodicals postage paid at New York, NY and additional mailing offices. Subscription prices are $350.00 per year (US individuals), $100.00 per year (US students), $659.00 per year (US institutions), $383.00 per year (Canadian individuals), $220.00 per year (Canadian students), $809.00 per year (Canadian institutions), $458.00 per year (international individuals), $220.00 per year (international students), and $809.00 per year (international institutions). Foreign air speed delivery is included in all *Clinics* subscription prices. All prices are subject to change without notice. **POSTMASTER**: Send address changes to *Gastroenterology Clinics of North America*, Elsevier Health Sciences Division, Subscription Customer Service, 3251 Riverport Lane, Maryland Heights, MO 63043. **Telephone: 1-800-654-2452 (U.S. and Canada); 314-447-8871 (outside U.S. and Canada). Fax: 314-447-8029. E-mail: journalscustomerservice-usa@elsevier.com (for print support); journalsonlinesupport-usa@elsevier.com (for online support).**

Reprints. For copies of 100 or more, of articles in this publication, please contact the Commercial Reprints Department, Elsevier Inc., 360 Part Avenue South, New York, New York 10010-1710. Tel. 212-633-3874, Fax: 212-633-3820, E-mail: reprints@elsevier.com.

Gastroenterology Clinics of North America is also published in Italian by Il Pensiero Scientifico Editore, Rome, Italy; and in Portuguese by Interlivros Edicoes Ltda., Rua Commandante Coelho 1085, 21250 Cordovil, Rio de Janeiro, Brazil.

Gastroenterology Clinics of North America is covered in *MEDLINE/PubMed (Index Medicus), Excerpta Medica, Current Contents/Clinical Medicine, Science Citation Index, ISI/BIOMED,* and *BIOSIS*.

Contributors

CONSULTING EDITOR

ALAN L. BUCHMAN, MD, MSPH, FACP, FACN, FACG, AGAF
Medical Director, Health Care Services Corporation; and Visiting Clinical Visiting Professor of Surgery and Medical Director, Intestinal rehabilitation and Transplant Center, University of Illinois at Chicago, Chicago, Illinois, USA

EDITORS

ENRICO BENEDETTI, MD, FACS
Warren H. Cole Chair in Surgery, Professor and Head, Department of Surgery, Division of Transplantation, The University of Illinois at Chicago, College of Medicine, Chicago, Illinois, USA

IVO G. TZVETANOV, MD, FACS
Carl H. & Billie M. Frese & Gerald S. Moss Professor in Transplant Surgery, Associate Professor and Chief, Department of Surgery, Division of Transplantation, The University of Illinois at Chicago, College of Medicine, Chicago, Illinois, USA

AUTHORS

KAREEM ABU-ELMAGD, MD, PhD, FACS
Professor of Surgery, Cleveland Clinic Lerner College of Medicine, Director, Center for Gut Rehabilitation and Transplantation, Cleveland Clinic, Cleveland, Ohio, USA

SAMIR ABU-GAZALA, MD
Department of Surgery, Transplantation Unit, Hadassah Hebrew University Medical Center, Jerusalem, Israel

SHERIF ARMANYOUS, MD
Research Fellow, Department of Nephrology, Cleveland Clinic, Cleveland, Ohio, USA

ENRICO BENEDETTI, MD, FACS
Warren H. Cole Chair in Surgery, Professor and Head, Department of Surgery, Division of Transplantation, The University of Illinois at Chicago, College of Medicine, Chicago, Illinois, USA

GEOFFREY J. BOND, MD
Assistant Professor, Department of Surgery, Division of Pediatric Transplantation, Hillman Center for Pediatric Transplantation, Children's Hospital of Pittsburgh of UPMC, Pittsburgh, Pennsylvania, USA

ALAN L. BUCHMAN, MD, MSPH, FACP, FACN, FACG, AGAF
Medical Director, Health Care Services Corporation; and Visiting Clinical Visiting Professor of Surgery and Medical Director, Intestinal rehabilitation and Transplant Center, University of Illinois at Chicago, Chicago, Illinois, USA

ROBERT E. CARROLL, MD
Department of Medicine, The University of Illinois at Chicago, Chicago Veterans
Administration Medical Center (West Side Division), Chicago, Illinois, USA

NESLIHAN CELIK, MD
Department of Surgery, Division of Pediatric Transplantation, Hillman Center for Pediatric
Transplantation, Children's Hospital of Pittsburgh of UPMC, Pittsburgh, Pennsylvania,
USA

GUILHERME COSTA, MD
Staff Surgeon, Center for Gut Rehabilitation and Transplantation, Cleveland Clinic,
Cleveland, Ohio, USA

GIUSEPPE D'AMICO, MD
Department of Surgery, Division of Transplantation, The University of Illinois at Chicago,
Chicago, Illinois, USA

CATERINA DI BELLA, MD
Department of Surgery, Division of Transplantation, The University of Illinois at Chicago,
Chicago, Illinois, USA

THOMAS M. FISHBEIN, MD
MedStar Georgetown University Hospital, Medtar Georgetown Transplant Institute,
Washington, DC, USA

MASATO FUJIKI, MD, PhD
Staff Surgeon, Center for Gut Rehabilitation and Transplantation, Cleveland Clinic,
Cleveland, Ohio, USA

ARMANDO GANOZA, MD
Assistant Professor, Department of Surgery, Division of Pediatric Transplantation,
Hillman Center for Pediatric Transplantation, Children's Hospital of Pittsburgh of UPMC,
Pittsburgh, Pennsylvania, USA

ANGELIKA C. GRUESSNER, MS, PhD, FAST
Department of Nephrology, SUNY Downstate Medical Center, Brooklyn, New York,
USA

RAINER W.G. GRUESSNER, MD
Department of Nephrology, SUNY Downstate Medical Center, Brooklyn, New York,
USA

JULIE K. HEIMBACH, MD
Chief, Division of Transplantation Surgery, Mayo Clinic, Rochester, Minnesota, USA

HOONBAE JEON, MD, FACS
Professor of Surgery, Tulane University, New Orleans, Louisiana, USA

BRENDAN KEATING, DPhil
Research Assistant Professor of Surgery, Division of Transplantation, Department
of Surgery, Penn Transplant Institute, University of Pennsylvania, Philadelphia,
Pennsylvania, USA

RUBEN KHAN, MD
Fellow, Department of Gastroenterology and Hepatology, The University of Illinois at
Chicago, Chicago, Illinois, USA

SEAN KOPPE, MD
Associate Professor of Medicine, Director of Hepatology, Department of Gastroenterology and Hepatology, The University of Illinois at Chicago, Chicago, Illinois, USA

ALEXANDRA LETO, BS
Division of Transplantation, Department of Surgery, Penn Transplant Institute, University of Pennsylvania, Philadelphia, Pennsylvania, USA

CAL S. MATSUMOTO, MD, FACS
MedStar Georgetown University Hospital, MedStar Georgetown Transplant Institute, Washington, DC, USA

GEORGE V. MAZARIEGOS, MD
Professor of Surgery and Critical Care Medicine, Department of Surgery, Division of Pediatric Transplantation, Hillman Center for Pediatric Transplantation, Children's Hospital of Pittsburgh of UPMC, Pittsburgh, Pennsylvania, USA

JOSE OBERHOLZER, MD, FACS
Department of Surgery, Division of Transplantation, University of Virginia Health System, Transplant Center, Charlottesville, Virginia, USA

KIM M. OLTHOFF, MD
Department of Surgery, Division of Transplant Surgery, Perelman School of Medicine, University of Pennsylvania, Philadelphia, Pennsylvania, USA

MOHAMMED OSMAN, MD
Staff Surgeon, Center for Gut Rehabilitation and Transplantation, Cleveland Clinic, Cleveland, Ohio, USA

NEHA PAREKH, MS, RD, LD, CNSC
Intestinal Transplant Coordinator, Center for Gut Rehabilitation and Transplantation, Cleveland Clinic, Cleveland, Ohio, USA

JEFFREY A. RUDOLPH, MD
Assistant Professor, Department of Pediatrics, Division of Gastroenterology, Children's Hospital of Pittsburgh of UPMC, Pittsburgh, Pennsylvania, USA

ABRAHAM SHAKED, MD, PhD
Eldridge L. Eliason Professor of Surgery, Division of Transplantation, Department of Surgery, Penn Transplant Institute, University of Pennsylvania, Philadelphia, Pennsylvania, USA

YANJUN SHI, MD, MS
Department of Surgery, Division of Pediatric Transplantation, Hillman Center for Pediatric Transplantation, Children's Hospital of Pittsburgh of UPMC, Pittsburgh, Pennsylvania, USA

RAKESH SINDHI, MD
Professor, Department of Surgery, Division of Pediatric Transplantation, Hillman Center for Pediatric Transplantation, Children's Hospital of Pittsburgh of UPMC, Pittsburgh, Pennsylvania, USA

KYLE SOLTYS, MD
Associate Professor, Department of Surgery, Division of Pediatric Transplantation, Hillman Center for Pediatric Transplantation, Children's Hospital of Pittsburgh of UPMC, Pittsburgh, Pennsylvania, USA

MARIO SPAGGIARI, MD
Department of Surgery, Division of Transplantation, The University of Illinois at Chicago, Chicago, Illinois, USA

SUKANYA SUBRAMANIAN, MD
MedStar Georgetown University Hospital, MedStar Georgetown Transplant Institute, Washington, DC, USA

KIARA A. TULLA, MD
Department of Surgery, Division of Transplantation, The University of Illinois at Chicago, Chicago, Illinois, USA

IVO G. TZVETANOV, MD, FACS
Carl H. & Billie M. Frese & Gerald S. Moss Professor in Transplant Surgery, Associate Professor and Chief, Department of Surgery, Division of Transplantation, The University of Illinois at Chicago, College of Medicine, Chicago, Illinois, USA

DANIEL ZAMORA-VALDES, MD
Division of Transplantation Surgery, Mayo Clinic, Rochester, Minnesota, USA

ANDREW ZHU, BSE
Division of Transplantation, Department of Surgery, Penn Transplant Institute, University of Pennsylvania, Philadelphia, Pennsylvania, USA

Contents

This article reviews the Adult-to-Adult Living Donor Liver Transplant Cohort Study (A2ALL). The findings show that the number of adult-to-adult living donor liver transplants is consistently increasing. Living donor liver transplant has an important benefit for patients with acute liver failure, does not compromise donor safety, and has lower rates of acute cellular rejection in biologically related donor and recipient. The conclusions from the A2ALL consortium have been critical in transplant advancement, supporting increased use to help decrease waitlist death and improve long-term survival of transplant recipients.

Acute liver failure is a rare but life-threatening disease that can lead to progressive encephalopathy, intracranial hypertension, and multiorgan failure. In the developed world, the most common cause remains acetaminophen overdose, but there are still many cases in which there is acute liver failure of unknown cause. The mainstay of acute liver failure management remains supportive care in the critical care setting. If supportive treatment does not stabilize the disease process, the patient may require emergent liver transplant. This article summarizes the current management of acute liver failure.

The rendering of proper care for the patient with intestinal failure requires the provider to have a functional understanding of digestion and absorption, nutrient requirements, and intestinal adaptation. Inherent in those concepts is that not only nutritional absorption but also medication absorption is compromised. The principles of the management of home parenteral nutrition must be mastered, and then proper and controlled weaning of parenteral nutrition may be commenced by use of dietary and pharmacologic means with appropriate clinical outcome measures followed. This complicated management requires a team experienced in both medical and surgical management of intestinal failure.

Adult intestinal transplant differs significantly from pediatric intestinal transplant. Although indications have remained largely consistent since 2000, indications for adults have expanded over the last 2 decades to include motility disorders and desmoid tumors. Graft type in adult recipients depends on the distinct anatomic characteristics of the adult recipient. Colonic inclusion, although initially speculated to portend unfavorable outcomes due to complex host-bacterial interactions, has increased over the past 2 decades with superior graft survival and improved patient quality of life. Overall, outcomes have steadily improved. For adult intestinal transplant candidates, intestinal transplantation remains a mainstay therapy for complicated intestinal failure and is a promising option for other life-threatening and debilitating conditions.

Pediatric intestinal transplantation has moved from the theoretic to an actual therapy for children with irreversible intestinal failure who are suffering from complications of total parenteral nutrition. Owing to significant advancement in the management of intestinal failure and prevention of parenteral nutrition–related complications that have led to a reduction in the incidence of parenteral nutrition–associated liver disease and improved intestinal adaptation, the indications for intestinal transplantation are evolving. Long-term outcomes have improved, but challenges in long-term graft function owing to chronic rejection and immunosuppressant-related complications remain the major opportunities for improvement.

Living donor intestinal transplant (LDIT) has been improved, leading to results comparable with those obtained with deceased donors. LDIT should be limited to specific indications and patient selection. The best indication is combined living donor intestinal/liver transplant in pediatric recipients with intestinal and hepatic failure; the virtual elimination of waiting time may avoid the high mortality experienced by candidates on the deceased waiting list. Potentially, LDIT could be used in highly sensitized recipients to allow the application of desensitization protocols. In the case of available identical twins or HLA-identical sibling, LDIT has a significant immunologic advantage and should be offered.

The growing population of intestinal transplant recipients present a unique challenge to the gastroenterologists responsible for their support and evaluation. Improvements in patient and graft survival are largely attributed to surgical advancements, refined antirejection therapy, and enhanced endoscopic surveillance protocols that better perceive rejection and other complications. This article reviews the endoscopic management and interventions provided for transplant recipients at the University of Illinois Hospital with complications, such as acute rejection, ischemia, bleeding, fistula, posttransplant lymphoproliferative disorder, and gastroparesis. Further research is needed on promising strategies currently used for related diseases to treat and sustain the intestinal graft.

GASTROENTEROLOGY
CLINICS OF NORTH AMERICA

Foreword

Transplantation of Abdominal Organs

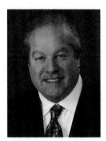

Alan L. Buchman, MD, MSPH, FACP, FACN, FACG, AGAF
Consulting Editor

Transplantation has encompassed many of the greatest recent advances in medicine. Now, all abdominal organs can be transplanted: liver, stomach, intestine, colon, pancreas, although spleen and gallbladder transplantation would not be particularly useful. The ultimate future goal is long-term functioning artificial organs. Transplantation, however, serves as an immediate bridge to that therapy, which is some time away from reality for most organs. Both graft and patient survival have improved dramatically due to advances in surgical technique and experience, immunosuppression and immunologic monitoring, and posttransplant care. Optimal patient outcome depends on an experienced team, each member with both defined and overlapping roles. Organ shortages have, to some degree, been alleviated by the use of the living donor. Most importantly, the best posttransplant outcomes are shaped by the selection of appropriate patients at the appropriate time. As pretransplant patient management improves, and in some cases transplantation can even be avoided, timing becomes even more important: avoiding premature transplantation, but also avoiding delayed transplantation when patient survival may be compromised.

In this issue of *Gastroenterology Clinics of North America*, Drs Benedetti and Tzvetanov have attempted to address these areas by engaging noted authors and investigators with substantial transplant experience to discuss the advancements in transplantation and patient care. Liver, intestine, pancreas, and multivisceral transplantation techniques, care, and outcome are discussed. Knowledge of the care of such patients is also important because it extends to the management of patients

Gastroenterol Clin N Am 47 (2018) xiii–xiv
https://doi.org/10.1016/j.gtc.2018.01.015
0889-8553/18/© 2018 Published by Elsevier Inc.

gastro.theclinics.com

outside the field of transplantation, namely the care of those with inflammatory bowel diseases.

Alan L. Buchman, MD, MSPH, FACP, FACN, FACG, AGAF
Intestinal Rehabilitation and Transplant Center
Department of Surgery
College of Medicine
The University of Illinois at Chicago
840 South Wood Street
Suite 402 Clinical Sciences Building, MC 958
Chicago, IL 60612, USA

Health Care Services Corporation
300 E. Randolph Street
Chicago, IL 60601, USA

E-mail address:
buchman@uic.edu

Preface

Gastrointestinal Transplantation

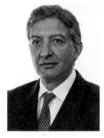
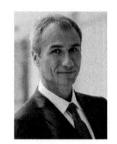

Enrico Benedetti, MD, FACS   Ivo G. Tzvetanov, MD, FACS
Editors

Organ transplantation plays an important role in the management of patients with end-stage organ diseases. Solid organ transplantation has experienced a steady development in surgical techniques as well as in immunosuppressive therapy; furthermore, the field has expanded in both volumes and indications. It is both challenging and important for practicing physicians without specific transplant training to be informed of the progress in the field.

The present issue of *Gastroenterology Clinics of North America* provides updated information on transplantation of the liver, pancreas, and intestine for practicing gastroenterologists.

Liver transplant recipients will be frequently seen by non-transplant-trained gastroenterologists and hepatologists for routine care. Recipients of less common transplants, such as the pancreas or the intestine, may be occasionally referred or identified within their practice. Information regarding gastrointestinal transplants will be certainly of interest for the audience of *Gastroenterology Clinics of North America*.

We have selected well-recognized specialists for each topic covered and requested them to provide the most relevant and up-to-date information. We trust that both transplant specialists and nonspecialists will find the information of interest.

Enrico Benedetti, MD, FACS
Department of Surgery
The University of Illinois at Chicago
College of Medicine
840 South Wood Street
Suite 402 (MC958)
Chicago, IL 60612, USA

Gastroenterol Clin N Am 47 (2018) xv–xvi
https://doi.org/10.1016/j.gtc.2018.01.014
0889-8553/18/© 2018 Published by Elsevier Inc.

Ivo G. Tzvetanov, MD, FACS
Division of Transplantation
Department of Surgery
The University of Illinois at Chicago
College of Medicine
840 South Wood Street
Suite 402 (MC958)
Chicago, IL 60612, USA

E-mail addresses:
Enrico@uic.edu (E. Benedetti)
itzveta@uic.edu (I.G. Tzvetanov)

Living Donor Liver Transplantation
Technical Innovations

Kiara A. Tulla, MD[a], Hoonbae Jeon, MD[b],*

KEYWORDS

- Living donor liver transplantation • Portal flow modulation
- Laparoscopic donor hepatectomy

KEY POINTS

- Selection of a donor and anatomic design of the allograft should be based on various factors of both the donor and the recipient.
- Small-for-size syndrome can be avoided by portal venous flow modulation in combination with careful calculation of required allograft volume.
- Large portosystemic collaterals may need to be obliterated to augment portal venous flow to the graft and to avoid portal venous steal.
- ABO-incompatible living donor liver transplantation can fail due to diffuse intrahepatic biliary strictures even with the use of optimal desensitization protocols.
- Minimally invasive approach for donor hepatectomy more common in high-volume living donor liver transplant programs.

INTRODUCTION

Liver transplantation has been serving as the best and the ultimate treatment for end-stage liver disease and certain hepatic malignant tumors for the past few decades. Striking developments in surgical technique, rapid acceptance of the procedure as the most sound treatment option, and outbreaks of hepatitis C related cirrhosis in the Western world created a wide gap between availability of livers from deceased donors for the ever-growing patient population that needed liver transplantation in the past 2 decades. For comparison, in 2010, Spain and the United States had the highest rates of deceased-donor liver transplantation (DDLT): 24.5 and 17.0 procedures per million compared with Taiwan and Korea at 4.0 and 6.0 per million, respectively.

Disclosure Statement: The authors have nothing to disclose.
[a] Department of Surgery, University of Illinois at Chicago, 840 South Wood Street, CSB 401, MC 958, Chicago, IL 60612, USA; [b] Department of Surgery, Tulane University, 1415 Tulane Avenue, #HC-5, New Orleans, LA 70112-2632, USA
* Corresponding author.
E-mail address: hjeon@tulane.edu

Gastroenterol Clin N Am 47 (2018) 253–265
https://doi.org/10.1016/j.gtc.2018.01.001
0889-8553/18/© 2018 Elsevier Inc. All rights reserved.

However, in that same year, Taiwan and Korea had the highest number of living donor liver transplantations (LDLTs) per million people, at 16.0 and 17.0 procedures, respectively, compared with 0.7 and 0.95 events per million in Spain and the United States, respectively,[1] This can be further understood because in Asia the issue with deceased organ donation has always been dire, with late legislation of brain death and lack of dedicated resources for organ recovery.[2] In response to such severe organ shortage, LDLTs between adults were started in a few leading institutions in Japan, Hong Kong, and Korea. Initial reluctance to support LDLT was seen, due to ethical concerns about donor safety and well-being, but was soon tempered by the obvious high demand for liver transplantation. Following by example, by 2000, many institutions in the United States started performing LDLT as well in response to worsening shortage of deceased-donor organs.[3–5]

With regard to the efficacy of living donor transplantation versus deceased-donor transplantation, a 14-year retrospective and prospective study of 1136 living and 464 deceased-donor liver recipients and their respective donors in the Adult-to-Adult Living Donor Liver Transplant Cohort Study in 2002 showed that after 10-year follow-up there is superior recipient survival with LDLT compared with undergoing or waiting for DDLT. This was further supported by data in which those with lower Model for End-Stage Liver Disease (MELD) scores still showed a benefit from having a living donor transplant.[6]

Despite widespread success and acceptance of LDLT, the procedure still has a steep learning curve and unresolved concern about donor safety.[7] A few well-publicized sets of donor mortalities in the early 2000s hampered enthusiasm for LDLT for the next few years.[8,9] Donation of a major portion of the liver is clearly a bigger undertaking for the donor than donating a kidney through a laparoscopic procedure. The transplant community continues to explore procedural endeavors to ensure the safety of the donor. The guidelines regarding donor selection criteria and selection of the surgical procedure are primarily dictated by donor safety; this is done at the potential expense of the transplant recipient. Therefore, careful selection of the recipient based on the best possible partial hepatic allograft provided by any given donor becomes of paramount importance for the successful LDLT.

SURGICAL CHALLENGES OF LIVING DONOR LIVER TRANSPLANTATION

Due to the anatomic nature of the liver being a single organ, partial hepatic allograft would pose some challenges in implantation because of the limited length of vascular pedicles and biliary ducts. Even with successful implantation, the small graft size may leave unmet metabolic demand of the recipient and may result in high morbidity and mortality. In the literature of hepatic resection of malignant tumors, it has been known that removal of healthy liver parenchyma up to 70% of the total volume is possible with traditionally reported mortality rate up to 8%.[10,11] However, that mortality risk in a healthy organ donors would be by no means acceptable. Initial attempts of LDLT used left lobe hepatic allograft, which removes approximately 40% to 45% of total liver volume of the donor to secure safe margins in the donor.[12] Most pioneering groups completing LDLT in Asia soon switched to a right lobe allograft to increase the size as they realized that left lobe allograft often becomes inadequate to meet the metabolic demand of the recipient.[13–15] Thus, all Western centers followed suit and started LDLT with right lobe allografts.

LDLT was conceptualized based on the regenerative capacity of the liver. Both the remnant liver in the donor and the hepatic allograft in the recipient grow bigger after the transplantation.[16] This regenerative process of the hepatic allograft may lead to dynamic changes in the spatial orientation of reconstructed blood vessels, especially the hepatic venous outflow.[17] Hepatic veins that become the draining basin of the vena cava are characterized by having very low pressure with a very high flow rate. Any disturbance of this state can lead to hepatic congestion, post-sinusoidal portal hypertension, and ascites.

Partial hepatic allografts inherently can only have short biliary stumps of intrahepatic ducts, making biliary reconstruction more technically demanding, and running a higher risk of leakage or stricture. This is especially true with right lobe grafts, which have higher incidences of biliary complications and a wider range of anatomic variations. For these reasons, the Roux-en-Y hepaticojejunostomy was used to ensure tension-free anastomosis of the biliary stump to a well-vascularized small bowel loop as the standard method of biliary reconstruction during early experiences in LDLT. Over time, for single-stump hepatic ducts, widespread use of duct-to-duct anastomosis in end-to-end fashion became standard. Various creative reconstruction methods are seen in the literature in hopes of achieving a salient duct-to-duct anastomosis. Concurrently, the donor procedure must be meticulous in identifying the exact locations of intrahepatic ducts near the confluence to obtain a single stump. Overzealous attempts to approach the biliary confluence may lead to stricture of the bile duct in the donor's remaining liver and thus, significant morbidity. The biliary anastomosis has always been considered the Achilles' heel of liver transplantation, and the incidence of biliary complication is proportional in frequency to the number of anastomosis to intrahepatic bile duct stumps. In nearly half of right lobe hepatic allografts, multiple hepatic duct stumps are present, and Roux-en-Y hepaticojejunostomy still is the anastomosis of choice for such situations.[18] Even with a single stump of the donor bile duct, there may be significant size mismatch with the recipient's duct. In such situations, more creative variations of anastomotic technique can be beneficial.[19]

Small-for-size syndrome (SFSS) is a relatively newly found entity observed in liver transplant recipients with small-sized hepatic allograft. The syndrome is characterized by persistent jaundice, ascites, and renal insufficiency. A small hepatic allograft appears unable to meet metabolic demand of the recipient, but also sustains damage from hyperperfusion from portal hypertension. These grafts often struggle with suboptimal function and can lead to high mortality from sepsis or renal failure.[20]

EARLY QUESTS FOR IDEAL GRAFT SIZE

In the quest for proper graft size, many studies estimate the standard total liver volume based on volumetric measurements using cross-sectional imaging studies that led to different formulas to calculate the liver volume in both the Asian population[21] and the Western population.[22] Regardless of different calculated formulas, the liver weighs approximately 2% of the body weight. In theory, the minimum size of the liver to maintain life is 0.6% (30% of the total liver weight) of total body weight. For surgical practice, early attempts of LDLT, used graft versus body weight ratios targeted to be greater than 0.8%.[23] Larger partial hepatic allografts of course offer greater benefit to recipients, but procurement of such a large portion of liver increases donor risk. Therefore, the selection of which type of partial hepatic allograft must be made with careful consideration of the age and anatomy of the donor, as well as the condition of the recipient.[24]

Removal of an arbitrary amount of hepatic parenchyma, while preserving anatomic integrity of the whole portion and workable vascular pedicles, is impossible. The size of hepatic allografts is determined by volume of each anatomic area and their combinations in the liver. Volume measurements of each anatomic section of the liver and evaluation of vascular anatomy are the first steps to the design a partial hepatic allograft. If there would be a significant difference in size between a smaller donor and a larger recipient, donation of the left lobe would be clearly out of consideration because of its small allograft size, and even the right lobe graft may not be adequate depending on volume distribution of hepatic parenchyma in different anatomic sections in the donor liver. Sufficient hepatic allograft size, which meets metabolic demand of the recipient, is also heavily dependent on the clinical status of the recipient. Therefore, all factors, including donor age, anatomic characteristics of the donor liver, degree of steatosis of the donor liver, and clinical severity of the recipient are evaluated for appropriation of the proper donor allograft for a particular recipient.[25] The Asan Medical Center group in Seoul, Korea, which has the largest LDLT experience in the world without a single donor mortality, uses specific donor selection guidelines that protect donors from hepatic failure, but also does not compromise recipient need for adequate liver volume and function for survival[26] (**Table 1**).

TECHNICAL BREAKTHROUGHS TO INCREASE GRAFT SIZE

Multiple groups continued to focus efforts on acquiring larger hepatic allograft size without compromising safety of the donor. In practice, full left lobe grafts including Couinaud segments 2, 3, and 4 with the middle hepatic vein were often inadequate in size for many recipients. The addition of the caudate lobe to the left lobe graft was proposed and attempted by Takayama and colleagues,[27] but the meager benefits from this small increase of the graft volume was challenged by the added complexity of implantation technique.

Lo and colleagues[28] first performed LDLT using an extended right lobe graft, which includes Couinaud segments 5, 6, 7, and 8 with the middle hepatic vein. That was the largest possible partial hepatic allograft that can be obtained from a living donor. Although the donor would have to undergo a potentially riskier procedure, this larger graft was clearly beneficial for patients. To mitigate this higher donor risk, some groups limited the right lobe allograft to not include the middle hepatic vein. The importance of venous outflow reconstruction during this early experience, prompted separate implantation of any short hepatic vein larger than 5 mm in diameter.[4] Lee and colleagues[29] reported venous congestion of the right anterior sector after transplantation. These patients characteristically had prolonged jaundice and ascites that mimiced SFSS despite larger size of the allograft. Although the right lobe allograft is larger than the left lobe allograft, it was found that the whole portion of the allograft may not function as expected, due to congestion of the drainage basin of the middle hepatic vein.[30] Segmental hepatic venous outflow leads to reversal of portal venous flow and eventually causes ischemia and atrophy of the corresponding sector.[31] The proposed solution for this venous congestion was reconstruction of hepatic

Table 1 Donor selection guideline by Asan Medical Center group in Seoul, Korea		
Donor Age, y	**Level of Fatty Infiltration**	**Donor Liver Volume Need**
≤35	No fatty changes	30% remnant liver volume
	<15% fatty changes	30%–35% remnant liver volume
	<30% fatty changes	>35% remnant liver volume
35–55	<15% fatty changes	>35% remnant liver volume

Data from Lee SG. A complete treatment of adult living donor liver transplantation: a review of surgical technique and current challenges to expand indication of patients. Am J Transplant 2016;15(1):17–38.

venous tributaries draining Couinaud segments 5 and 8 using saphenous vein. This technique of a routed reconstruction of hepatic venous tributaries was not initially embraced by some groups. In Hong Kong and Toronto, groups continued to use extended right lobe grafts that included the middle hepatic vein to avoid hepatic venous congestion. Others disregarded this issue with venous congestion of the right anterior sector, and achieved inferior outcomes. In retrospect, venous outflow reconstruction of the right anterior sector appears mandatory in 15% to 20% of cases.

An innovative way to cope with the size limitation of partial hepatic grafts, was described by Lee and colleagues[32] where a dual graft transplantation from 2 individual living donors was devised. Even with 2 small donors, 2 partial allografts can offer enough hepatic parenchyma to fulfill metabolic demand of the recipient. Besides the technical complexity of the procedure, logistic issues, and health insurance coverage issues, this potentially useful procedure has not been widely accepted in the Western world. Further work has persisted with this technique in a large series improving the surgical technique and its viability as a solution for issues with graft size.[33]

Conversely, in the rare situation with a donor who has a very large right hemi-liver and a small left hemi-liver, a partial hepatic allograft can be obtained from the right posterior section. And this right posterior section allograft can be larger than the full left lobe.[34]

PORTAL VENOUS FLOW OPTIMIZATION

Once the implantation of the graft is in place, there is a delicate balance between liver regeneration and the increasing demand of the liver to function. When a balance is not achieved between the graft and the recipient, manifestations of transplant failure can ensue. This phenomenon is described as SFSS,[35] in which the balance between the functional mass of the liver, the inflow of the portal vasculature, and the outflow of the hepatic vein are not harmonious, presenting postoperatively as primary hepatocyte dysfunction. Since the early experience of LDLT in pediatric recipients, inferior outcomes from small-for-size grafts (SFSGs) were noticed. Concerning histopathologic features (low mitosis rate, enhanced cholestasis and necrosis) were described by Emond et al[36] in a small series of SFSG transplantations in larger children. The Kyoto group first reported in 1999 a significantly lower graft survival in cases of LDLT using small grafts.[37] The combination of prolonged cholestasis, intractable ascites, encephalopathy, and persistent coagulopathy were thereafter acknowledged and reported as a specific clinical-anatomic-pathologic entity termed SFSS. To date, there is no universal definition, but rather a collection of signs and symptoms that may presuppose SFSS before hepatic failure. Furthermore, SFSS as an entity has been described as more than the direct consequence of SFSG because of the recipient factors that influence the vascular flow to and from the graft. The first proposal for parameters on the diagnosis of SFSS came from Dahm and colleagues,[38] who proposed a dysfunction of a partial graft with a graft-to-recipient body weight ratio (GRBWR) less than 0.8% during the first postoperative week after the exclusion of other causes, by the presence of 2 of the following parameters on 3 consecutive days: international normalized ratio greater than 2, total bilirubin greater than 5.8 mg/dL, and encephalopathy grade 3 or 4. They furthermore defined the "small-for-size nonfunction" as the failure of a small graft, with graft loss, retransplantation, or death during the first postoperative week after the exclusion of other causes. The most recent definition was proposed by Ikegami and colleagues[39] who depicted SFSS as an evolving situation of graft dysfunction termed "delayed functional hyperbilirubinemia": a condition with a total bilirubin greater than 20 mg/dL for more than 7 consecutive days after the first postoperative week, excluding technical, immunologic, and infectious factors. Currently, a donor liver is considered an SFSG when the GRBWR is less than 0.8 or when the ratio between graft volume and standard liver volume (GV/SLV) is less than 40%.[40]

Knowing excessive portal venous pressure and hyperperfusion of the hepatic allograft can cause shear injury to lining endothelium of hepatic sinusoid, various efforts have been made to decrease portal venous inflow to prevent SFSS.[41] To achieve the ideal flow rate in the portal vein and promote regeneration of partial hepatic allograft, splenic artery embolization or ligation has been described to decrease the portal venous flow rate by 30%. Splenic artery embolization or ligation in either the pretransplant or posttransplant period has been used to prevent or treat SFSS.[42,43] As devascularization of spleen may carry the risk of infarction and abscess of spleen, splenectomy was also proposed as a viable preventive measure.[44] Creation of a partial portosystemic shunt, such as mesocaval or splenorenal shunt, which diverts a modest amount of portal venous blood also has been proposed.[45–47] To prevent persistent steal of portal venous blood, endovascular technique to obliterate the shunt also has been described. All these strategies have been attempted to provide a favorable environment of for allograft hypertrophy and normal synthetic hepatocyte function.[48]

Cases with chronic portal vein thrombosis and stenosis are often associated with massive portosystemic collaterals, such as coronary or splenorenal varices and insufficient flow to the liver. As a result of the higher resistance in the portal vein, these collaterals often divert a very large amount of circulating blood. Even after transplantation, these collaterals may persist and continue to maintain flow, especially in a patient with high hepatic resistance, as a result of receiving a small partial graft. Moreover, these collaterals may cause excessive steal of portal venous flow and even lead to hepatic allograft ischemia secondary to hepatofugal flow.[49] Allograft edema from such an ischemic condition may increase the resistance even higher and create a vicious cycle leading to more ischemia and necrosis of the hepatic allograft. Such a disastrous consequence of persistent large portosystemic collateral has been described.[50] Therefore, in these cases, attention should be paid to obliterate these collaterals through ligation of the left renal vein or coronary vein,[51,52] meanwhile employing strategies such as thrombectomy, stenting, or venous bypass graft to improve the flow through the portal vein to the hepatic allograft.[53]

Optimal portal venous inflow should follow the principles: (1) avoidance of excessive inflow that may cause hepatic allograft damage, (2) obliteration of large portosystemic collaterals, and (3) creation of a large-diameter portal inflow conduit.

SIMPLIFICATION OF HEPATIC ALLOGRAFT CREATION

Despite widespread usage of right lobe allografts in most centers, a few Japanese institutions consistently used left lobe grafts in their relatively small patients with lower MELD scores <20.[54] Left lobe living donor hepatectomy is less risky for the donor and also produces a single hepatic duct stump in most cases, making the biliary reconstruction less technically challenging.[55] These are the clear benefits of left lobe allograft despite their small size, which with improper patient selection can increase the risk for SFSS. With accumulation of experience in patient selection (graft-recipient body weight ratio [GRBWR] >0.8, MELD <20, <2 predictive biliary anastomoses) and perioperative management, left lobe LDLT has utility if one uses proper selection criteria and portal venous flow optimization. Recently, more usage of left lobe allograft has been reported by Halazun et al.[56] and Botha et al.[57] where in they demonstrate comparable outcome with right lobe LDLT.

ABO-INCOMPATIBLE LIVING DONOR LIVER TRANSPLANTATION

ABO blood group compatibility was one of the essential requirements for successful adult LDLT until the early 2010s when the ever-changing landscape of immunosuppression opened the door to ABO-incompatible transplantation, especially in Asia. A small sample was first treated by Song and colleagues[58] in 2010 with anti–CD-20 (rituximab) infusions and plasmapheresis preoperatively and hepatic artery infusion, which resulted in no antibody-mediated rejection, no biliary complications, and survival for all 3 patients to 9.5 months of follow-up. The same group was able to reproduce results with a large sample size, making the ABO-incompatible LDLT a viable therapeutic option with an ever-growing demand for liver transplantation.[59] The success of this experience did bring to light in the past 4 years that these patients have dire complications that need to be further evaluated and studied, namely antibody-mediated rejection, manifested as diffuse intrahepatic biliary stricture. The largest single-center experience with ABO-incompatible adult living donor transplantation of 235 patients followed a desensitization protocol (including rituximab and total plasma exchange) that showed promising outcomes in comparison with the ABO-compatible groups.[60] Patient and surgical characteristics have been evaluated but no significant risk factors were identified for patients who would eventually succumb to diffuse intrahepatic biliary strictures. The biliary stricture–free survival was similar among all transplant patients; graft and patient survival rates were significantly reduced only when the ABO-incompatible recipients acquired diffuse intrahepatic biliary stricture, a devastating complication.[61] With vigilance and proper patient vetting, ABO-incompatible LDLT is a player in the organ pool available to many suffering from end-stage liver disease.

MINIMALLY INVASIVE DONOR HEPATECTOMY

Because of the size and the location of the liver, living donor hepatectomy traditionally requires a bilateral subcostal incision and constant retraction of the rib cage throughout the procedure. Besides cosmetically negative consequences, weakening of abdominal musculature and sensory changes can cause a sense of disfigurement, especially in young and active individuals. This may lead to compromise in quality of life after the donation. Laparoscopic living donor nephrectomy created a high impact on kidney transplantation in the late 1990s through elimination of the necessity for flank incision, which had been required for open donor nephrectomy, so donation of a kidney became significantly easier with minimal scar and shorter recovery.[62] Laparoscopic liver resection has gained popularity with accumulation of operator experience.[63,64] After assessing outcomes after the 20th case learning curve at a center, only bile leaks were recorded more often in living donors rather than deceased-donor recipients.[65] To cope with problems from a large and potentially disfiguring incision, the minimally invasive approach to donor hepatectomy has been attempted for the past decade. Soubrane and colleagues[66] demonstrated feasibility of laparoscopic harvest of left lateral sector from an adult donor for pediatric LDLT. Koffron and colleagues[67] described a "hybrid" technique that uses a laparoscopic technique to mobilize ligamentous attachments of the liver and conventional open technique to resect hepatic parenchyma through an upper midline incision. This hand-assisted technique is applicable to various major hepatic resection procedures, including right lobe living donor hepatectomy.

The initial application of the total laparoscopic technique to donor hepatectomy of the left lateral section for pediatric liver transplantation was extended to harvest full left or right lobe allografts with timely success. Samstein and colleagues[68] published their first series of LDLTs using the left lobe allograft, obtained laparoscopically. Following, Suh and colleagues[69,70] reported their early series of totally laparoscopic right lobe living donor hepatectomy. Although the operative time and frequency of biliary duct openings was higher, the length of stay and complication rates were similar to donors undergoing open surgery, making these small studies further extend the application of this minimally invasive technique.[69] In these series, the allograft after hepatic transection was delivered through a Pfannenstiel incision, which is much more cosmetically desirable and causes less pain postoperatively.

Minimally invasive hepatic resection is still an evolving procedure with a very steep learning curve. Any premature attempts at laparoscopic living donor hepatectomy can easily lead to a surgical disaster and donor mortality.[71] So far, this procedure is performed only in highly experienced large volume institutions in donors with favorable anatomy. Depending on skill level and experience of each individual in a liver transplant program, there has to be a tailored approach to donor hepatectomies, which finds the balance between rapid favorable recovery of the donor and potential risk of catastrophic complications.

STEATOSIS AND AGE OF DONOR CANDIDATES

The rapid epidemic of obesity in the developed world has become a global public health issue affecting morbidity and mortality of overweight patients. This is not an exception in patients with end-stage liver disease who are in need of a DDLT or LDLT. Deceased-donor livers with excessive steatosis are associated with increased incidence of primary nonfunction and delayed graft function in recipients. In LDLT, hepatic steatosis can compromise the safety of the donor and the quality of the partial allograft, which is already smaller in size than the whole deceased-donor organ. Many LDLT programs have been including liver biopsy as a part of preoperative evaluation of the donor. Excessive hepatic steatosis has been one of major causes of donor disqualification.[72]

Hwang and colleagues[73] demonstrated that active short-term reduction of body weight could resolve hepatic steatosis in most previously disqualified donor candidates. Donor obesity and hepatic steatosis can be especially problematic in the United States. Living donor transplant programs should be able to provide donor candidates with nutritional counseling, and an active weight loss program to improve donor availability.

Limited regeneration capacity of the liver in older individuals has been deduced from a known higher mortality rate from major hepatic resections for malignancy whereby older generations are not able to adequately meet the functional demand of the remnant liver. Most LDLT programs have been limiting the donor age to younger than 50; however, there have been recent reports demonstrating comparable outcomes of recipients without increasing the risk of donation in the older population both to the donor and recipient. The graft function and patient survival data were similar and the complications in both the recipient and donor groups were low regardless of donor age.[74–76] This has further expanded the pool of potential donor organs available for transplantation, exploiting the further potential to decrease the mortality rate of those age-matched patients on the waiting list.

SUMMARY

To date, LDLT is the only realistic alternative to DDLT, which can generate a significant number of additional transplantable hepatic allografts. From the accumulated global and American experiences, mortality and morbidity risks of donors have been elucidated. Donor candidates are able to make an informed decision based on this information. Donor safety is still of paramount importance in LDLTs, and the transplant program must continue endeavors to maintain the highest possible technical and safety standards for donor procedures.[77]

Anatomic tailoring of partial hepatic allograft should be based on the clinical severity of the recipient. Portal venous flow optimization always needs to be considered based on GRBWR and MELD score to evaluate recipient resiliency, and knowing the existence of large portosystemic collaterals. Avoiding devastating complications like SFSS and rejection manifested as biliary stenosis is paramount to continue to serve the very patients that will continue to benefit from properly vetted LDLT.

REFERENCES

1. Chen CL, Kabiling CS, Concejero AM. Why does living donor liver transplantation flourish in Asia? Nat Rev Gastroenterol Hepatol 2013;10(12):746–51.
2. Kawasaki S, Hashikura Y, Ikegami T, et al. First case of cadaveric liver transplantation in Japan. J Hepatobiliary Pancreat Surg 1999;6(4):387–90.
3. Wachs ME, Bak TE, Karrer FM, et al. Adult living donor liver transplantation using a right hepatic lobe. Transplantation 1998;66(10):1313–6.
4. Marcos A, Fisher RA, Ham JM, et al. Right lobe living donor liver transplantation. Transplantation 1999;68(6):798–803.
5. Miller CM, Delmonico FL. Transplantation of liver grafts from living donors into adults. N Engl J Med 2001;345(12):923 [author reply: 924].
6. Berg CL, Gillespie BW, Merion RM, et al, A2ALL Study Group. Improvement in survival associated with adult-to-adult living donor liver transplantation. Gastreoenterology 2007;133(6):1806–13.
7. Malago M, Testa G, Marcos A, et al. Ethical considerations and rationale of adult-to-adult living donor liver transplantation. Liver Transpl 2001;7(10):921–7.
8. Makuuchi M, Miller CM, Olthoff K, et al. Adult-adult living donor liver transplantation. J Gastrointest Surg 2004;8(3):303–12.
9. Miller C, Florman S, Kim-Schluger L, et al. Fulminant and fatal gas gangrene of the stomach in a healthy live liver donor. Liver Transpl 2004;10(10):1315–9.
10. Belghiti J, Hiramatsu K, Benoist S, et al. Seven hundred forty-seven hepatectomies in the 1990s: an update to evaluate the actual risk of liver resection. J Am Coll Surg 2000;191(1):38–46.
11. Strong RW, Lynch SV, Wall DR, et al. The safety of elective liver resection in a special unit. Aust N Z J Surg 1994;64(8):530–4.
12. Hashikura Y, Makuuchi M, Kawasaki S, et al. Successful living-related partial liver transplantation to an adult patient. Lancet 1994;343(8907):1233–4.
13. Lo CM, Fan ST, Liu CL, et al. Adult-to-adult living donor liver transplantation using extended right lobe grafts. Ann Surg 1997;226(3):261–9 [discussion: 269–70].
14. Lee SG, Park KM, Lee YJ, et al. 157 adult-to-adult living donor liver transplantation. Transplant Proc 2001;33(1–2):1323–5.
15. Kiuchi T, Inomata Y, Uemoto S, et al. Evolution of living donor liver transplantation in adults: a single center experience. Transpl Int 2000;13(Suppl 1):S134–5.
16. Kawasaki S, Makuuchi M, Ishizone S, et al. Liver regeneration in recipients and donors after transplantation. Lancet 1992;339(8793):580–1.

17. Lee SG. Techniques of reconstruction of hepatic veins in living-donor liver transplantation, especially for right hepatic vein and major short hepatic veins of right-lobe graft. J Hepatobiliary Pancreat Surg 2006;13(2):131–8.
18. Chok KS, Lo CM. Biliary complications in right lobe living donor liver transplantation. Hepatol Int 2016;10(4):553–8.
19. Kim SH, Lee KW, Kim YK, et al. Tailored telescopic reconstruction of the bile duct in living donor liver transplantation. Liver Transpl 2010;16(9):1069–74.
20. Graham JA, Samstein B, Emond JC. Early graft dysfunction in living donor liver transplantation and the small for size syndrome. Curr Transplant Rep 2014; 1(1):43–52.
21. Urata K, Kawasaki S, Matsunami H, et al. Calculation of child and adult standard liver volume for liver transplantation. Hepatology 1995;21(5):1317–21.
22. Vauthey JN, Abdalla EK, Doherty DA, et al. Body surface area and body weight predict total liver volume in Western adults. Liver Transpl 2002;8(3):233–40.
23. Sugawara Y, Makuuchi M, Takayama T, et al. Small-for-size grafts in living-related liver transplantation. J Am Coll Surg 2001;192(4):510–3.
24. Kokudo N, Sugawara Y, Imamura H, et al. Tailoring the type of donor hepatectomy for adult living donor liver transplantation. Am J Transplant 2005;5(7):1694–703.
25. Kurihara T, Yoshizumi T, Yoshida Y, et al. Graft selection strategy in adult-to-adult living donor liver transplantation: when both hemiliver grafts meet volumetric criteria. Liver Transpl 2016;22(7):914–22.
26. Lee SG. A complete treatment of adult living donor liver transplantation: a review of surgical technique and current challenges to expand indication of patients. Am J Transpl 2015;15(1):17–38.
27. Takayama T, Makuuchi M, Kubota K, et al. Living-related transplantation of left liver plus caudate lobe. J Am Coll Surg 2000;190(5):635–8.
28. Lo CM, Fan ST, Liu CL, et al. Extending the limit on the size of adult recipient in living donor liver transplantation using extended right lobe graft. Transplantation 1997;63(10):1524–8.
29. Lee S, Park K, Hwang S, et al. Congestion of right liver graft in living donor liver transplantation. Transplantation 2001;71(6):812–4.
30. Maema A, Imamura H, Takayama T, et al. Impaired volume regeneration of split livers with partial venous disruption: a latent problem in partial liver transplantation. Transplantation 2002;73(5):765–9.
31. Sano K, Makuuchi M, Miki K, et al. Evaluation of hepatic venous congestion: proposed indication criteria for hepatic vein reconstruction. Ann Surg 2002;236(2): 241–7.
32. Lee SG, Hwang S, Park KM, et al. Seventeen adult-to-adult living donor liver transplantations using dual grafts. Transpl Proc 2001;33(7–8):3461–3.
33. Song GW, Lee SG, Moon DB, et al. Dual-graft adult living donor liver transplantation: an innovative surgical procedure for live liver donor pool expansion. Ann Surg 2017;266(1):10–8.
34. Sugawara Y, Makuuchi M. Right lateral sector graft as a feasible option for partial liver transplantation. Liver Transpl 2004;10(9):1156–7.
35. Rajakumar A, Kaliamoorthy I, Rela M, et al. Small-for-size syndrome: bridging the gap between liver transplantation and graft recovery. Semin Cardiothorac Vasc Anesth 2017;21(3):252–61.
36. Emond JC, Renz JF, Ferrell LD, et al. Functional analysis of grafts from living donors. Implications for the treatment of older recipients. Annals of surgery 1996;224(4):544–52.

37. Kiuchi T, Kasahara M, Uryuhara K, et al. Impact of graft size mismatching on graft prognosis in liver transplantation from living donors. Transplantation 1999;67(2): 321–7.
38. Dahm F, Georgiev P, Clavien PA. Small-for-size syndrome after partial liver transplantation: definition, mechanisms of disease and clinical implications. Am J Transpl 2005;5(11):2605–10.
39. Ikegami T, Shirabe K, Yoshizumi T, et al. Primary graft dysfunction after living donor liver transplantation is characterized by delayed functional hyperbilirubinemia. Am J Transpl 2012;12(7):1886–97.
40. Yonemura Y, Taketomi A, Soejima Y, et al. Validity of preoperative volumetric analysis of congestion volume in living donor liver transplantation using three-dimensional computed tomography. Liver Transpl 2005;11:1556–62.
41. Man K, Lo CM, Ng IO, et al. Liver transplantation in rats using small-for-size grafts: a study of hemodynamic and morphological changes. Arch Surg 2001; 136(3):280–5.
42. Umeda Y, Yagi T, Sadamori H, et al. Preoperative proximal splenic artery embolization: a safe and efficacious portal decompression technique that improves the outcome of live donor liver transplantation. Transpl Int 2007;20(11):947–55.
43. Humar A, Beissel J, Crotteau S, et al. Delayed splenic artery occlusion for treatment of established small-for-size syndrome after partial liver transplantation. Liver Transpl 2009;15(2):163–8.
44. Shimada M, Ijichi H, Yonemura Y, et al. The impact of splenectomy or splenic artery ligation on the outcome of a living donor adult liver transplantation using a left lobe graft. Hepatogastroenterology 2004;51(57):625–9.
45. Takada Y, Ueda M, Ishikawa Y, et al. End-to-side portocaval shunting for a small-for-size graft in living donor liver transplantation. Liver Transpl 2004;10(6):807–10.
46. Troisi R, Ricciardi S, Smeets P, et al. Effects of hemi-portocaval shunts for inflow modulation on the outcome of small-for-size grafts in living donor liver transplantation. Am J Transpl 2005;5(6):1397–404.
47. Sampietro R, Ciccarelli O, Wittebolle X, et al. Temporary transjugular intrahepatic portosystemic shunt to overcome small-for-size syndrome after right lobe adult split liver transplantation. Transpl Int 2006;19(12):1032–4.
48. Botha JF, Campos BD, Johanning J, et al. Endovascular closure of a hemiportocaval shunt after small-for-size adult-to-adult left lobe living donor liver transplantation. Liver Transpl 2009;15(12):1671–5.
49. Kita Y, Harihara Y, Sano K, et al. Reversible hepatofugal portal flow after liver transplantation using a small-for-size graft from a living donor. Transpl Int 2001; 14(4):217–22.
50. Moon DB, Lee SG, Ahn C, et al. Application of intraoperative cine-portogram to detect spontaneous portosystemic collaterals missed by intraoperative doppler exam in adult living donor liver transplantation. Liver Transpl 2007;13(9):1279–84.
51. Lee SG, Moon DB, Ahn CS, et al. Ligation of left renal vein for large spontaneous splenorenal shunt to prevent portal flow steal in adult living donor liver transplantation. Transpl Int 2007;20(1):45–50.
52. Gupta A, Klintmalm GB, Kim PT. Ligating coronary vein varices: an effective treatment of "coronary vein steal" to increase portal flow in liver transplantation. Liver Transpl 2016;22(7):1037–9.
53. Kim YJ, Ko GY, Yoon HK, et al. Intraoperative stent placement in the portal vein during or after liver transplantation. Liver Transpl 2007;13(8):1145–52.
54. Ikegami T, Yoshizumi T, Sakata K, et al. Left lobe living donor liver transplantation in adults: what is the safety limit? Liver Transpl 2016;22(12):1666–75.

55. Campos BD, Botha JF. Strategies to optimize donor safety with smaller grafts for adult-to-adult living donor liver transplantation. Curr Opin Organ Transplant 2012; 17(3):230–4.

56. Halazun KJ, Przybyszewski EM, Griesemer AD, et al. Leaning to the left: increasing the donor pool by using the left lobe, outcomes of the largest single-center North American experience of left lobe adult-to-adult living donor liver transplantation. Ann Surg 2016;264(3):448–56.

57. Botha JF, Langnas AN, Campos BD, et al. Left lobe adult-to-adult living donor liver transplantation: small grafts and hemiportocaval shunts in the prevention of small-for-size syndrome. Liver Transpl 2010;16(5):649–57.

58. Song GW, Lee SG, Hwang S, et al. Dual living donor liver transplantation with ABO-incompatible and ABO-compatible grafts to overcome small-for-size graft and ABO blood group barrier. Liver Transpl 2010;16(4):491–8.

59. Song GW, Lee SG, Hwang S, et al. Successful experiences of ABO-incompatible adult living donor liver transplantation in a single institute: no immunological failure in 10 consecutive cases. Transpl Proc 2013;45(1):272–5.

60. Song S, Kwon CH, Kim JM, et al. Single-center experience of living donor liver transplantation in patients with portal vein thrombosis. Clin Transplant 2016; 30(9):1146–51.

61. Song GW, Lee SG, Hwang S, et al. Biliary stricture is the only concern in ABO-incompatible adult living donor liver transplantation in the rituximab era. J Hepatol 2014;61(3):575–82.

62. Kuo PC, Johnson LB. Laparoscopic donor nephrectomy increases the supply of living donor kidneys: a center-specific microeconomic analysis. Transplantation 2000;69(10):2211–3.

63. Wakabayashi G, Cherqui D, Geller DA, et al. Recommendations for laparoscopic liver resection: a report from the second international consensus conference held in Morioka. Ann Surg 2015;261(4):619–29.

64. Buell JF, Cherqui D, Geller DA, et al, World Consensus Conference on Laparoscopic Surgery. The international position on laparoscopic liver surgery: the Louisville Statement, 2008. Ann Surg 2009;250(5):825–30.

65. Freise CE, Gillespie BW, Koffron AJ, et al. Recipient morbidity after living and deceased donor liver transplantation: findings from the A2ALL Retrospective Cohort Study. Am J Transpl 2008;8(12):2569–79.

66. Soubrane O, Cherqui D, Scatton O, et al. Laparoscopic left lateral sectionectomy in living donors: safety and reproducibility of the technique in a single center. Ann Surg 2006;244(5):815–20.

67. Koffron AJ, Kung R, Baker T, et al. Laparoscopic-assisted right lobe donor hepatectomy. Am J Transpl 2006;6(10):2522–5.

68. Samstein B, Cherqui D, Rotellar F, et al. Totally laparoscopic full left hepatectomy for living donor liver transplantation in adolescents and adults. Am J Transpl 2013;13(9):2462–6.

69. Suh KS, Hong SK, Lee KW, et al. Pure laparoscopic living donor hepatectomy: focus on 55 donors undergoing right hepatectomy. Am J Transpl 2017. https://doi.org/10.1111/ajt.14455.

70. Suh KS, Yi NJ, Kim J, et al. Laparoscopic hepatectomy for a modified right graft in adult-to-adult living donor liver transplantation. Transpl Proc 2008;40(10): 3529–31.

71. Soubrane O, Gateau V, Lefeve C. Is laparoscopic live donor hepatectomy justified ethically? J Hepatobiliary Pancreat Sci 2016;23(4):209–11.

72. Tamura S, Sugawara Y, Kokudo N. Donor evaluation and hepatectomy for living-donor liver transplantation. J Hepatobiliary Pancreat Surg 2008;15(2):79–91.
73. Hwang S, Lee SG, Jang SJ, et al. The effect of donor weight reduction on hepatic steatosis for living donor liver transplantation. Liver Transpl 2004;10(6):721–5.
74. Akamatsu N, Sugawara Y, Tamura S, et al. Impact of live donor age (>or=50) on liver transplantation. Transpl Proc 2007;39(10):3189–93.
75. Goldaracena N, Sapisochin G, Spetzler V, et al. Live donor liver transplantation with older (>/=50 years) versus younger (<50 years) donors: does age matter? Ann Surg 2016;263(5):979–85.
76. Yoshizumi T, Taketomi A, Soejima Y, et al. Impact of donor age and recipient status on left-lobe graft for living donor adult liver transplantation. Transpl Int 2008; 21(1):81–8.
77. Miller CM, Quintini C, Dhawan A, et al. The International Liver Transplantation Society living donor liver transplant recipient guideline. Transplantation 2017; 101(5):938–44.

Liver Transplant for Cholangiocarcinoma

Daniel Zamora-Valdes, MD, Julie K. Heimbach, MD*

KEYWORDS

- Liver transplantation • Liver cancer • Neoadjuvant radiotherapy
- Hilar cholangiocarcinoma • Intrahepatic cholangiocarcinoma

KEY POINTS

- The outcome for patients who undergo liver transplant (LT) for malignancy should be similar to outcomes that are observed in patients with chronic liver disease without cancer.
- Neoadjuvant chemoradiotherapy followed by LT is an established treatment strategy for selected patients with early-stage, unresectable hilar cholangiocarcinoma and achieves 5-year survival of approximately 65% to 70%.
- Operative staging before transplant and avoidance of transperitoneal biopsy of the primary tumor are essential for reducing risk of recurrence following LT.
- Data on LT for intrahepatic cholangiocarcinoma are preliminary.

INTRODUCTION

Cholangiocarcinoma (CCA) is a group of heterogeneous malignancies that originate from any portion of the bile ducts and exhibit biliary epithelial differentiation. The disease can be classified anatomically in 3 categories. Intrahepatic CCA (ICC) originates proximal to the second-degree bile ducts; hilar CCA is localized between the second-degree bile ducts and the cystic duct; and distal CCA originates distal to the cystic duct.[1]

The relative frequency of ICC, CCA, and distal CCA has been widely cited as 8%, 50%, and 42%, respectively.[2] However, the national incidence of ICC increased significantly in the United States during the last 4 decades (0.44–1.18 cases per 100,000; 128% increase from 1973 to 2012), with an annual increase of 2.3%. It is unclear whether this increase is reflective of an actual increase or an improved detection and classification of ICC. During the same period, the incidence of CCA increased by 5% (0.95–1.02 per 100,000; annual increase 0.14%).[3] The incidences of CCA and ICC in the United States are now similar (1.02 and 1.18 per 100,000, respectively).

Disclosure: The authors have nothing to disclose.
Division of Transplantation Surgery, Mayo Clinic, 200 First Street, Rochester, MN 55905, USA
* Corresponding author.
E-mail address: heimbach.julie@mayo.edu

Most CCAs arise de novo, and no risk factor is identified. Risk factors for CCA described worldwide (fluke infestation and congenital biliary abnormalities) are rare in the United States, where primary sclerosing cholangitis (PSC) is a well-established risk factor. Among a high-incidence population in Thailand, ultrasonography screening (but not tumor markers) can detect early-stage disease and premalignant lesions.[4]

Resection is the standard of care, but most lesions are detected at an unresectable stage. CCA and ICC require the resection of affected bile ducts and associated liver parenchyma, whereas distal CCA is treated through pancreaticoduodenectomy. Resection for CCA and ICC is also limited by the presence of chronic liver disease, the need to preserve vascular inflow and outflow, as well as adequate liver volume. To overcome this problem, liver transplant (LT) alone was attempted with dismal results. However, the use of neoadjuvant radiotherapy followed by LT in patients with early-stage, unresectable CCA is now an established therapy with excellent results. The role of LT for ICC is not yet clearly established, although there are preliminary data for patients with solitary ICC less than or equal to 2 cm, which suggests a benefit for LT.

This article focuses on LT following neoadjuvant therapy for CCA as well as the limited data on LT alone for ICC.

Liver Transplant for Hilar Cholangiocarcinoma

Attempts at LT alone for the treatment of CCA were faced with high rates of early disease recurrence and poor patient survival.[5–7] Outcomes were dismal even on incidental CCA detected in explanted livers of patients who underwent LT for PSC.[8,9] A small number of patients with negative surgical margins and no nodal disease can reach long-term survival.[10]

The lack of impact of adjuvant therapy on overall survival (OS) after curative resection for CCA (including LT),[11,12] along with the need for an effective therapy while awaiting LT, paved the way to neoadjuvant therapy as a new paradigm. CCA generally shows unsustained responses to conventional chemotherapy. Although CCA is radiosensitive, its location in the liver hilum prevents its widespread application with a curative intent because of hepatotoxicity. The introduction and modification of catheter-based brachytherapy[13] led to favorable response among unresectable patients.[14–17] These results, along with the outcome after curative resections for de novo CCA,[18] and the pioneer experience at the University of Nebraska,[19] led to the development of the Mayo Clinic protocol. LT achieves a radical resection and eliminates risk of long-term hepatic failure caused by high-dose radiotherapy, plus it treats underlying liver disease (PSC).

The protocol includes (1) selection of patients without evidence of metastatic or nodal disease; (2) neoadjuvant high-dose radiotherapy; (3) operative staging; and (4) LT.[20]

Selection

All patients with nodal or metastatic disease are excluded. Biliary drainage is performed to alleviate symptoms, treat cholangitis, and enable the liver to tolerate neoadjuvant therapy.[21] The association between percutaneous drainage and seeding metastases among patients undergoing biliary drainage before liver resection is controversial,[22,23] but has been rarely observed in patients undergoing LT (2 patients out of 181); therefore, endoscopic drainage is preferred in our center, but percutaneous drainage is not an exclusion criterion.

Exclusion criteria include CCA below the cystic duct, radial (perpendicular to duct axis) tumor diameter greater than 3 cm (**Fig. 1**), and violation of the tumor plane

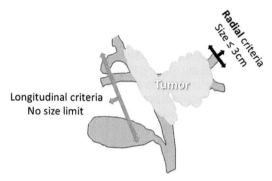

Fig. 1. Exclusion criteria based on tumor size (if mass is present). There is no limit in longitudinal size (along the bile duct). The limit on radial size is 3 cm (perpendicular to the bile duct).

(surgical exploration or diagnostic transperitoneal biopsy).[24] Endoscopic ultrasonography with lymphatic sampling is performed before neoadjuvant therapy.

Neoadjuvant therapy

Intravenous 5-fluorouracil is given for radiosensitization (500 mg/m^2 daily bolus for 3 days). External beam radiotherapy is administered with a target dose of 4500 cGy in 30 fractions delivered over a 3-week period. Brachytherapy is then delivered using iridium-192 (2000–3000 cGy) to encompass a 2-cm margin above and below the radiographic extent of the tumor. Patients receive 2000 mg/m^2 of oral capecitabine per day in 2 divided doses, 2 out of every 3 weeks, as tolerated until transplant.

Acute cholangitis and cholecystitis are a major source of morbidity in patients awaiting LT. Liver abscesses may be misdiagnosed as intrahepatic metastasis and vice versa. Other complications include gastroduodenal ulceration and delayed gastric emptying. Patients with advanced liver disease are at risk of decompensation caused by radiation damage (**Fig. 2**).

Operative staging

Staging is essential to avoid transplanting patients with lymphatic and/or peritoneal disease after completion of neoadjuvant therapy. Approximately 20% of patients

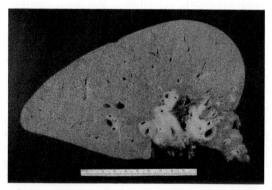

Fig. 2. Liver explant from a patient with de novo perihilar CCA showing radiation-induced damage in the parenchyma around the portal pedicles. Note the atrophy of the left hemiliver caused by prolonged biliary obstruction and portal vein encasement.

have positive staging, with lymphatic and peritoneal spread being the most common sites. Among living donor LT recipients, staging is timed just before the transplant, whereas, in deceased donor LT recipients, staging is performed as time for transplant nears based on the patient's appealed model for end-stage liver disease (MELD) score and anticipated time of transplant. Staging in advance avoids the need for reallocation of the deceased donor organ and allows pathology adequate time for interpretation. Minimally invasive operative staging is performed in most cases. Any suspicious lesion is biopsied and perihilar lymph nodes are routinely sampled even if they appear normal.

If a patient is too ill to tolerate the operation without LT, staging can be deferred until an allograft is available, although this requires an experienced pathologist and possible reallocation in case of metastatic disease. Around 30% of the patients included in the protocol drop out either based on detection of metastatic disease before or during operative staging or because of complications of portal hypertension caused by underling liver disease. The outcomes of these patients are similar to those of patients who undergo palliative therapy.[25]

Liver transplant

The liver hilum is not dissected during hepatectomy in order to avoid tumor dissemination; it is resected en bloc with the liver. The hepatic artery, portal vein, and bile duct are transected as close to the duodenum as possible. The dissection between the liver and the vena cava is challenging; it frequently leads to suspicion of tumor invasion, but explant studies have shown radiation injury rather than malignant invasion as the cause of the loss of the dissection plane between the liver capsule and the caval adventitia. The common bile duct margin is sent for frozen section in patients with PSC and, if positive, pancreaticoduodenectomy is performed.

The portal vein in living donor recipients is reconstructed with an ABO-compatible deceased donor iliac vein graft; this allows a tension-free anastomosis and provides length for the placement of a stent if radiation-induced portal vein stenosis occurs later. Radiation vascular injury is progressive over time; therefore, patients awaiting deceased donor LT with a lengthy period between neoadjuvant therapy and LT undergo aortic infrarenal jump graft for arterial reconstruction, whereas the native hepatic artery is typically used in living donor liver transplants. The bile duct is reconstructed with a Roux-en-Y in all cases.

Recognition of the effects of neoadjuvant therapy on vascular complications after LT is essential for optimizing outcomes,[26] and our group has recently updated our experience on its management.[27]

The incidence of hepatic artery complications is higher among living donor recipients compared with deceased donor recipients (thrombosis 8.3% vs 20.3%, $P = .041$; stenosis 5% vs 16.7%, $P = .018$). The short interval between the completion of neoadjuvant radiation and LT in living donor recipients makes it possible to use the native hepatic artery, whereas most deceased donor recipients have no other option but jump graft reconstruction.[27]

Portal vein stenosis is common among patients with CCA (deceased donor recipients 22.8%, living donor recipients 35%), whereas it is very rare in patients undergoing transplant for other indications, and thus it is likely caused by radiation injury. Stenting is very successful (94% overall patency; n = 35). Screening for portal vein stenosis at 4 months has reduced the incidence of thrombosis over time from 9% (1993–2005) to 2.8% (2006–2015).[27]

The response to neoadjuvant therapy predicts OS. Among 152 patients, the overall percentage of residual viable CCA was calculated and classified into 4 main categories: complete/near-complete response ($\leq$1% viable tumor; 56.6% of patients), marked response (>1 to <10% viable tumor; 16.4% of patients), moderate response (>10 to <30% viable tumor; 17.8% of patients), and minimal response ($\geq$30% viable tumor; 9.2% of patients). The percentage of residual disease according to this classification is independently associated with the probability of disease-free survival.[28]

Patients with high-risk features for disease recurrence are currently enrolled in an adjuvant therapy protocol including conversion from tacrolimus to sirolimus followed by adjuvant chemotherapy (gemcitabine and cisplatin) given from months 4 to 10 posttransplant, although it is too early to determine the efficacy of this therapy. Recurrence screening with computed tomography and serum cancer antigen (CA) 19-9 is performed 4 and 12 months after LT and yearly thereafter. The incidence of recurrence is 25% (45 out of 181 patients), most often local initially ($\sim$70%). Failure from distant metastatic disease is less likely than local or regional disease.

PRIMARY SCLEROSING CHOLANGITIS–ASSOCIATED CHOLANGIOCARCINOMA

The association between PSC and CCA is well established.[29] The reported lifetime incidence of CCA in these patients is 6.8% to 13%,[30,31] but as high as 26% among those with dominant strictures.[32,33] Half of the patients who develop CCA do so within 1 year of diagnosis of PSC.[34,35] Patients with PSC-associated CCA are diagnosed at a younger age (47 $\pm$ 9 years) than patients with de novo disease (64 $\pm$ 10 years).[36,37] Patients with PSC are at high risk of multifocal CCA; therefore, even in the absence of advanced liver disease, they are considered candidates for neoadjuvant therapy followed by LT rather than liver resection.

CCA screening among patients with PSC is performed by magnetic resonance cholangiopancreatography (MRCP) and serum CA 19-9. The use of CA 19-9 as a screening tool has been debated for many years.[36,38–40] At present, our group screens patients with PSC through laboratory tests (including liver function tests and CA 19-9) every 3 to 6 months and MRCP every year. Biliary obstruction, worsening laboratory results (including CA 19-9 $\geq$100 U/mL in the absence of cholangitis), or a dominant stricture on MRCP are indicators for further diagnostic work-up.

Patients with a new dominant stricture or focal bile duct thickening, irregularity, or contrast-enhancement are assessed through endoscopic retrograde cholangiopancreatography with cytology/biopsy. Pathologic confirmation of CCA is difficult and not always possible in these patients. Microscopic features of PSC,[41,42] along with the desmoplastic nature of CCA (resulting in paucicellular cytology specimens), obscure the diagnosis. A meta-analysis of 11 studies assessing brush cytology for the diagnosis of CCA in 747 patients with PSC identified a pooled sensitivity of 43% and specificity of 97%.[43] Targeted intraluminal biopsies of biliary strictures improve accuracy.[44,45] A recent meta-analysis of 4 studies showed that single-operator cholangioscopy had a pooled sensitivity of 65% and specificity of 95%.[46]

To further aid cytology, fluorescence in situ hybridization (FISH; UroVysion) can be performed on the epithelial cells obtained. FISH identifies aneusomy (numerical abnormalities of selected chromosomes or chromosomal foci), which is considered equivalent to aneuploidy (a term restricted to assays examining the whole genome). The presence of an increased number of copies of chromosomes 3, 7, or 17 and/or deletion of 9p21 (p16) on FISH increases the sensitivity of brush cytology to 89%.[47] A more specific set of pancreatobiliary FISH probes (gain of 1q21, 7p12, and/or 8q24 and/or loss of 9p21) has recently been tested in patients with and without PSC, showing better diagnostic performance.[48]

At present, listing criteria for CCA under the Organ Procurement and Transplantation Network (OPTN) criteria are[49]:

1. Diagnostic luminal cytology/biopsy (via endoluminal or percutaneous transhepatic route; not transperitoneal); or
2. Malignant-appearing stricture and at least 1 of the following:
   a. CA-19.9 greater than 100 UI/mL in the absence of cholangitis; or
   b. Aneuploidy by FISH; or
   c. Mass on cross-sectional imaging at site of stricture

Absence of pathologic confirmation of CCA in the liver explant has been cited as an argument against the diagnosis of CCA in patients undergoing LT following neoadjuvant therapy. However, complete pathologic response has also been observed after liver resection following neoadjuvant radiation for CCA,[50] and is frequently observed in LT following liver-directed therapy for other forms of liver cancer, such as hepatocellular carcinoma.[51] Furthermore, lack of pathologic response is predictive of an increased risk of recurrence.[28]

The decision to proceed to neoadjuvant therapy and LT without confirmed histologic diagnosis among patients with PSC has been controversial, but it is based on the following facts: (1) the absence of positive cytology does not exclude cancer; (2) patients with PSC and dominant strictures have a 26% risk of CCA at 10 years[31,33]; (3) the possibility of progression of CCA beyond criteria; (4) the diagnostic performance of combined rather than individual diagnostic strategies; and (5) the observation that 53% of patients with PSC and without pathologic confirmation before the initiation of neoadjuvant therapy have a positive surgical staging after neoadjuvant therapy, residual CCA in the explant, or recurrence after LT.[52]

After the enrollment of 171 patients with PSC from 1993 to March 2016, the Mayo Clinic protocol shows intention-to-treat 5-year survival rates of 60%, with a 77% 5-year survival rate following transplant (n = 113).

DE NOVO CHOLANGIOCARCINOMA

Preoperative evaluation and definition of the anatomic location and extent is critical among patients with de novo CCA. The Bismuth-Corlette classification has been widely adopted to describe tumor location and biliary involvement.[53] The strength of the Bismuth-Corlette classification is its ability to conceptualize CCA into operative approaches.

Standard criteria for resectability on early CCA include bilateral segmental ductal involvement; unilateral atrophy with contralateral segmental ductal or vascular inflow involvement (not amenable to vascular reconstruction), and unilateral segmental ductal involvement with contralateral atrophy or vascular involvement (not amenable to reconstruction); and an insufficient future liver remnant even after portal inflow modulation.[54–56] Associated liver partition and portal vein ligation for staged hepatectomy is associated with high 90-day mortality (48%) and is currently not recommended for patients with CCA.[57] Resectability criteria are constantly challenged, because a progressively higher rate of R0 and lower perioperative mortality are obtained with multistep procedures including vascular reconstructions[37]; however, the decision to resect a vascular structure should be based on evidence of involvement during exploration.

If lymph node involvement is identified on imaging studies, LT is no longer an option and aggressive surgical resections could be offered, although long-term survival is poor.[58] The survival of patients undergoing resection with positive margins, even microscopic, is drastically reduced.[59] Patients who undergo surgical exploration with violation of the tumor plane can no longer be considered candidates for LT. For patients with unresectable de novo CCA (n = 112), the Mayo Clinic protocol shows intention-to-treat 5-year survival rates of 37%, with a 5-year survival rate after transplant of 56% (n = 68) primarily caused by being diagnosed with larger tumors than those with underlying PSC. These outcomes in unresectable patients who have no other therapeutic option are comparable with or slightly superior to the rate that can be achieved for those who present with resectable disease and undergo an R0 resection without lymph node involvement.[60] Whether the survival of patients with resectable disease can be improved by neoadjuvant therapy followed by LT is under investigation (Liver Resection Versus Radio-chemotherapy-Transplantation for Hilar Cholangiocarcinoma (TRANSPHIL) study, to be completed on 2021). At present, OPTN criteria for an exception score for CCA requires the tumor to be considered unresectable.[49]

Liver Transplant for Intrahepatic Cholangiocarcinoma

ICC originates from the intrahepatic biliary epithelium. Risk factors for ICC are similar to those for CCA (hepatobiliary flukes, PSC, choledochal cysts, hepatolithiasis), and for hepatocellular carcinoma (cirrhosis hepatitis B, hepatitis C, alcohol use, diabetes, and obesity).[61] The incidence of ICC has increased in the United States[62,63]; between 1973 and 2012, the number of cases of ICC per year increased more than 150%.[3] A similar trend has been observed in other countries.[64,65]

At present, ICC can only be diagnosed through biopsy. Distinctive imaging features of ICC include surface retraction, peritumoral biliary dilatation, and absence of capsule formation.[66,67] Lesions less than or equal to 3 cm tend to have a diffuse arterial enhancement and lesions larger than 3 cm tend to have a peripheral or rimlike arterial enhancement (**Fig. 3**).[68] Portal and venous phases show progressive or stable enhancement, whereas contrast washout is exceedingly rare.[68,69] Gadoxetic acid–enhanced MRI shows peripheral washout on delayed phases; hepatobiliary phases show well-demarcated tumor-to-liver interface and target appearance with a hypointense rim.[66,70]

ICC is located in the central areas of the liver.[71-73] Survival after resection depends on tumor size, multinodularity, CA 19-9, vascular invasion, margin status, and nodal disease.[74-77] Long-term disease-free survival is rarely achieved after resection (9.7% for all patients), even among patients with favorable predictive factors (25.8%

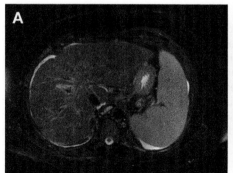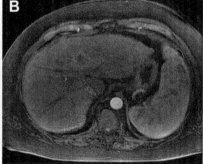

Fig. 3. Magnetic resonance images of a solitary, 3-cm, biopsy-proven, intrahepatic CCA in a patient with cirrhosis in segment 4. The lesion shows early peripheral enhancement (*A*) with progressive enhancement of the rest of the lesion (*B*). This pattern is observed in lesions larger than 2 cm. Smaller lesions tend to present an early diffuse enhancement pattern followed by persistence of enhancement in later sequences.

among patients with solitary, well-differentiated, ≤5-cm ICC without vascular/periductal/lymphatic involvement).[78] Until 2011, there was no specific ICC American Joint Committee On Cancer staging system and the HCC system was used.[79] Furthermore, the rarity of patients with small ICC undergoing liver resection has led most surgical series to establish a cutoff of 5 cm.[76,80] Recently, a Japanese group reported a 100% 5-year survival among patients with solitary ICC less than or equal to 2 cm with no vascular invasion or nodal disease.[81] Although encouraging, this finding was infrequent (15 out of 419 patients; 3.5%) and the survival of patients with solitary ICC less than or equal to 2 cm with vascular invasion was only 60% at 2 years.[81]

The limited data to support LT for ICC in the setting of cirrhosis come from 2 recent retrospective multicenter studies from liver explants. Twenty-three patients with incidental very early ICC (solitary, ≤2 cm) were identified in 2 studies (first cohort of 7876 LTs[82,83]; and a second cohort of 25,016 LTs).[84,85] The 5-year recurrence after LT among patients with very early ICC (15 patients) was 12% (compared with 77% among patients with ICC >2 cm or multinodularity) and 5-year OS was 65% (compared with 45%).[84]

LT for early unresectable ICC in the setting of a noncirrhotic liver has infrequently been reported and is currently limited to reports from small, single-center case series. The University of California, Los Angeles group published a series comparing LT and resection using neoadjuvant chemotherapy in some patients. In more than 2 decades, they performed 25 LTs for locally advanced ICC, with 5-year OS after LT of 32%.[86] However, the OS was calculated for both ICC and CCA and granular data on each type of cancer are unavailable.[86] The same group identified multifocal tumors, perineural invasion, infiltrative subtype, and lack of neoadjuvant and adjuvant therapies, but not tumor size, as factors associated with poor prognosis on multivariate analysis.[87] The small number of patients who received neoadjuvant treatment and the lack of a standardized protocol makes these results hard to interpret.[87] It is also unclear how many patients they listed for transplant and how they decided whether to use LT or resection.[86]

A promising strategy among patients with unresectable ICC is radioembolization with yttrium-90 (Y^{90}). Rayar and colleagues[88,89] showed that this therapy may reduce the size of unresectable ICCs, allowing surgical resection in selected cases and LT in 1 case.

SUMMARY

CCA is an accepted indication for LT, under strict selection criteria and a neoadjuvant therapy protocol, including extensive preoperative diagnostic work-up and operative staging to rule out nodal and peritoneal disease. The 5-year OS of patients undergoing LT following neoadjuvant therapy is similar to that of patients undergoing resection with negative margins and no nodal disease.

ICC is not a standard indication for LT outside of experimental studies. Further studies are necessary to assess the impact of transperitoneal biopsy on ICC. Whether radioembolization can be used as neoadjuvant therapy for ICC will be the subject of future studies.

REFERENCES

1. Banales JM, Cardinale V, Carpino G, et al. Expert consensus document: cholangiocarcinoma: current knowledge and future perspectives consensus statement from the European Network for the Study of Cholangiocarcinoma (ENS-CCA). Nat Rev Gastroenterol Hepatol 2016;13(5):261–80.

2. DeOliveira ML, Cunningham SC, Cameron JL, et al. Cholangiocarcinoma: thirty-one-year experience with 564 patients at a single institution. Ann Surg 2007; 245(5):755–62.

3. Saha SK, Zhu AX, Fuchs CS, et al. Forty-year trends in cholangiocarcinoma incidence in the U.S.: intrahepatic disease on the rise. Oncologist 2016;21(5): 594–9.

4. Sungkasubun P, Siripongsakun S, Akkarachinorate K, et al. Ultrasound screening for cholangiocarcinoma could detect premalignant lesions and early-stage diseases with survival benefits: a population-based prospective study of 4,225 subjects in an endemic area. BMC Cancer 2016;16:346.

5. Ringe B, Wittekind C, Bechstein WO, et al. The role of liver transplantation in hepatobiliary malignancy. A retrospective analysis of 95 patients with particular regard to tumor stage and recurrence. Ann Surg 1989;209(1):88–98.

6. Meyer CG, Penn I, James L. Liver transplantation for cholangiocarcinoma: results in 207 patients. Transplantation 2000;69(8):1633–7.

7. Robles R, Figueras J, Turrion VS, et al. Spanish experience in liver transplantation for hilar and peripheral cholangiocarcinoma. Ann Surg 2004;239(2):265–71.

8. Goss JA, Shackleton CR, Farmer DG, et al. Orthotopic liver transplantation for primary sclerosing cholangitis. A 12-year single center experience. Ann Surg 1997; 225(5):472–81 [discussion: 481–3].

9. Ghali P, Marotta PJ, Yoshida EM, et al. Liver transplantation for incidental cholangiocarcinoma: analysis of the Canadian experience. Liver Transpl 2005;11(11): 1412–6.

10. Iwatsuki S, Todo S, Marsh JW, et al. Treatment of hilar cholangiocarcinoma (Klatskin tumors) with hepatic resection or transplantation. J Am Coll Surg 1998;187(4):358–64.

11. Goldstein RM, Stone M, Tillery GW, et al. Is liver transplantation indicated for cholangiocarcinoma? Am J Surg 1993;166(6):768–71 [discussion: 771–2].

12. Fuller CD, Wang SJ, Choi M, et al. Multimodality therapy for locoregional extrahepatic cholangiocarcinoma: a population-based analysis. Cancer 2009;115(22): 5175–83.

13. Conroy RM, Shahbazian AA, Edwards KC, et al. A new method for treating carcinomatous biliary obstruction with intracatheter radium. Cancer 1982;49(7): 1321–7.

14. Buskirk SJ, Gunderson LL, Adson MA, et al. Analysis of failure following curative irradiation of gallbladder and extrahepatic bile duct carcinoma. Int J Radiat Oncol Biol Phys 1984;10(11):2013–23.

15. Alden ME, Mohiuddin M. The impact of radiation dose in combined external beam and intraluminal Ir-192 brachytherapy for bile duct cancer. Int J Radiat Oncol Biol Phys 1994;28(4):945–51.

16. Buskirk SJ, Gunderson LL, Schild SE, et al. Analysis of failure after curative irradiation of extrahepatic bile duct carcinoma. Ann Surg 1992;215(2):125–31.

17. Foo ML, Gunderson LL, Bender CE, et al. External radiation therapy and transcatheter iridium in the treatment of extrahepatic bile duct carcinoma. Int J Radiat Oncol Biol Phys 1997;39(4):929–35.

18. Nagorney DM, Donohue JH, Farnell MB, et al. Outcomes after curative resections of cholangiocarcinoma. Arch Surg 1993;128(8):871–7 [discussion: 877–9].

19. Sudan D, DeRoover A, Chinnakotla S, et al. Radiochemotherapy and transplantation allow long-term survival for nonresectable hilar cholangiocarcinoma. Am J Transplant 2002;2(8):774–9.

20. Heimbach JK, Gores GJ, Nagorney DM, et al. Liver transplantation for perihilar cholangiocarcinoma after aggressive neoadjuvant therapy: a new paradigm for liver and biliary malignancies? Surgery 2006;140(3):331–4.

21. Al Mahjoub A, Menahem B, Fohlen A, et al. Preoperative biliary drainage in patients with resectable perihilar cholangiocarcinoma: is percutaneous transhepatic biliary drainage safer and more effective than endoscopic biliary drainage? A meta-analysis. J Vasc Interv Radiol 2017;28(4):576–82.

22. Wiggers JK, Groot Koerkamp B, Coelen RJ, et al. Percutaneous preoperative biliary drainage for resectable perihilar cholangiocarcinoma: no association with survival and no increase in seeding metastases. Ann Surg Oncol 2015; 22(Suppl 3):S1156–63.

23. Komaya K, Ebata T, Yokoyama Y, et al. Verification of the oncologic inferiority of percutaneous biliary drainage to endoscopic drainage: a propensity score matching analysis of resectable perihilar cholangiocarcinoma. Surgery 2017; 161(2):394–404.

24. Heimbach JK, Sanchez W, Rosen CB, et al. Trans-peritoneal fine needle aspiration biopsy of hilar cholangiocarcinoma is associated with disease dissemination. HPB (Oxford) 2011;13(5):356–60.

25. Sio TT, Martenson JA Jr, Haddock MG, et al. Outcome of transplant-fallout patients with unresectable cholangiocarcinoma. Am J Clin Oncol 2016;39(3):271–5.

26. Mantel HT, Rosen CB, Heimbach JK, et al. Vascular complications after orthotopic liver transplantation after neoadjuvant therapy for hilar cholangiocarcinoma. Liver Transpl 2007;13(10):1372–81.

27. Zamora-Valdes D, Rosen CB, Heimbach JK, et al. Vascular complications are common following liver transplantation for hilar cholangiocarcinoma after neoadjuvant chemoradiotherapy. HPB (Oxford) 2016;18(S1):e127.

28. Lehrke HD, Heimbach JK, Wu TT, et al. Prognostic significance of the histologic response of perihilar cholangiocarcinoma to preoperative neoadjuvant chemoradiation in liver explants. Am J Surg Pathol 2016;40(4):510–8.

29. Rosen CB, Nagorney DM, Wiesner RH, et al. Cholangiocarcinoma complicating primary sclerosing cholangitis. Ann Surg 1991;213(1):21–5.

30. Bergquist A, Ekbom A, Olsson R, et al. Hepatic and extrahepatic malignancies in primary sclerosing cholangitis. J Hepatol 2002;36(3):321–7.

31. Claessen MM, Vleggaar FP, Tytgat KM, et al. High lifetime risk of cancer in primary sclerosing cholangitis. J Hepatol 2009;50(1):158–64.

32. Chapman R, Fevery J, Kalloo A, et al. Diagnosis and management of primary sclerosing cholangitis. Hepatology 2010;51(2):660–78.

33. Chapman MH, Webster GJ, Bannoo S, et al. Cholangiocarcinoma and dominant strictures in patients with primary sclerosing cholangitis: a 25-year single-centre experience. Eur J Gastroenterol Hepatol 2012;24(9):1051–8.

34. Boberg KM, Bergquist A, Mitchell S, et al. Cholangiocarcinoma in primary sclerosing cholangitis: risk factors and clinical presentation. Scand J Gastroenterol 2002;37(10):1205–11.

35. Weismuller TJ, Trivedi PJ, Bergquist A, et al. Patient age, sex, and inflammatory bowel disease phenotype associate with course of primary sclerosing cholangitis. Gastroenterology 2017;152(8):1975–84.e8.

36. Chalasani N, Baluyut A, Ismail A, et al. Cholangiocarcinoma in patients with primary sclerosing cholangitis: a multicenter case-control study. Hepatology 2000; 31(1):7–11.

37. Nagino M, Ebata T, Yokoyama Y, et al. Evolution of surgical treatment for perihilar cholangiocarcinoma: a single-center 34-year review of 574 consecutive resections. Ann Surg 2013;258(1):129–40.
38. Levy C, Lymp J, Angulo P, et al. The value of serum CA 19-9 in predicting cholangiocarcinomas in patients with primary sclerosing cholangitis. Dig Dis Sci 2005;50(9):1734–40.
39. Charatcharoenwitthaya P, Enders FB, Halling KC, et al. Utility of serum tumor markers, imaging, and biliary cytology for detecting cholangiocarcinoma in primary sclerosing cholangitis. Hepatology 2008;48(4):1106–17.
40. Sinakos E, Saenger AK, Keach J, et al. Many patients with primary sclerosing cholangitis and increased serum levels of carbohydrate antigen 19-9 do not have cholangiocarcinoma. Clin Gastroenterol Hepatol 2011;9(5):434–9.e1.
41. Katabi N, Albores-Saavedra J. The extrahepatic bile duct lesions in end-stage primary sclerosing cholangitis. Am J Surg Pathol 2003;27(3):349–55.
42. Lewis JT, Talwalkar JA, Rosen CB, et al. Precancerous bile duct pathology in end-stage primary sclerosing cholangitis, with and without cholangiocarcinoma. Am J Surg Pathol 2010;34(1):27–34.
43. Trikudanathan G, Navaneethan U, Njei B, et al. Diagnostic yield of bile duct brushings for cholangiocarcinoma in primary sclerosing cholangitis: a systematic review and meta-analysis. Gastrointest Endosc 2014;79(5):783–9.
44. Tischendorf JJ, Kruger M, Trautwein C, et al. Cholangioscopic characterization of dominant bile duct stenoses in patients with primary sclerosing cholangitis. Endoscopy 2006;38(7):665–9.
45. Arnelo U, von Seth E, Bergquist A. Prospective evaluation of the clinical utility of single-operator peroral cholangioscopy in patients with primary sclerosing cholangitis. Endoscopy 2015;47(8):696–702.
46. Njei B, McCarty TR, Varadarajulu S, et al. Systematic review with meta-analysis: endoscopic retrograde cholangiopancreatography-based modalities for the diagnosis of cholangiocarcinoma in primary sclerosing cholangitis. Aliment Pharmacol Ther 2016;44(11–12):1139–51.
47. Gonda TA, Glick MP, Sethi A, et al. Polysomy and p16 deletion by fluorescence in situ hybridization in the diagnosis of indeterminate biliary strictures. Gastrointest Endosc 2012;75(1):74–9.
48. Barr Fritcher EG, Voss JS, Brankley SM, et al. An optimized set of fluorescence in situ hybridization probes for detection of pancreatobiliary tract cancer in cytology brush samples. Gastroenterology 2015;149(7):1813–24.e1.
49. Gores GJ, Gish RG, Sudan D, et al. Model for end-stage liver disease (MELD) exception for cholangiocarcinoma or biliary dysplasia. Liver Transpl 2006;12(12 Suppl 3):S95–7.
50. McMasters KM, Tuttle TM, Leach SD, et al. Neoadjuvant chemoradiation for extrahepatic cholangiocarcinoma. Am J Surg 1997;174(6):605–8 [discussion: 608–9].
51. Agopian VG, Morshedi MM, McWilliams J, et al. Complete pathologic response to pretransplant locoregional therapy for hepatocellular carcinoma defines cancer cure after liver transplantation: analysis of 501 consecutively treated patients. Ann Surg 2015;262(3):536–45 [discussion: 543–5].
52. Rosen CB, Darwish Murad S, Heimbach JK, et al. Neoadjuvant therapy and liver transplantation for hilar cholangiocarcinoma: is pretreatment pathological confirmation of diagnosis necessary? J Am Coll Surg 2012;215(1):31–8 [discussion: 38–40].
53. Bismuth H, Corlette MB. Intrahepatic cholangioenteric anastomosis in carcinoma of the hilus of the liver. Surg Gynecol Obstet 1975;140(2):170–8.

54. Mansour JC, Aloia TA, Crane CH, et al. Hilar cholangiocarcinoma: expert consensus statement. HPB (Oxford) 2015;17(8):691–9.
55. Hwang S, Lee SG, Ko GY, et al. Sequential preoperative ipsilateral hepatic vein embolization after portal vein embolization to induce further liver regeneration in patients with hepatobiliary malignancy. Ann Surg 2009;249(4):608–16.
56. Hyodo R, Suzuki K, Ebata T, et al. Assessment of percutaneous transhepatic portal vein embolization with portal vein stenting for perihilar cholangiocarcinoma with severe portal vein stenosis. J Hepatobiliary Pancreat Sci 2015;22(4):310–5.
57. Olthof PB, Coelen RJ, Wiggers JK, et al. High mortality after ALPPS for perihilar cholangiocarcinoma: case-control analysis including the first series from the international ALPPS registry. HPB (Oxford) 2017;19(5):381–7.
58. Aoba T, Ebata T, Yokoyama Y, et al. Assessment of nodal status for perihilar cholangiocarcinoma: location, number, or ratio of involved nodes. Ann Surg 2013; 257(4):718–25.
59. Tsukahara T, Ebata T, Shimoyama Y, et al. Residual carcinoma in situ at the ductal stump has a negative survival effect: an analysis of early-stage cholangiocarcinomas. Ann Surg 2017;266(1):126–32.
60. Croome KP, Rosen CB, Heimbach JK, et al. Is liver transplantation appropriate for patients with potentially resectable de novo hilar cholangiocarcinoma? J Am Coll Surg 2015;221(1):130–9.
61. Palmer WC, Patel T. Are common factors involved in the pathogenesis of primary liver cancers? A meta-analysis of risk factors for intrahepatic cholangiocarcinoma. J Hepatol 2012;57(1):69–76.
62. Yang JD, Kim B, Sanderson SO, et al. Biliary tract cancers in Olmsted County, Minnesota, 1976-2008. Am J Gastroenterol 2012;107(8):1256–62.
63. Yao KJ, Jabbour S, Parekh N, et al. Increasing mortality in the United States from cholangiocarcinoma: an analysis of the National Center for Health Statistics Database. BMC Gastroenterol 2016;16(1):117.
64. Taylor-Robinson SD, Foster GR, Arora S, et al. Increase in primary liver cancer in the UK, 1979-94. Lancet 1997;350(9085):1142–3.
65. Kato I, Kuroishi T, Tominaga S. Descriptive epidemiology of subsites of cancers of the liver, biliary tract and pancreas in Japan. Jpn J Clin Oncol 1990;20(3):232–7.
66. Kim R, Lee JM, Shin CI, et al. Differentiation of intrahepatic mass-forming cholangiocarcinoma from hepatocellular carcinoma on gadoxetic acid-enhanced liver MR imaging. Eur Radiol 2016;26(6):1808–17.
67. Iavarone M, Piscaglia F, Vavassori S, et al. Contrast enhanced CT-scan to diagnose intrahepatic cholangiocarcinoma in patients with cirrhosis. J Hepatol 2013;58(6):1188–93.
68. Huang B, Wu L, Lu XY, et al. Small intrahepatic cholangiocarcinoma and hepatocellular carcinoma in cirrhotic livers may share similar enhancement patterns at multiphase dynamic MR imaging. Radiology 2016;281(1):150–7.
69. Rimola J, Forner A, Reig M, et al. Cholangiocarcinoma in cirrhosis: absence of contrast washout in delayed phases by magnetic resonance imaging avoids misdiagnosis of hepatocellular carcinoma. Hepatology 2009;50(3):791–8.
70. Choi SH, Lee SS, Kim SY, et al. Intrahepatic cholangiocarcinoma in patients with cirrhosis: differentiation from hepatocellular carcinoma by using gadoxetic acid-enhanced MR imaging and dynamic CT. Radiology 2017;282(3):771–81.
71. Lang H, Sotiropoulos GC, Fruhauf NR, et al. Extended hepatectomy for intrahepatic cholangiocellular carcinoma (ICC): when is it worthwhile? Single center experience with 27 resections in 50 patients over a 5-year period. Ann Surg 2005;241(1):134–43.

72. Ali SM, Clark CJ, Zaydfudim VM, et al. Role of major vascular resection in patients with intrahepatic cholangiocarcinoma. Ann Surg Oncol 2013;20(6):2023–8.
73. Reames BN, Ejaz A, Koerkamp BG, et al. Impact of major vascular resection on outcomes and survival in patients with intrahepatic cholangiocarcinoma: a multi-institutional analysis. J Surg Oncol 2017;116(2):133–9.
74. Hyder O, Marques H, Pulitano C, et al. A nomogram to predict long-term survival after resection for intrahepatic cholangiocarcinoma: an Eastern and Western experience. JAMA Surg 2014;149(5):432–8.
75. Wang Y, Li J, Xia Y, et al. Prognostic nomogram for intrahepatic cholangiocarcinoma after partial hepatectomy. J Clin Oncol 2013;31(9):1188–95.
76. Ali SM, Clark CJ, Mounajjed T, et al. Model to predict survival after surgical resection of intrahepatic cholangiocarcinoma: the Mayo Clinic experience. HPB (Oxford) 2015;17(3):244–50.
77. Bergquist JR, Ivanics T, Storlie CB, et al. Implications of CA19-9 elevation for survival, staging, and treatment sequencing in intrahepatic cholangiocarcinoma: a national cohort analysis. J Surg Oncol 2016;114(4):475–82.
78. Spolverato G, Vitale A, Cucchetti A, et al. Can hepatic resection provide a long-term cure for patients with intrahepatic cholangiocarcinoma? Cancer 2015; 121(22):3998–4006.
79. Farges O, Fuks D, Le Treut YP, et al. AJCC 7th edition of TNM staging accurately discriminates outcomes of patients with resectable intrahepatic cholangiocarcinoma: by the AFC-IHCC-2009 study group. Cancer 2011;117(10):2170–7.
80. Spolverato G, Kim Y, Ejaz A, et al. Conditional probability of long-term survival after liver resection for intrahepatic cholangiocarcinoma: a multi-institutional analysis of 535 patients. JAMA Surg 2015;150(6):538–45.
81. Sakamoto Y, Kokudo N, Matsuyama Y, et al. Proposal of a new staging system for intrahepatic cholangiocarcinoma: analysis of surgical patients from a nationwide survey of the Liver Cancer Study Group of Japan. Cancer 2016;122(1):61–70.
82. Sapisochin G, Rodriguez de Lope C, Gastaca M, et al. "Very early" intrahepatic cholangiocarcinoma in cirrhotic patients: should liver transplantation be reconsidered in these patients? Am J Transplant 2014;14(3):660–7.
83. Sapisochin G, de Lope CR, Gastaca M, et al. Intrahepatic cholangiocarcinoma or mixed hepatocellular-cholangiocarcinoma in patients undergoing liver transplantation: a Spanish matched cohort multicenter study. Ann Surg 2014;259(5): 944–52.
84. Sapisochin G, Facciuto M, Rubbia-Brandt L, et al. Liver transplantation for "very early" intrahepatic cholangiocarcinoma: international retrospective study supporting a prospective assessment. Hepatology 2016;64(4):1178–88.
85. Groeschl R, Zamora-Valdes D, Bergquist J, et al. Survival after liver transplantation for intrahepatic cholangiocarcinoma: analysis of the National Cancer Data Base. J Am Coll Surg 2016;223(4S2):e191–192.
86. Hong JC, Jones CM, Duffy JP, et al. Comparative analysis of resection and liver transplantation for intrahepatic and hilar cholangiocarcinoma: a 24-year experience in a single center. Arch Surg 2011;146(6):683–9.
87. Hong JC, Petrowsky H, Kaldas FM, et al. Predictive index for tumor recurrence after liver transplantation for locally advanced intrahepatic and hilar cholangiocarcinoma. J Am Coll Surg 2011;212(4):514–20 [discussion: 520–1].
88. Rayar M, Sulpice L, Edeline J, et al. Intra-arterial yttrium-90 radioembolization combined with systemic chemotherapy is a promising method for downstaging unresectable huge intrahepatic cholangiocarcinoma to surgical treatment. Ann Surg Oncol 2015;22(9):3102–8.

89. Rayar M, Levi Sandri GB, Houssel-Debry P, et al. Multimodal therapy including yttrium-90 radioembolization as a bridging therapy to liver transplantation for a huge and locally advanced intrahepatic cholangiocarcinoma. J Gastrointestin Liver Dis 2016;25(3):401–4.

Immunologic Monitoring to Personalize Immunosuppression After Liver Transplant

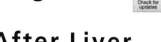

Andrew Zhu, BSE, Alexandra Leto, BS, Abraham Shaked, MD, PhD*,
Brendan Keating, DPhil

KEYWORDS

- Liver transplantation • Immunosuppression • Biomarker monitoring
- Personalization • Pharmacogenetics

KEY POINTS

- Immunosuppressive drugs exhibit a wide array of side effects, and current methods of immunosuppressive monitoring are unable to adequately account for individual variation to these drugs.
- Ongoing research in biomarker monitoring has produced promising results in early diagnosis of graft damage or immune response.
- In particular, microRNA biomarkers and regulatory T lymphocytes are leading candidates as biomarkers of organ damage and immune response, respectively.
- Introduction and improvement of genetic sequencing techniques has allowed more powerful, statistically significant results in the identification of drug-specific and nonspecific genes.

INTRODUCTION

In the past few decades, advances in pharmacologic immunosuppressive agents have led to large improvements in overall outcomes of liver transplants. However, there are still significant issues with risks for long-term drug adverse events for transplant recipients. Current immunosuppressive drug regimens are one-size-fits-all, with many recipients being either oversuppressed (leading to drug toxicity) or undersuppressed (leading to adverse immune reaction): preliminary general findings from clinical trials (iWITH and A-WISH) indicate that more than half of

---

Disclosure Statement: The authors have nothing to disclose.
Division of Transplantation, Department of Surgery, Penn Transplant Institute, The University of Pennsylvania, 3400 Spruce Street, Two Dulles Pavilion, Philadelphia, PA 19104, USA
* Corresponding author.
E-mail address: abraham.shaked@uphs.upenn.edu

Gastroenterol Clin N Am 47 (2018) 281–296
https://doi.org/10.1016/j.gtc.2018.01.003
0889-8553/18/© 2018 Elsevier Inc. All rights reserved.

individuals can tolerate a 50% reduction in standard immunosuppressive therapy and more than one-third of individuals can tolerate a 75% reduction.[1] Because much of the risk in transplantation stems from the difficulty of predicting individual patient response to drug regimens, the transplant community continues to seek out methods of personalized dosing to balance adequate immune suppression while reducing harmful side effects of pharmacotherapy. This article presents a brief background into the current repertoire of immunosuppressive management in liver transplantation before focusing on the developing efforts for personalized immuno-suppression in liver transplantation via biomarkers.

CURRENT IMMUNOSUPPRESSION MANAGEMENT
Contemporary Monitoring Methods in Liver Transplantation

Many immunosuppressive drugs exhibit a wide variability in pharmacokinetic behavior combined with a narrow therapeutic index, making it challenging for physicians to administer the optimal dosages of immunosuppressive agents during and after transplant. Therefore, to ensure best patient outcomes, close therapeutic drug monitoring becomes essential to minimize adverse effects of immunosuppressive drug regimens while avoiding chronic or acute organ rejection. Although calcineurin inhibitors (CNIs) and mammalian target of rapamycin (mTOR) inhibitors are closely monitored because of their narrow therapeutic range and potential for adverse pleiotropic effects, corticosteroids and costimulatory blockers (belatacept) do not usually require therapeutic drug monitoring.[2] For nearly all immunosuppressive drugs, specimen collection occurs at the trough level or predose level, immediately before the next round of drug administration. Known as C0 trough monitoring, this approach serves to standardize measurements and results (**Fig. 1**). The 1 exception is cyclosporine A (CsA) monitoring, which occurs 2 hours postdosing, also known as C2 monitoring.[3] Most of these techniques require pre-treatment of whole blood to determine the relevant drug concentrations.[2] Blood plasma is usually not sufficient for analysis, per se, because most immunosuppressants are distributed unevenly throughout blood, leading to differences in drug concentration within the various blood components. Mycophenolic acid (MPA) measurements remain an exception, because nearly all MPA is found in plasma, so therapeutic drug monitoring for MPA can be conducted with only blood serum or plasma.[4]

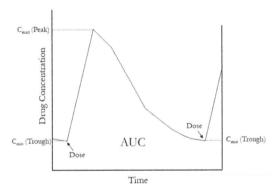

Fig. 1. Drug levels over dosing interval. Drug concentrations decrease to minimum trough level (C0) before increasing to peak concentration C_{max}. The area under the concentration-time curve (AUC) gives total drug exposure in the timespan.

Immunoassays

Although liquid chromatography (LC) and mass spectrometry (MS) are considered the gold standard in therapeutic monitoring, immunoassays represent a widely used option within the transplant community because of their ease of use and speed. At present, a variety of immunoassays are widely available for each immunosuppressant,[2] but there exists a positive bias with immunoassay results compared with those of LC and tandem MS (LC-MS/MS). Using high-performance LC values as a baseline, one study found that the enzyme multiplied immunoassay technique (EMIT) CsA assay resulted in 43% and 34% positive bias in C0 and C2 specimens, respectively,[2] whereas tacrolimus immunoassays had an average overestimation ranging from 16.6% antibody conjugate magnetic immunoassay (ACMIA) to 33.1% cloned enzyme donor immunoassay (CEDIA).[5,6] A major factor contributing to the range in results is cross reactivity between various metabolites of tacrolimus and the immunoassays: testing the chemiluminescent microparticle immunoassay (CMIA), Bazin and colleagues[7] determined that the active form of M-II and inactive form of M-III, two primary metabolites of tacrolimus, show 94% and 45% cross reactivity, respectively. Nevertheless, because of the large disparity in immunoassay results, there exists a pressing need for tacrolimus standardization. Another class of immunosuppressive drugs, mTOR inhibitors, show similarly increased immunoassay readings. In particular, 41-O-demethyl-sirolimus, the major metabolite found in whole blood, can lead to mean positive biases of at least 20% compared with the LC-MS/MS method.[8,9] Analysis of everolimus molecules using the Innofluor Certican assay revealed only 1% cross reactivity among the major metabolites, but cross reactivity of minor metabolites ranged from 16.3% to 142%.[10]

Chromatography and mass spectroscopy Given effects of metabolic cross reaction in immunoassay therapeutic drug monitoring, the transplant community has targeted nonimmunoassay techniques to monitor immunosuppressive drugs. Although these methods include solid phase extraction and laser diode desorption technologies,[11] most nonimmunoassay approaches are based in chromatography and MS.[12] In general, LC is used in therapeutic drug monitoring; it involves passing a solution of interest through a chromatographic column consisting of the stationary phase, and separating the analytes through differences in chemical and physical properties. The separated substances are ionized and subjected to a mass spectrometer before entering a mass spectrometer.[12] Several factors can limit LC-MS/MS efficiency. Crosstalk, when ions linger in the collision cell, can lead to false-positives,[12,13] and components in the spectrometric matrix can influence the charge of ions that reach the mass detectors.[12] Nevertheless, with intraday and interday measurement errors of less than or equal to 12.2% over a wide calibration range,[14] LC-MS/MS provides significant advantages in accuracy and precision compared with immunoassays.[14] Therefore, LC-MS/MS has great potential for identifying novel biomarkers in transplantation.[2,12]

Immunosuppression-Related Adverse Events Following Liver Transplant

Although allograft rejection remains a concern posttransplant, alloimmune response is typically only one of many factors deciding the fate of the transplanted liver. Acute rejection usually occurs without long-term tissue damage, whereas chronic rejection is unlikely to result in graft loss.[15–18] Immunosuppression can lead to adverse events such as kidney injury, metabolic syndrome, and acute infection.[15] Therefore, there exists a balance between limiting an allograft immune response and controlling the negative effects of immunosuppressive drugs, eventually weaning the patient off the immunosuppressive regimen to allow the immune system to regain its supervisory role.

Kidney injury
Although the introduction of CNIs into posttransplant care revolutionized long-term patient outcomes, they are associated with a multitude of adverse outcomes. Both cyclosporine and tacrolimus are associated with a wide variety of long-term complications, including nephrotoxicity leading to chronic renal failure (CRF) or end-stage renal disease.[19] A population-based cohort analysis of liver transplants from 1990 to 2000 showed frequencies of CRF of 13.9% at 3 years and 18.1% after 5 years.[20]

Given the toxicology concerns, current studies are designed to turn toward other immunosuppressive methods to reduce exposure to CNIs immediately after transplant. Recent studies involving antibody induction indicate a higher glomerular filtration rate (GFR) in the short term, but long-term results are inconclusive.[15] In addition, recent studies indicate benefits to replacing or supplementing CNIs with mTOR inhibitors: a multicenter prospective study covering 370 patients supported the hypothesis that, compared with a standard tacrolimus regimen, administering everolimus with reduced tacrolimus levels results in significant renal benefit, attenuating the rate of GFR decline by approximately 55%.[21]

Infectious complications
Improved immunosuppressive regimens have greatly improved graft and patient survival but leave a risk for opportunistic infections. Bacterial infections account for up to 70% of posttransplant infections, with viral and fungal infections comprising most of the remainder.[22] Physicians generally administer prophylactic treatments immediately following operation; the bacterial infection rate is highest in the first month and, by 6 months after the transplant, opportunistic bacterial infections are uncommon because the immunosuppression dosages are lowered.[23]

Metabolic syndrome
Metabolic syndrome is an important set of risk factors associated with risk in development of type 2 diabetes (T2D) and cardiovascular disease. In a clinical trial conducted by First and colleagues,[24] new-onset diabetes after transplant (NODAT) was measured at up to 45% of at-risk liver transplant recipients, although literature values vary widely on the incidence rate because of differences in diagnostic criteria, study design, and patient characteristics.[15] An analysis of the United Network for Organ Sharing database revealed differences between NODAT incidence in deceased versus living donor transplants, indicating that donor characteristics may contribute to NODAT.[25] Among the immunosuppressive drugs within the immunosuppressive regimen, both glucocorticoids and CNIs are recognized as causing hypertension. In addition to its other effects, CNIs promote sympathetic activity and the renin-angiotensin system, inducing vasoconstriction and sodium reabsorption in the kidneys,[26] and the incidence of hypertension/use of antihypertensive drugs increases from a pretransplant prevalence of between ∼15% and 60% to 70% posttransplant.[27–29]

By adjusting the levels of CNI administered in the immunosuppression regimen, this complication can be alleviated with little or no risk to patient and graft health.[30] Furthermore, mTOR inhibitors can carry significant metabolic and hematologic side effects,[31] because they reduce lipase activity, which results in decreased catabolism of circulating lipoproteins and leads to dyslipidemia.[32] In one study, hypertriglyceridemia levels were significantly higher ($P<.01$) for patients on sirolimus compared with patients on CsA, at 51% versus 12%. Hypercholesterolemia was also found to be significantly associated ($P<.01$) in sirolimus patients as opposed to CsA patients, at 44% versus 14%.[33] This condition is usually managed by further introduction of statins, a widely used class of lipid level–lowering medications,[34] and stopping mTOR inhibitor administration also reverses these effects.[30]

BIOMARKER MONITORING

Even with close monitoring of immunosuppressive drugs within established therapeutic ranges, clinical experience shows a broad range of outcomes among patients. Moreover, therapeutic drug monitoring does not apply to corticosteroids (eg, prednisone) or biologics (eg, belatacept), and it provides no information on minimization and weaning of the immunosuppressive regimen. Although biomarkers such as creatinine, proteinuria, and bilirubin are readily available to complement contemporary analytical methods, they are not effective at predicting rejection or immune response.[35] Thus, more accurate biomarkers are needed in transplantation; these biomarkers need to be cost-effective, quick to use, and accurate.[36] Biomarkers in transplantation can be divided into 2 general categories: drug-specific biomarkers, which monitor drug pharmacology; and drug nonspecific biomarkers, which provide a picture of generalized immunosuppressive effect.[36] Drug-specific biomarkers include biomarkers for immunosuppressive drugs and pharmacogenetic biomarkers, whereas drug nonspecific biomarkers include biomarkers of immune response and organ function, as seen in **Fig. 2**.

Immunosuppressive Biomarkers

Immunosuppressive regimens typically comprise combinations of steroids, CNIs, antibody inductors, antimetabolites, and mTOR inhibitors. In recent years, research on biomarkers for immunosuppressive drug pharmacology has shifted toward CNIs, mTOR inhibitors, and mycophenolate.[37]

Biomarkers for calcineurin inhibitors

Although most transplant patients use tacrolimus, most research regarding the pharmacodynamic influence of CNIs has been performed with CsA.[38] Studies suggest that calcineurin phosphatase activity in peripheral blood mononuclear cells (PBMCs) is closely related to CsA concentrations.[39–41] In a longitudinal study with 107 lung transplant patients, calcineurin activity was inversely correlated to increased levels of graft-versus-host disease, with the optimal enzyme activity ranging from 12 to 102 pmol/mg/min within the study sample.[39] Within liver transplant patients, there is evidence that patients on tacrolimus show a link between low calcineurin activity and nephrotoxicity,[40] whereas Blanchet and colleagues[41] observed that decreased

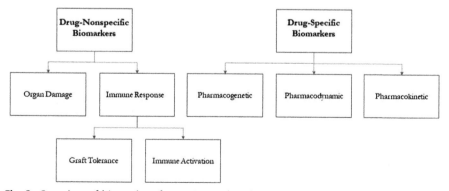

Fig. 2. Overview of biomarkers for posttransplant immunosuppression monitoring.

pretransplant levels of calcineurin activity correlated with increased rates of hepato-cellular carcinoma. These studies provide a motivation for therapy optimization in transplantation.

Nuclear factor of activated T (NFAT) lymphocytes is another promising biomarker for monitoring CNI pharmacodynamics. Of the 5 NFAT proteins, *NFAT1*, *NFAT2*, and *NFAT4* regulate downstream immune response of calcineurin[42]; dephosphorylation of NFAT prevents the nuclear translocation and transcription required for activation of T-cell mobilization. Current methods of measuring NFAT activity involve reverse transcription polymerase chain reaction[43,44] or flow cytometry.[45] Although preliminary results appear compelling, further studies are required to elucidate the effects of NFAT translocation in transplantation.[42]

Biomarkers for mammalian target of rapamycin inhibitors

Compared with the work completed on CNI biomarkers, research on drug-specific biomarkers of mTOR inhibitors remains in a preliminary phase.[36] In addition to standard Western blot analysis,[46,47] enzyme-linked immunosorbent assay (ELISA)[46] and phosphoflow cytometry have been used to analyze p70S6 kinase and S6 protein phosphorylation, respectively.[48]

Biomarkers for mycophenolic acid

MPA acts as an inhibitor of inosine monophosphate dehydrogenase (IMPDH) I and II within PBMCs, and numerous pharmacodynamic studies have logically targeted IMPDH as a biomarker candidate of MPA.[37] Glander and colleagues[49] were instrumental in developing an accurate, reproducible assay measuring conversion of IMP to xanthosine 5'-monophosphate, and later researchers modified the assay to measure IMPDH activity in CD4+ T cells.[50] In a study conducted with 48 renal transplant recipients, Glander and colleagues[51] observed large interindividual variability in pretransplant IMPDH activity at 9.35 ± 4.22 nmol/mg/h. Further investigating mycophenolate mofetil (MMF), the ester prodrug form of MPA, the team found that patient age, extent of MMF dose reduction posttransplant, and high IMPDH activity were all significant contributors to rejection.[51] Moreover, significantly lower IMPDH expression levels were found to be associated with patients with T2D.[52] IMPDH biomarkers for MPA offer promising potential, but large-scale implementation is hindered by the time-intensive and labor-intensive aspects of collecting IMPDH measurements.[37]

Drug-specific Pharmacogenetic Biomarkers

With the rapid advances in genotyping and sequencing technologies over the last decade, the advent of genotype-based personalized dosing is approaching integration into clinical practice. Studies on immunosuppressive drugs, particularly on the CNI and mTOR inhibitor classes, have the potential for genetics to predict individual response to specific ISTs.[53,54] Even with the potential for precision medicine in genomic testing, very few contemporary transplant programs use genetic tests to identify genetic polymorphisms relevant to the pharmacokinetics and pharmacodynamics of drugs. The hesitance at incorporating genotype-based dosing stems from the dearth of scientific research showing added benefit to current therapeutic drug monitoring approaches. Nevertheless, several widely studied genes show clinical promise as complementary tools in therapeutic drug monitoring.[55] A summary of the most relevant pharmacogenetic studies with patients on tacrolimus is given in **Table 1**.[56]

Cytochrome P450–related enzymes

Numerous studies have shown that tacrolimus pharmacokinetics depend significantly on the *CYP3A5*1/3* (*rs776746*) allele, a genetic polymorphism relating to poor

Table 1
Pharmacogenetic studies on tacrolimus pharmacokinetics in liver transplantation

Gene	Variant	PMID	Sample Size	Results
ABCB1	rs1128503	17885626	150D	rs1128503T and rs2032582T hepatic C greater than CC and GG (P<.035)
CYP3A5	rs776746, rs10264272	17885626	150D	rs776746G higher D than AA (P<.05)
CYP3A7	*1/*3	17885626	150D	NA

Abbreviations: NA, not available; PMID, PubMed identifier.

metabolization of tacrolimus.[55,57] *CYP3A5*1/3* shows ethnic differences in allele frequencies; in white people, the polymorphism is mostly absent, whereas 73% of African Americans have at least 1 functional copy.[58] Although there has been no randomized controlled trial to date showing that *CYP3A5* has affected a clinical end point, perhaps because of the alleviating effects of other immunosuppressive drugs such as MPA and steroids,[55] a growing number of transplant pharmacy practitioners suggest that *CYP3A5* should be taken into account during therapeutic drug monitoring of tacrolimus.

Sharing 85% of its genetic sequence with *CYP3A5*,[59] *CYP3A4* offers intriguing effects on immunosuppressive drug metabolism. Initial research focused on its impact on the pharmacodynamics of CNIs such as cyclosporine and tacrolimus,[55] and the *CYP3A4*22* variant may significant affect tacrolimus clearance.[32] Studies have also indicated that *CYP3A4* may also moderate mTOR inhibitor effects in patients, including associations with decreased cyclosporine and sirolimus clearance as well as increased risk of nephrotoxicity.[60–62] In addition to *CYP3A5* and *CYP3A4*, cytochrome P450 (CYP) oxidoreductase (*POR*) has been studied extensively. A diflavin reductase, *POR* provides CYPs with electrons by which to metabolize drugs.[55] Studies have shown that, in patients carrying the *CYP3A5*1* variant, the *POR*28* allele induces *CYP3A5* activity to speed up CNI metabolism.[3]

Adenosine triphosphate-binding cassette subfamily B member 1

Adenosine triphosphate-binding cassette subfamily B member 1 (*ABCB 1*), also known by its classic name *P-gp 1*, is an efflux pump lining many tissues of the body, including the lining of epithelial cells and hepatocytes.[54] Using adenosine triphosphate (*ATP*), it actively transports xenobiotics into bile ducts within the liver.[55] Most studies involving *ABCB-1* have focused on its effects on the bioavailability of such drugs as tacrolimus and sirolimus. By targeting P-gp, researchers expect to both improve oral bioavailability and decrease intraindividual variability of immunosuppressive drugs. Several single nucleotide polymorphisms (SNPs) have been identified within *ABCB-1*, including *ABCB1 3435TT* (*rs 1045642*), a variant that leads to a 1.7-fold decrease in the drug-removal efficiency of CsA,[63] and *ABCB1 3435CC* (*rs 1045642*), a variant that results in an improved action of *ABCB-1* for tacrolimus removal.[55]

Nonspecific Biomarkers

As opposed to drug-specific biomarkers, nonspecific biomarkers give information regarding general transplant status. These nonspecific biomarkers can be subdivided into biomarkers of organ damage and biomarkers of immune response.[55] Although termed nonspecific, these biomarkers nonetheless hold the potential for personalizing approaches to posttransplant therapeutics.

Biomarkers of organ damage

Among liver recipients, nephrotoxicity leading to end-stage renal disease remains one of the major complications of patient survival, affecting 5% of recipients 13 years after transplant.[15,19] Much of these outcomes are attributable to chronic kidney disease (CKD). Therefore, there exists a need for accurate, noninvasive biomarkers to monitor and predict renal damage in addition to the liver allograft. However, although contemporary clinical practice does incorporate biomarkers such as creatinine, proteinuria, and bilirubin, these markers do not suggest ongoing injury or forewarn of potential graft injury; instead, they only corroborate the presence of an already advanced graft injury.[55]

In the weeks, months, and years after liver transplant, recipients undergo liver function tests (LFTs) to screen for hepatic dysfunction and damage; commonly screened values include bilirubin and aminotransferase levels. Although a combined bevy of many LFTs can provide sensitive indications of liver damage, they possess non-negligible false-positive rates.[64] Therefore, there is active research ongoing for alternative biomarkers for liver damage. In particular, microRNAs (miRNAs), a class of noncoding RNAs, have been investigated for assessment of graft quality. Compared with traditional substances measured in LFTs, miRNA offers superior detection of liver injury because of earlier increases and stabilization of miRNA levels.[65] An investigation into hepatocyte-derived miRNAs (HDmiRs) as biomarkers of ischemic liver injury and liver rejection revealed that serum HDmiRs miR-122, miR-148a, and miR-194 were associated with posttransplant hepatic injury.[66] In a study to diagnose acute cellular rejection (ACR) with high specificity and sensitivity, Shaked and colleagues[67] performed miRNA profiling in 318 serum samples from 69 liver transplant recipients on tacrolimus. Levels of 31 miRNAs were significantly associated with ACR diagnosis, with 2 of these miRNAs predicting ACR up to 40 days before biopsy-proven rejection. Thus, there is significant potential for personalizing immunosuppression via facilitating minimization and preemptive adjustment of drug levels based on levels of these prognostic/diagnostic miRNA markers. Furthermore, 2 hierarchical clusters of miRNA were discovered, showing association with hepatic injury and immune function, respectively.[67] Further studies have identified additional miRNA biomarkers in pretransplant prefusates, lymphocytes, and posttransplant bile **(Table 2)**.[65,68–70] Although miRNA test results have not yet translated into clinical practice in the management of individual transplant patients,[71] the continuing development of increasingly sensitive miRNA assays, with sequence specificity down to a single base, will soon allow techniques suitable for clinical use.[72]

Urine-based measurement of protein and mRNA biomarkers provides a noninvasive alternative to method such as biopsies. In a study of 262 urine samples covering both healthy and nephropathic allografts, Sigdel and colleagues[73] used two-dimensional LC-MS/MS to identify 6379 unique peptides ($P<.001$). Several biomarkers, including calreticulin (CALR), F-box and leucine-rich repeat protein (FBXL 19), and antigenic protein DPP4, were found to be strongly associated with acute rejection (AR), chronic injury, and BK virus nephritis.[73] Various studies have also identified numerous biomarkers associated with CKD, including kidney injury molecule (KIM-1)[74] and neutrophil gelatinase-associated lipocalin (NGAL).[75,76]

Graft-derived cell-free DNA (cfDNA) represents another approach to analyzing graft integrity and rejection. cfDNA is released via necrotic and apoptotic cells into the bloodstream, where it can be measured using a droplet digital polymerase chain reaction (ddPCR) assay.[71,77] Known as a liquid biopsy, the ddPCR assay provides quick, cost-effective results and has the potential to standardize the methodology of solid organ graft integrity measurement.[71] Beck and colleagues[78] determined that monitoring

Table 2
Summary of identified microRNA biomarkers of liver injury

PMID	Medium	miRNAs	Summary of Results
21932376[65]	Peritransplant liver tissue, posttransplant serum	miR-122 miR-148a miR-194	miR-122 and miR-148a reduction in liver tissue negatively correlated with ischemia time length miR-122, miR-148a, miR-194 levels correlated with levels of transaminases
23466638[69]	Plasma and portal lymphocytes	miR-122 miR-146a miR-192	Increased plasma levels in all miRNAs during AR
24648209[70]	Posttransplant bile	miR-106a miR-517a miR-892a	Increased in bile after development of ischemic cholangiopathy posttransplant
23928409[68]	Pretransplant graft perfusates	miR-30e miR-122 miR-146a miR-148a miR-192 miR-222 miR-296	Profiles of cholangiocyte-derived and hepatocyte-derived miRNAs predictive for development of posttransplant ischemic cholangiopathy

Abbreviation: AR, acute rejection.

of cfDNA identifies rejection episodes earlier than either LFT monitoring of aspartate transaminase or bilirubin. Schütz and colleagues[77] reached a similar conclusion: cfDNA showed superior identification of AR than did any LFT, with an area under the curve of 97.1 (95% confidence interval, 93.4%–100%). Moreover, whole-genome, shotgun, or targeting sequencing technologies can also be used to identify SNPs to calculate the percentage of donor DNA. The percentage of the cell-specific (graft) DNA can be closely monitored over time, and disturbances in the percentage can be identified to indicate graft damage.[71] Nevertheless, the liver poses a specific problem for cfDNA and cell-specific cfDNA monitoring with its remarkable ability to regenerate and replace lost tissue[79]; hundreds of millions of hepatocytes are shed each day, which cause issues with sensitivity and specificity of monitoring.

Biomarkers of immune response

Despite advances in surgical techniques and the introduction of more efficient immunosuppressant therapies, nearly one-fifth (17%) of liver recipients experience rejection. When genetic disparities exist between the donor-recipient pair, the recipient's immune system may recognize polymorphic peptides of the donor as nonself.[56] A well-established system method of therapeutic drug monitoring is screening of anti–human leukocyte antigen (anti-HLA) antibodies via ELISA and LUMINEX-based assessments.[36] Key HLA loci have been generally considered to be the main contributors to allograft rejection in solid organ transplants, although the high genetic variability within HLA loci means that detailed characterization of donor-recipient HLA mismatches is not routinely achieved[56]; furthermore, the incidence of transplant rejection among HLA-matching siblings suggests noncompatibility between non-HLA loci.[80] Therefore, a major area of intense research within the transplant community is the use of large-scale genetic maps, such as the International HapMap Project,[81] to investigate factors of genetic variation associated with outcomes including rejection, graft failure, and delay graft function.[56] To identify important genomic variants across thousands of potential candidates, a large pool of genetic information is required to bolster statistical power by facilitating ease of cross-cohort meta-analyses among high-priority genomic candidates.[82] As part of the International Genetics & Translational Research in Transplantation Network (iGeneTRAiN), a major international consortium on transplantation genomics,[83] Li and colleagues[82] designed a customized genome-wide genotyping array (TxArray) consisting of approximately 782,000 markers to capture SNPs of natural killer cell immunoglobulinlike receptor (KIR) region, HLA, pharmacogenomic, and metabolic loci. With the introduction of a cost-effective, comprehensive, genome-wide genotyping tool that provides accurate results with high statistical power, large-scale genotyping of transplant-related studies is likely to constitute a significant portion of future transplantation research.

Given that immunosuppression influences rejection and elicits toxicity, a major focus within transplantation is induction of operational tolerance, which can be defined as the absence of acute and chronic rejection with indefinite graft survival within an immunosuppressant-free host.[84] Regulatory T lymphocytes (T_{regs}) have been known to prevent allograft rejection for more than 3 decades and have the potential to identify patients who need additional immunosuppression as well as patients who have achieved operational tolerance.[36,85] Typical clinical practice involves close immunologic profiling of the de novo donor-recipient encounter in the early posttransplant period to detect rejection; in the long term, tolerance assays identify T-cell regulation patterns and presence of operational tolerance.[84] Forkhead/winghead helix transcription factor P3 (FoxP3) has been identified as a key transcriptional factor to elucidate the immunologic characteristics of T_{regs} in liver transplants, with increases in $CD4^+$ $CD25^+$ $FoxP3^+$ T_{regs} transcripts associated with operational tolerance during immunosuppressant withdrawal[84]; liver transplant patients being weaned off a CNI-based immunosuppression regimen showed a 3.5-fold increase in relative expression of FoxP3 mRNA.[15,86] Furthermore, both in vitro and in vivo experimental models have shown that FoxP3 transfection and subsequent T_{regs} production in naive T cells can lead to tolerance induction and graft acceptance.[84,87,88] With intense and continuing research, T_{reg} technology is progressing rapidly. TRACT (T_{reg} Adoptive Cell Transfer) therapeutics, a biotechnology firm, has already received US Food and Drug Administration approval to start phase 2 clinical trials to investigate T_{reg} therapy for kidney transplant recipients, which involves pretransplant in vitro isolation and proliferation of each patient's own T_{reg} cells; after transplant, the patient is infused with these laboratory-grown cells, drastically reducing the need for immunosuppressive drugs.[89,90]

In addition to T_{regs}, dendritic cells (DCs) have shown promise in transplant rejection research. Tolerogenic DCs, a specific type of immature DC, serve to help promote T_{reg} development to help mediate their suppressive functions.[91] From a clinical perspective, in vitro propagation of DCs will be necessary to generate sufficient numbers of DCs for therapeutic applications.[84]

SUMMARY

Although the introduction of immunosuppressive agents has been responsible for the great success of liver transplantation, there is significant long-term morbidity because of off-target effects of these immunosuppressive drugs. Moreover, current immunosuppressive methods are not sufficiently specific or sensitive to account for the large variability in interindividual response to transplantation and drug therapeutics. Considering these facts, it is necessary to develop new strategies for personalized care in liver transplantation; current research in biomarkers of organ damage and immune response reveals compelling methods of minimally invasive, precise approaches for posttransplant monitoring of drug regimens and liver health.

REFERENCES

1. Feng S, Ekong UD, Lobritto SJ, et al. Complete immunosuppression withdrawal and subsequent allograft function among pediatric recipients of parental living donor liver transplants. JAMA 2012;307(3). https://doi.org/10.1001/jama.2011. 2014.
2. Dasgupta A. Limitations of immunoassays used for therapeutic drug monitoring of immunosuppressants. In: Personalized immunosuppression in transplantation: role of biomarker monitoring and therapeutic drug monitoring. 2015. p. 29–56. https://doi.org/10.1016/B978-0-12-800885-0.00002-3.
3. de Jonge H, Geerts I, Declercq P, et al. Apparent elevation of cyclosporine whole blood concentrations in a renal allograft recipient. Ther Drug Monit 2010;32(5): 529–31.
4. Langman LJ, LeGatt DF, Yatscoff RW. Blood distribution of mycophenolic acid. Ther Drug Monit 1994;16(6):602–7.
5. Tempestilli M, Di Stasio E, Basile MR, et al. Low plasma concentrations of albumin influence the affinity column-mediated immunoassay method for the measurement of tacrolimus in blood during the early period after liver transplantation. Ther Drug Monit 2013;35(1):96–100.
6. Westley IS, Taylor PJ, Salm P, et al. Cloned enzyme donor immunoassay tacrolimus assay compared with high-performance liquid chromatography-tandem mass spectrometry and microparticle enzyme immunoassay in liver and renal transplant recipients. Ther Drug Monit 2007;29(5):584–91.
7. Bazin C, Guinedor A, Barau C, et al. Evaluation of the Architect® tacrolimus assay in kidney, liver, and heart transplant recipients. J Pharm Biomed Anal 2010;53(4):997–1002.
8. Westley IS, Morris RG, Taylor PJ, et al. CEDIA sirolimus assay compared with HPLC-MS/MS and HPLC-UV in transplant recipient specimens. Ther Drug Monit 2005;27(3):309–14.
9. Schmid RW, Lotz J, Schweigert R, et al. Multi-site analytical evaluation of a chemiluminescent magnetic microparticle immunoassay (CMIA) for sirolimus on the Abbott ARCHITECT analyzer. Clin Biochem 2009;42(15):1543–8.
10. Strom T, Haschke M, Boyd J, et al. Crossreactivity of isolated everolimus metabolites with the Innofluor Certican immunoassay for therapeutic drug monitoring of everolimus. Ther Drug Monit 2007;29(6):743–9.
11. Jourdil J-F, Picard P, Meunier C, et al. Ultra-fast cyclosporin A quantitation in whole blood by laser diode thermal desorption-tandem mass spectrometry; comparison with high performance liquid chromatography-tandem mass spectrometry. Anal Chim Acta 2013;805:80–6.
12. Johnson-Davis KL, McMillin GA. Application of liquid chromatography combined with mass spectrometry or tandem mass spectrometry for therapeutic drug monitoring of immunosuppressants. Chapter 3. In: Personalized immunosuppression in transplantation. 2016. p. 57–81. https://doi.org/10.1016/B978-0-12-800885-0. 00003-5.
13. Vogeser M, Seger C. Pitfalls associated with the use of liquid chromatography-tandem mass spectrometry in the clinical laboratory. Clin Chem 2010;56(8): 1234–44.

14. Sallustio BC, Noll BD, Morris RG. Comparison of blood sirolimus, tacrolimus and everolimus concentrations measured by LC-MS/MS, HPLC-UV and immunoassay methods. Clin Biochem 2011;44(2–3):231–6.

15. Porrett PM, Hashmi SK, Shaked A. Immunosuppression: trends and tolerance? Clin Liver Dis 2014;18(3):687–716.

16. Demetris AJ. Liver biopsy interpretation for causes of late liver allograft dysfunction. Hepatology 2006;44(2):489–501.

17. Jain A, Demetris AJ, Kashyap R, et al. Does tacrolimus offer virtual freedom from chronic rejection after primary liver transplantation? Risk and prognostic factors in 1,048 liver transplantations with a mean follow-up of 6 years. Liver Transpl 2001;7(7):623–30.

18. Shepherd RW, Turmelle Y, Nadler M, et al. Risk factors for rejection and infection in pediatric liver transplantation. Am J Transplant 2008;8(2):396–403.

19. Gonwa TA, Mai ML, Melton LB, et al. End-stage renal disease (ESRD) after orthotopic liver transplantation (OLTX) using calcineurin-based immunotherapy: risk of development and treatment. Transplantation 2001;72(12):1934–9.

20. Ojo AO, Held PJ, Port FK, et al. Chronic renal failure after transplantation of a nonrenal organ. N Engl J Med 2003;349(10):931–40.

21. Fischer L, Saliba F, Kaiser GM, et al. Three-year outcomes in de novo liver transplant patients receiving everolimus with reduced tacrolimus: follow-up results from a randomized, multicenter study. Transplantation 2015;99(7):1455–62.

22. Hernandez MDP, Martin P, Simkins J. Infectious complications after liver transplantation. Gastroenterol Hepatol (N Y) 2015;11(11):741–53. Available at: http://www.pubmedcentral.nih.gov/articlerender.fcgi?artid=4849501&tool=pmcentrez&rendertype=abstract.

23. del Pozo JL. Update and actual trends on bacterial infections following liver transplantation. World J Gastroenterol 2008;14(32):4977–83.

24. First MR, Dhadda S, Croy R, et al. New-onset diabetes after transplantation (NODAT): an evaluation of definitions in clinical trials. Transplantation 2013;96(1):58–64.

25. Yadav AD, Chang Y-H, Aqel BA, et al. New onset diabetes mellitus in living donor versus deceased donor liver transplant recipients: analysis of the UNOS/OPTN database. J Transplant 2013;2013:269096.

26. Mells G, Neuberger J. Reducing the risks of cardiovascular disease in liver allograft recipients. Transplantation 2007;83:1141–50.

27. Watt KDS, Pedersen RA, Kremers WK, et al. Evolution of causes and risk factors for mortality post-liver transplant: results of the NIDDK long-term follow-up study. Am J Transplant 2010;10(6):1420–7.

28. Laryea M, Watt KD, Molinari M, et al. Metabolic syndrome in liver transplant recipients: prevalence and association with major vascular events. Liver Transpl 2007;13(8):1109–14.

29. Pfitzmann R, Nüssler NC, Hippler-Benscheidt M, et al. Long-term results after liver transplantation. Transpl Int 2008;21(3):234–46.

30. Segev DL, Sozio SM, Shin EJ, et al. Steroid avoidance in liver transplantation: meta-analysis and meta-regression of randomized trials. Liver Transpl 2008;14(4):512–25.

31. Taylor AL, Watson CJE, Bradley JA. Immunosuppressive agents in solid organ transplantation: mechanisms of action and therapeutic efficacy. Crit Rev Oncol Hematol 2005;56(1 SPEC. ISS.):23–46.

32. Pallet N, Legendre C. Adverse events associated with mTOR inhibitors. Expert Opin Drug Saf 2013;12(2):177–86.

33. Trotter JF, Wachs ME, Trouillot TE, et al. Dyslipidemia during sirolimus therapy in liver transplant recipients occurs with concomitant cyclosporine but not tacrolimus. Liver Transpl 2001;7(5):401–8.
34. Kaplan B, Qazi Y, Wellen JR. Strategies for the management of adverse events associated with mTOR inhibitors. Transplant Rev (Orlando) 2014;28(3):126–33.
35. Sood S, Testro AG. Immune monitoring post liver transplant. World J Transplant 2014;4(1):30–9.
36. Shipkova M. Biomarker monitoring in immunosuppressant therapy: an overview. In: Personalized immunosuppression in transplantation: role of biomarker monitoring and therapeutic drug monitoring. 2015. p. 125–52. https://doi.org/10.1016/B978-0-12-800885-0.00006-0.
37. Shipkova M, Schütz E, Besenthal I, et al. Investigation of the crossreactivity of mycophenolic acid glucuronide metabolites and of mycophenolate mofetil in the Cedia MPA assay. Ther Drug Monit 2010;32(1):79–85.
38. Yano I. Pharmacodynamic monitoring of calcineurin phosphatase activity in transplant patients treated with calcineurin inhibitors. Drug Metab Pharmacokinet 2008;23(3):150–7.
39. Sanquer S, Amrein C, Grenet D, et al. Expression of calcineurin activity after lung transplantation: a 2-year follow-up. PLoS One 2013;8(3). https://doi.org/10.1371/journal.pone.0059634.
40. Fukudo M, Yano I, Katsura T, et al. A transient increase of calcineurin phosphatase activity in living-donor kidney transplant recipients with acute rejection. Drug Metab Pharmacokinet 2010;25(5):411–7.
41. Blanchet B, Hurtova M, Roudot-Thoraval F, et al. Deficiency in calcineurin activity in liver transplantation candidates with alcoholic cirrhosis or hepatocellular carcinoma. Liver Int 2009;29(8):1152–7.
42. Bremer S, Vethe NT, Bergan S. Monitoring calcineurin inhibitors response based on NFAT-regulated gene expression. Chapter 11. Elsevier Inc; 2016. https://doi.org/10.1016/B978-0-12-800885-0.00011-4.
43. Billing H, Giese T, Sommerer C, et al. Pharmacodynamic monitoring of cyclosporine A by NFAT-regulated gene expression and the relationship with infectious complications in pediatric renal transplant recipients. Pediatr Transplant 2010;14(7):844–51.
44. Giese T, Zeier M, Schemmer P, et al. Monitoring of NFAT-regulated gene expression in the peripheral blood of allograft recipients: a novel perspective toward individually optimized drug doses of cyclosporine A. Transplantation 2004;77(3):339–44.
45. Maguire O, Tornatore KM, O'Loughlin KL, et al. Nuclear translocation of nuclear factor of activated T cells (NFAT) as a quantitative pharmacodynamic parameter for tacrolimus. Cytometry A 2013;83(12):1096–104.
46. Hartmann B, He X, Keller F, et al. Development of a sensitive phospho-p70 S6 kinase ELISA to quantify mTOR proliferation signal inhibition. Ther Drug Monit 2013;35(2):233–9.
47. Leogrande D, Teutonico A, Ranieri E, et al. Monitoring biological action of rapamycin in renal transplantation. Am J Kidney Dis 2007;50(2):314–25.
48. Dieterlen MT, Bittner HB, Klein S, et al. Assay validation of phosphorylated S6 ribosomal protein for a pharmacodynamic monitoring of mTOR-inhibitors in peripheral human blood. Cytometry B Clin Cytom 2012;82 B(3):151–7.
49. Glander P, Patrick Braun K, Hambach P, et al. Non-radioactive determination of inosine 5′-monophosphate dehydro-genase (IMPDH) in peripheral mononuclear cells. Clin Biochem 2001;34(7):543–9.

50. Vethe NT, Bergan S. Determination of inosine monophosphate dehydrogenase activity in human CD4+ cells isolated from whole blood during mycophenolic acid therapy. Ther Drug Monit 2006;28(5):608–13.

51. Glander P, Hambach P, Braun K-P, et al. Pre-transplant inosine monophosphate dehydrogenase activity is associated with clinical outcome after renal transplantation. Am J Transplant 2004;4(12):2045–51.

52. Dostalek M, Gohh RY, Akhlaghi F. Inosine monophosphate dehydrogenase expression and activity are significantly lower in kidney transplant recipients with diabetes mellitus. Ther Drug Monit 2013;35(3):374–83.

53. Birdwell KA, Decker B, Barbarino JM, et al. Clinical pharmacogenetics implementation consortium (CPIC) guidelines for CYP3A5 genotype and tacrolimus dosing. Clin Pharmacol Ther 2015;98(1):19–24.

54. Roden DM. Cardiovascular pharmacogenomics: the future of cardiovascular therapeutics? Can J Cardiol 2013;29(1):58–66.

55. Langman L, Van Gelder T, Van Schaik RHN. Pharmacogenomics aspect of immunosuppressant therapy. In: Personalized immunosuppression in transplantation: role of biomarker monitoring and therapeutic drug monitoring. 2015. p. 109–24. https://doi.org/10.1016/B978-0-12-800885-0.00005-9.

56. Almoguera B, Shaked A, Keating BJ. Transplantation genetics: current status and prospects. Am J Transplant 2014;14(4):764–78.

57. Hesselink DA, Van Schaik RHN, Van Der Heiden IP, et al. Genetic polymorphisms of the CUP3A4, CUP3A5, and MDR-1 genes and pharmacokinetics of the calcineurin inhibitors cyclosporine and tacrolimus. Clin Pharmacol Ther 2003;74(3): 245–54.

58. Hustert E, Haberl M, Burk O, et al. The genetic determinants of the CYP3A5 polymorphism. Pharmacogenetics 2001;11(9):773–9.

59. Hamosh A, Scott AF, Amberger J, et al. Online Mendelian Inheritance in Man (OMIM). Hum Mutat 2000;15(1):57–61.

60. Moes DJ, Swen JJ, den Hartigh J, et al. Effect of CYP3A4*22, CYP3A5*3, and CYP3A combined genotypes on cyclosporine, everolimus, and tacrolimus pharmacokinetics in renal transplantation. CPT Pharmacometrics Syst Pharmacol 2014;3:e100.

61. Woillard JB, Kamar N, Coste S, et al. Effect of CYP3a4*22, POR*28, and PPARA RS4253728 on sirolimus in vitro metabolism and trough concentrations in kidney transplant recipients. Clin Chem 2013;59(12):1761–9.

62. Elens L, Bouamar R, Hesselink DA, et al. The new CYP3A4 intron 6 C>T polymorphism (CYP3A4*22) is associated with an increased risk of delayed graft function and worse renal function in cyclosporine-treated kidney transplant patients. Pharmacogenet Genomics 2012;6:1.

63. Crettol S, Venetz J-P, Fontana M, et al. Influence of ABCB1 genetic polymorphisms on cyclosporine intracellular concentration in transplant recipients. Pharmacogenet Genomics 2008;18(4):307–15.

64. Thapa BR, Walia A. Liver function tests and their interpretation. Indian J Pediatr 2007;74(7):67–75.

65. Farid WRR, Pan Q, Van Der Meer AJP, et al. Hepatocyte-derived microRNAs as serum biomarkers of hepatic injury and rejection after liver transplantation. Liver Transpl 2012;18(3):290–7.

66. Farid WRR, Verhoeven CJ, De Jonge J, et al. The ins and outs of microRNAs as biomarkers in liver disease and transplantation. Transpl Int 2014;27(12):1222–32.

67. Shaked A, Chang BL, Barnes MR, et al. An ectopically expressed serum miRNA signature is prognostic, diagnostic, and biologically related to liver allograft rejection. Hepatology 2017;65(1):269–80.
68. Verhoeven CJ, Farid WRR, De Ruiter PE, et al. MicroRNA profiles in graft preservation solution are predictive of ischemic-type biliary lesions after liver transplantation. J Hepatol 2013;59(6):1231–8.
69. Hu J, Wang Z, Tan C-J, et al. Plasma microRNA, a potential biomarker for acute rejection after liver transplantation. Transplantation 2013;95(8):991–9.
70. Lankisch TO, Voigtländer T, Manns MP, et al. MicroRNAs in the bile of patients with biliary strictures after liver transplantation. Liver Transpl 2014;20(6):673–8.
71. Oellerich M, Beck J, Kanzow P, et al. Graft-derived cell-free DNA as a marker of graft integrity after transplantation. In: Personalized immunosuppression in transplantation: role of biomarker monitoring and therapeutic drug monitoring. 2015. p. 153–76. https://doi.org/10.1016/B978-0-12-800885-0.00007-2.
72. Rissin DM, López-Longarela B, Pernagallo S, et al. Polymerase-free measurement of microRNA- 122 with single base specificity using single molecule arrays: detection of drug-induced liver injury. PLoS One 2017;1–15. https://doi.org/10.1371/journal.pone.0179669.
73. Sigdel TK, Salomonis N, Nicora CD, et al. The identification of novel potential injury mechanisms and candidate biomarkers in renal allograft rejection by quantitative proteomics. Mol Cell Proteomics 2014;13(2):621–31.
74. Krolewski AS, Niewczas MA, Skupien J, et al. Early progressive renal decline precedes the onset of microalbuminuria and its progression to macroalbuminuria. Diabetes Care 2014;37(1):226–34.
75. Bolignano D, Coppolino G, Campo S, et al. Neutrophil gelatinase-associated lipocalin in patients with autosomal-dominant polycystic kidney disease. Am J Nephrol 2007;27(4):373–8.
76. Lopez-Giacoman S, Madero M. Biomarkers in chronic kidney disease, from kidney function to kidney damage. World J Nephrol 2015;4(1):57–73.
77. Schütz E, Fischer A, Beck J, et al. Graft-derived cell-free DNA, a noninvasive early rejection and graft damage marker in liver transplantation: a prospective, observational, multicenter cohort study. PLoS Med 2017;14(4). https://doi.org/10.1371/journal.pmed.1002286.
78. Beck J, Bierau S, Balzer S, et al. Digital droplet PCR for rapid quantification of donor DNA in the circulation of transplant recipients as a potential universal biomarker of graft injury. Clin Chem 2013;59(12):1732–41.
79. Michalopoulos GK. Liver regeneration. J Cell Physiol 2007;213(2):286–300.
80. Gratwohl A, Döhler B, Stern M, et al. H-Y as a minor histocompatibility antigen in kidney transplantation: a retrospective cohort study. Lancet 2008;372:49–53.
81. International HapMap Consortium. The international HapMap project. Nature 2003;426(6968):789–96.
82. Li YR, van Setten J, Verma SS, et al. Concept and design of a genome-wide association genotyping array tailored for transplantation-specific studies. Genome Med 2015;7(1):90.
83. International Genetics & Translational Research in Transplantation Network (iGeneTRAiN). Design and implementation of the international genetics and translational research in transplantation network. Transplantation 2015;99(11):2401–12.
84. Wieers G, Gras J, Bourdeaux C, et al. Monitoring tolerance after human liver transplantation. Transpl Immunol 2007;17(2):83–93.
85. Baroja-Mazo A, Revilla-Nuin B, Parrilla P, et al. Tolerance in liver transplantation: biomarkers and clinical relevance. World J Gastroenterol 2016;22(34):7676–91.

86. Pons JA, Revilla-Nuin B, Baroja-Mazo A, et al. FoxP3 in peripheral blood is associated with operational tolerance in liver transplant patients during immunosuppression withdrawal. Transplantation 2008;86(10):1370–8.

87. Yong Z, Chang L, Mei YX, et al. Role and mechanisms of CD4+CD25+ regulatory T cells in the induction and maintenance of transplantation tolerance. Transpl Immunol 2007;17(2):120–9.

88. Chai JG, Xue SA, Coe D, et al. Regulatory T cells, derived from naive CD4+CD25- T cells by in vitro Foxp3 gene transfer, can induce transplantation tolerance. Transplantation 2005;79(10):1310–6.

89. Conti F, Dahlqvist G, Brisson H, et al. Regulatory T cell therapy: an option to induce operational tolerance in liver transplantation. Clin Res Hepatol Gastroenterol 2016;40(6):660–5.

90. Barker CF, Markmann JF. Historical overview of transplantation. Cold Spring Harb Perspect Med 2013;3(4):1–18.

91. Jonuleit H, Schmitt E, Schuler G, et al. Induction of interleukin 10-producing, non-proliferating CD4(+) T cells with regulatory properties by repetitive stimulation with allogeneic immature human dendritic cells. J Exp Med 2000;192(9):1213–22.

Status of Adult Living Donor Liver Transplantation in the United States

Results from the Adult-To-Adult Living Donor Liver Transplantation Cohort Study

Samir Abu-Gazala, MD[a],*, Kim M. Olthoff, MD[b]

KEYWORDS

- Adult living donor liver transplantation • Cohort study • Acute liver failure

KEY POINTS

- The number of adult-to-adult living donor liver transplants (ALDLT) is consistently increasing.
- Living donor liver transplantation (LDLT) has an important benefit for patients with acute liver failure, without compromising donor safety.
- Lower rates of acute cellular rejection can be found after LDLT in biologically related donor and recipient.

INTRODUCTION

The first adult-to-adult living donor liver transplant (ALDLT) in the United States was reported in 1998[1] as a response to the shortage of organ donors. Since then, ALDLT has been performed in more than 4500 patients in 89 centers across the United States. Although it remains a small percentage of total transplants, there has been a steady increase in ALDLT over the past 5 years (**Fig. 1**). This growth has been slow in coming to the United States. Initial reports were mainly single-center experiences, limiting the applicability of ALDLT. In 2002, the Adult-to-Adult Living Donor Liver Transplant Cohort Study (A2ALL) was launched, with funding mainly by the National Institutes of Health. The A2ALL was the first multicenter consortium aimed at providing accurate information on outcomes for both donors and recipients of ALDLT. Nine North American

Disclosure: The authors have nothing to disclose.
[a] Department of Surgery, Transplantation Unit, Hadassah Hebrew University Medical Center, Kiryat Hadassah, POB 12000, Jerusalem 91120, Israel; [b] Department of Surgery, Division of Transplant Surgery, Perelman School of Medicine, University of Pennsylvania, 3400 Spruce Street, Philadelphia, PA 19104, USA
* Corresponding author.
E-mail address: samirski11@yahoo.com

Gastroenterol Clin N Am 47 (2018) 297–311
https://doi.org/10.1016/j.gtc.2018.01.004
0889-8553/18/© 2018 Elsevier Inc. All rights reserved.

Liver Transplant Volumes – Living Donor and Total Liver Transplants

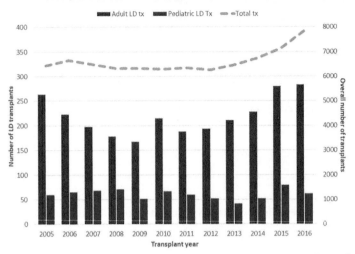

Fig. 1. Annual number of adult-to-adult and adult-to-pediatric living donor liver trans-plants, and total number of liver transplants in the United States from 2005 to 2016. Adult LD tx, adult-to-adult living donor liver transplant; Pediatric LD Tx, pediatric living donor liver transplant; Total tx, total number of liver transplants.

liver transplant centers comprised the first A2ALL consortium, initiating retrospective and prospective studies with donor and recipient outcomes over a decade (1998–2008). In 2009, the study was continued as 3 new centers joined the renewed study with additional funding from the National Institutes of Health (see Acknowledgments).

The Adult-to-Adult Living Donor Liver Transplant Cohort Study Database and Publications

The A2ALL study was carried out in 2 phases: A2ALL-1 enrolled potential liver donors and recipients evaluated for ALDLT between January 1, 1998, and August 31, 2009, and A2ALL-2 enrolled ALDLT donors and recipients who received transplant between September 1, 2009, and January 31, 2014, or were previously enrolled in A2ALL-1. Before February 28, 2003, data were collected retrospectively (retrospective cohort), and prospective data collection started thereafter (prospective cohort). In total, data from 2742 donors and 2182 recipients were collected for A2ALL, including the main study and numerous ancillary and substudies. The first publication from the consortium was in 2005. Since then, 41 articles have been published. The entire A2ALL list of publications is shown at this link: https://www.nih-a2all.org/publications.aspx.

Gillespie and colleagues[2] compared Scientific Registry of Transplant Recipients (SRTR) data with data from the A2LL and found that most submitted Organ Procurement and Transplant Network (OPTN)/SRTR data were consistent with the A2ALL, demonstrating the accuracy of the A2ALL database in comparison with the OPTN/SRTR database.

Initial Landmark Findings of the Adult-to-Adult Living Donor Liver Transplant Cohort Study

The first publication to come out of the A2ALL retrospective data examined postoperative outcomes of 385 ALDLT recipients. A primary finding was the identification of a significant learning curve for ALDLT, with more graft and patient loss reported in the first 15 to 20 living donor liver transplantation (LDLT) recipients at most centers, and survival improving with experience. Overall graft survival rates of 81% at 1 year were demonstrated[3] in this initial US experience.

A distinctive feature of the A2ALL was the consortium's decision to enroll and gather recipient data from the time of evaluation for liver transplantation and consideration of LDLT (**Fig. 2**). In 2007, Berg and colleagues[4] published the benefit of undergoing LDLT by comparing it to waiting for a deceased donor or remaining on the list without a transplant. This was among the first studies demonstrating superiority of LDLT over deceased donor liver transplantation (DDLT).

Characteristics of the Liver Transplant in the Adult-to-Adult Living Donor Liver Transplant Cohort Study and Non–Adult-to-Adult Living Donor Liver Transplant Cohort Study Centers

The A2ALL experience (9 centers, 702 LDLTs) was compared with that of other non-A2ALL US transplant centers performing LDLT[5] (67 centers, 1664 LDLTs).

Similar rates of mortality were found between A2ALL and non-A2ALL centers. Also, older recipient age, hepatocellular carcinoma (HCC) diagnosis, cold ischemia time greater than 4.5 hours, higher serum creatinine, and in-patient or intensive care unit (ICU) hospitalization were significant predictors of mortality. Again, early center experience was a predictor of higher mortality or graft failure in both A2ALL and non-A2ALL centers. Current trends in LDLT show that ALDLT is concentrating in relatively few centers across the country, with only 12 centers currently performing more than 10 ALDLT in 2016 (**Fig. 3**).

RECIPIENT AND GRAFT OUTCOMES
Graft and Patient Survival: Comparing Living Donor Liver Transplant with Deceased Donor Liver Transplant

The A2ALL consortium was able to demonstrate a significant and sustained benefit of LDLT compared with DDLT, with 70% versus 64% unadjusted survival probability at 10 years posttransplant, respectively. After adjusting for risk factors (lower Model for End-stage Liver Disease [MELD] score), fewer patients who received transplants were inpatient or in the ICU, were ventilated, were on dialysis, or had ascites. LDLT and DDLT showed similar survival rates.

Risk factors for mortality after LDLT included older age of recipients (>55 years), older donors (>50 years), dialysis at transplant, and HCC. Risk factors for reduced

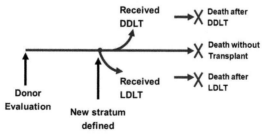

Fig. 2. Sequential stratification approach: analysis from the time of potential donor's evaluation. Recipients of LDLT were associated with the least adjusted mortality. (*Data from* Olthoff KM, Smith AR, Abecassis M, et al. Defining long-term outcomes with living donor liver transplantation in North America. Ann Surg 2015;262(3):465–75.)

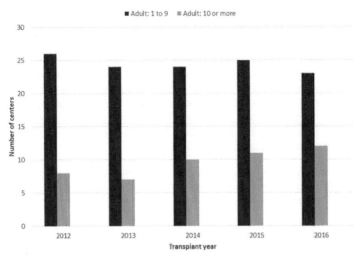

Fig. 3. Number of transplant centers performing adult LDLT in the United States based on the number of LDLT performed in a certain year. Dark bars: number of centers performing 1 to 9 adult LDLT cases in that year; light bars: number of centers performing 10 or more adult LDLT cases in that year.

graft survival also included a high MELD score, whereas female sex and diagnosis of autoimmune hepatitis or primary sclerosing cholangitis were associated with better graft survival (**Fig. 4**). Right and left donated lobes had similar graft survival.[6] These findings from the A2ALL were compatible with other published data from large registry studies comparing LDLT with DDLT.[7,8] The improved outcomes demonstrated with LDLT provided the needed support to encourage increased use in North America.

Survival Benefit with Living Donor Liver Transplant

The survival benefit of LDLT as demonstrated by the early A2ALL findings is applicable to the counseling of candidates who are contemplating pursuit of LDLT as an alternative to DDLT alternative. This survival benefit was seen across the range of MELD scores, including MELD less than 15 group (which was shown not to significantly benefit from DDLT[9]), except for when HCC was present (no survival benefit of LDLT for patients with HCC when MELD <15). These results continue to justify the role LDLT in the United States in times of limited supply of deceased organs for transplantation and the substantial waitlist mortality.

Outcomes of Living Donor Liver Transplant in Specific Patient Cohorts: The Adult-to-Adult Living Donor Liver Transplant Cohort Study Experience

Acute hepatic failure

In an A2ALL study by Campsen and colleagues[10] acute hepatic failure (ALF) was an indication for transplantation in only 1% of potential recipients considered for LDLT. The survival rate of LDLT and DDLT recipients was lower but statistically comparable (70% vs 82%, respectively) at a median follow-up of 5 years after transplant. The rate of recipient and donor complications was similar to the rate experienced overall in the A2ALL study.[11,12] Additionally, none of the patients with ALF who were evaluated for LDLT died while waiting for transplantation. This may represent an important benefit for LDLT as centers gain additional experience with ALDLT. Although this study

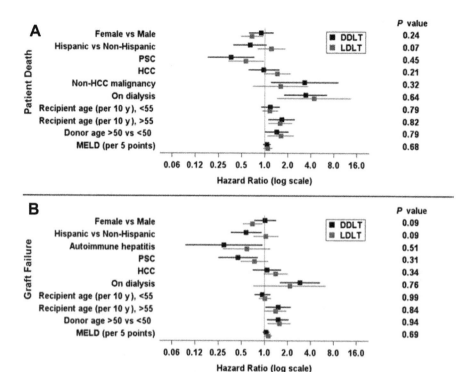

Fig. 4. Estimated hazard ratios associated with (*A*) patient mortality and (*B*) graft failure from separate Cox models for LDLT (gray boxes) and DDLT (black boxes) recipients; whiskers show 5% confidence intervals for true log hazard ratios. *P* values are from tests of interaction between each covariate and LDLT versus DDLT in a combined model. Note that all *P* values greater than 0.05 imply no significant differences in log hazard ratios between LDLT and DDLT. PSC, primary sclerosing cholangitis. (*From* Olthoff KM, Smith AR, Abecassis M, et al. Defining long-term outcomes with living donor liver transplantation in North America. Ann Surg 2015;262(3):470; with permission.)

represented a relatively limited number of cases, it was similar to the worldwide experience of LDLT in ALF.[13–15]

Recipients with the hepatitis C virus

Previous reports of poorer outcomes of LDLT for recipients with hepatitis C virus (HCV) infection[16,17] led the A2ALL to publish several studies aimed at investigating that risk, keeping in mind the risks that healthy donors have to take to enable LDLT. All of these studies were conducted before the era of direct antiviral medications for HCV.

In 2007, Terrault and colleagues[18] found similar overall 3-year patient and graft survival between LDLT and DDLT HCV-infected recipients after the first 20 LDLT cases. A study published in 2014, with a larger LDLT cohort and with a longer median posttransplant follow-up (~5 years), again showed similar results.[19] The A2ALL also showed that pretransplant treatment of HCV (with pegylated interferon α-2a or 2b and ribavirin (Peg-IFN-a2b/RBV)) prevented recurrence of HCV posttransplant in selected patients.[20] With today's treatment options for HCV, there should be no hesitation to perform LDLT in this patient population. LDLT allows the timing of transplant to coincide with the successful completion of therapy and eradication of the virus.

Recipients with hepatocellular carcinoma

In the first report from the A2ALL by Fisher and colleagues,[21] results were disappointing. They found a higher rate of HCC recurrence among LDLT recipients compared with their DDLT counterparts at 3 years (29% vs 0%, $P = .002$), similar to previously published single-center results.[22] An expedited evaluation and transplant process, termed fast-tracking, may have provided inadequate time to assess the tumor's biological behavior.

A more recent study of the A2ALL,[23] with double the number of recipients in the A2ALL cohort, and more in the MELD-era (64% vs 57%),with a longer follow-up period (median of 4.9 years), confirmed similar survival rates but still significantly higher overall recurrence of HCC after LDLT (38% vs 11% for DDLT, $P = .0004$). However, after controlling for tumor characteristics there were similar adjusted tumor recurrence rates.

Reports from Asia, where LDLT is more abundant than in Western countries, have focused on biological markers, rather than size criteria, that could predict HCC recurrence after LDLT.[24,25] If LDLT is to be used for tumors beyond current accepted criteria, these types of markers, as well as tumor differentiation, may be the best way to determine prognosis when considering risk to the donor.

Recipient Complications

Early reports from the A2ALL detailed recipient complications mainly in the early posttransplant period, similar in scope to previous single-center reports.[3,26] Infections (32%) and bile leaks (30%) were the most commonly reported early complications, whereas biliary strictures were the most common late complications (10%). Center experience correlated with the occurrence of technical complications, with reduced rate of complications after 20 cases, again demonstrating the relatively steep learning curve for LDLT.

A follow-up study reported overall long-term (up to 10 years of follow-up) complications and resolution in recipients of both DDLT and LDLT[27] (Table 1). There was a qualitative difference in the types of complications between LDLT and DDLT, with a higher probability of technical complications after LDLT, specifically biliary and vascular complications; whereas ascites, intraabdominal bleeding, cardiac complications, pulmonary edema, and the development of chronic kidney disease were more common after DDLT, reflecting a sicker group of patients. There were no differences in the rates of Clavien grade 4 complications.

Biliary complications

Biliary complications remain the Achilles heel of LDLT. The overall incidence varies widely among transplant centers and ranges between 5% and 40%, a higher incidence than DDLT.[28–30] This difference may be attributed to donor ductal size and anatomy, and biliary ischemia. The A2ALL consortium found a higher rate of a biliary complication (leak or stricture) among LDLT recipients (40%), significantly more than the 25% with DDLT. Biliary leak was the most common (64.5%) complication in the LDLT group, whereas a stricture was the most common (59.6%) in DDLT. Despite the higher incidence of biliary complication after LDLT, treatment requirements and the time to resolution was similar in both groups (1.3 months vs 2.3 months for leaks, $P = .29$; 2.3 months vs 4.9 months for strictures, $P = .61$).

Vascular complications

Initially, the A2ALL reported significantly higher rates of vascular complications in LDLT compared with DDLT.[11] These included hepatic artery thrombosis (6.5% vs 2.3%) and portal vein thrombosis (2.9% vs 0.0). The later study by Samstein and

Table 1
Probability of specific complications in recipients of living or deceased donor liver transplantation

	Complication	Overall Complication Rate		Log-Rank P Value
		LDLT	DDLT	
Significantly higher in LDLT	Bile leak or biloma	0.26	0.09	<0.0001
	Blood infection	0.26	0.15	0.0091
	Biliary stricture	0.32	0.21	0.0002
	Biliary tree infection	0.14	0.06	0.0062
	Hepatic artery thrombosis	0.06	0.04	0.0378
Significantly higher in DDLT	Pulmonary edema	0.1	0.36	<0.0001
	Ascites	0.21	0.25	0.0151
	Cardiac complication	0.02	0.06	0.0008
	Intraabdominal bleeding	0.05	0.08	0.0190

Adapted from Samstein B, Smith AR, Freise CE, et al. Complications and their resolution in recipients of deceased and living donor liver transplants: findings from the A2ALL cohort study. Am J Transplant 2016;16(2):597; with permission.

colleagues[27] found that the probability for hepatic artery thrombosis was still significantly higher in LDLT compared with DDLT, emphasizing that a higher rate of technical complications remains in LDLT. The possible causes for these complications included greater technical demand of LDLT and the donor caliber of LDLT donor vessels.

Early allograft dysfunction
In LDLT, early allograft dysfunction (EAD) has been termed small-for-size syndrome and was initially defined in the A2ALL as the presence of jaundice (bilirubin >10 mg/dL on day 7) or coagulopathy (international normalized ratio [INR] >1.6 on day 7), without technical complications.[31] Because all grafts in ALDLT are essentially small for size, the term segmental graft dysfunction was also introduced.[31] A more appropriate term is probably EAD after LDLT (EAD-LDLT). EAD-LDLT is often associated with grafts that do not meet recipient metabolic needs and is seen in grafts smaller than 0.8% graft weight to recipient body weight (<0.8%) or less than 40% of standard liver volume.[32] In addition to graft size and other donor factors, such as age and steatosis, recipient factors, such as preoperative disease severity and excessive venous flow and/or pressure, also contribute to EAD-LDLT.

In a recent study of the A2ALL, Pomposelli and colleagues[32] investigated the incidence and risk of EAD-LDLT and found EAD to occur in 16% to 19% of grafts. Risk factors associated with EAD-LDLT included graft type (left lobe grafts), size (lower graft weight among left lobes), higher preoperative bilirubin, higher portal perfusion pressure, higher donor age, and higher donor body mass index. Most importantly, LDLT recipients who met the criteria of EAD[31] were at a much higher risk for graft loss within 90 days than recipients without EAD (24% vs 5%, $P<.001$).

Liver regeneration after living donor liver transplant
Numerous single-center reports have documented the regeneration of the liver following donation and transplantation.[33–35] The patterns of liver regeneration after LDLT were comprehensively studied in the A2ALL prospective multicenter study. Everson and colleagues[20] showed that the maximal liver regeneration happened during the first 2 weeks of surgery and slowed in the next few months to reach 84% to 92% of its baseline volume by 6 months.

Regeneration was studied in detail in the prospective part of the A2ALL.[31] Among donors, mean liver growth was 80% plus or minus 13% of baseline total liver volume whereas a higher rate of regeneration was seen among recipients, with 3-month percentage reconstitution of 93% plus or minus 18% of standard liver volume.

Emond and colleagues[36] showed that donor liver volumes reached 79% and 88% of predonation volumes at 3 months and 1 year postsurgery, respectively. Enlarged spleen (which could explain postdonation thrombocytopenia) was seen in 92% and 88% of donors, at 3 months and 1 year postdonation, respectively.

Allograft rejection after living donor liver transplant

Historical single-center reports indicated a lower rate of rejection in LDLT compared with DDLT, implying an immunologic advantage of LDLT.[16,37] Shaked and colleagues[38] showed similar rates of biopsy-proven and clinically treated acute cellular rejection episodes among LDLT and DDLT recipients. Levitsky and colleagues[39] analyzed 2 comparable large cohorts from the A2ALL and SRTR that showed, contrary to older data,[40,41] graft failure and death were at an increased risk following an acute rejection episode, most significantly after the first year posttransplant. Additionally, the risk of acute rejection was lower when the donor and recipient were biologically related. In another recent study from the A2ALL, preformed donor specific antibodies (DSA) was associated with higher graft failure in DDLT.[42]

Cost-effectiveness of living donor liver transplant based on the Adult-to-Adult Living Donor Liver Transplant Cohort Study

The A2ALL presented an extensive cost-effectiveness model of adding the option of LDLT to a program performing DDLT, demonstrating increased cost but improved recipient survival and reduced deaths on the waitlist. Medical management of cirrhosis was the least cost-effective compared with DDLT and LDLT.[43]

Merion and colleagues[44] examined resource utilization by LDLT compared with DDLT by analyzing the A2ALL data and found that the overall hospitalization rates, from the time a potential donor was initially evaluated, was higher for eventual LDLT recipients. Center experience also influenced admission rates. More experienced centers (>20 LDLT cases) had fewer hospitalizations.

DONOR OUTCOMES
Predonation Evaluation and Selection

It is important to remember that donor safety must take priority over all else in LDLT. Many single centers have published on the appropriate components of the donor evaluation process, which can be exhaustive.[45,46] The A2ALL conducted different studies aimed at assessing decision-making and improving the donor evaluation process.[47,48] In a study by Trotter and colleagues[47], 1101 donor candidates were evaluated, yielding 405 (40%) actual donors. Both donor and recipient factors influenced the acceptance rate of a donor, including younger donor and recipient age, lower body mass index of the donor, biological or spousal relationship between the donor and the recipient, shorter listing time, and lower recipient MELD score.

Donor Complications and Mortality

The most common donor complications reported by the A2ALL are shown in **Table 2**.

Most donor complications were Clavien grade 1 (minor) and 2 (possibly life-threatening) complications but 1.1% of donors developed grade 3 (residual disability, n = 5) or grade 4 (leading to death, n = 3) complications, thus a mortality rate of 0.4%.[49]

Table 2		
Type of complications of donors in the Adult-to-Adult Living Donor Liver Transplant Cohort Study		
A2ALL Study, Year of Publication	**Number of Donors Who Successfully Donated**[a]	**Reported Common Complications**
Ghobrial et al,[12] 2008	393	• Bacterial infections (12%) • Biliary leaks (9%) • Incisional hernias (6%) • Pleural effusions requiring intervention (5%) • Neuropraxia (4%) • Wound infections (3%) • Reexplorations (3%) • Intraabdominal abscess (2%).
Abecassis et al,[49] 2012	740	• Bacterial infections (12.5%) • Biliary complications (9.7%) • Intraoperative complications (6%) • Incisional hernias (5.6%) • Pleural effusions (5.3%) • Psychological difficulties (4.1%) • Reexplorations (3%)

[a] Note: Donors who successfully donated plus those with graft resected but not transplanted (n = 1,[12] and n = 2[49]).

Risk factors for postdonation complications were blood transfusion, intraoperative hypotension (systolic blood pressure <100 mm Hg), and higher donor body weight (each increment of 10 kg in body weight increased the risk by 22%). Older age, male gender, and high basic metabolic index were found to be risk factors for incisional hernia formation. Most (95%) donor complications were shown to resolve by 1 year; however, some complications, such as neuropraxia, hernias, and psychological complications, remained unresolved for as long as 3 to 5 years.

In a world-wide survey, an A2ALL center reported[50] a 24% rate of donor complications (most were Clavien grade 1 or 2), 0.04% rate of need for transplantation, and a 0.2% mortality rate. Programs that performed 50 or fewer LDLTs had more aborted hepatectomies and near-miss events; hoever, center experience did not affect the incidence of donor morbidity and mortality, as seen by the A2ALL experience.[12,49]

Long-Term Postdonation Outcomes

Most donor health-related quality of life studies demonstrated results at or above US norms, and found that nearly all donors would donate again, regardless of recipient outcomes.[51,52] However, psychological distress is common in both liver and kidney donors,[53] and approximately 70% of liver donors have symptoms attributed to donation for as long as several months postdonation.[43]

The A2ALL conducted several studies aimed at postdonation outcomes and follow-up.

Long-term donor follow-up

The intensity and duration of the A2ALL donor follow-up protocol was beyond the standard follow-up at most LDLT centers: follow-up at 1 week, 1 month, 3 months, 12 months, and annually thereafter. Brown and colleagues[54] found several donor factors that influenced donor follow-up, such as donor age and race. Additionally, recipient factors, such as recipients with HCV or HCC, also decreased donor follow-up.

The A2ALL also described the long-term changes in common laboratory tests for living liver donors that may reflect their underlying health.[55] Most laboratory test values returned to normal within 3 months after donation. However, platelet counts were significantly decreased at every time point compared with baseline.

Psychological, social, and financial outcomes after donation

The A2ALL consortium has examined the psychological, social, and financial effects on donors after undergoing this procedure.[56–59] Early findings identified 16 out of 392 (4.1%) donors who had at least 1 psychiatric complication after donation. Three severe psychiatric complications were identified, including suicide, suicide attempt, and an accidental drug overdose.[56] In a follow-up report on the long-term donation, psychosocial effects, and physical health problems or concerns related to donation were found in 15% to 48% of donors, and up to 60% expressed socioeconomic concerns (financial expenditures, insurance difficulties). However, 90% felt positively about their donation and most donors experienced high psychosocial growth.[57]

Among the largest multicenter prospective studies of live liver donors' well-being, Butt and colleagues[58] showed that nearly 95% of donors reported they would make the decision to donate again if they could. Donors whose recipients had died were more likely to report unwillingness to donate again, and one-third had feelings of guilt or responsibility for the recipient's death. Up to approximately 10% of donors reported impaired mental well-being.

Another A2ALL study examined social and financial issues following donation,[59] surveying 271 live donors over a 2-year postdonation period. Among these donors, only a few (2%–8%) had worsening of family, spouse, or recipient relationships following donation, and most donors had stable or even improved relationships postdonation. This was in contrast to previous single-center studies on kidney and liver donors that found worsening of such relationships in up to 10% to 20% of donors.[60]

Sexual function after liver donation

One study from the A2LL examined the sexual functioning of donors across the donation process and up to 1 year after surgery.[61] When surveyed about their sexual functioning, most donors, of both sexes, reported poorer functioning at the evaluation phase and at 3 months after surgery, but they were least likely to report problems at 1 year.

SUMMARY

LDLT has been performed as a response to the shortage of organ donors and despite the steady increase in numbers in recent years, it still remains a small percentage of total transplants. The findings from the A2ALL consortium have been critical in the advancement of LDLT in North America. They support increased use to help decrease waitlist death and improve long-term survival of transplant recipients:

- The A2ALL multi-center cohort study was distinct in that it enrolled data on the recipient from the time of evaluation of a potential live donor, demonstrating a benefit of decreased death on the waitlist.
- A learning curve was identified, and more graft and patient loss was identified in the first 15 to 20 LDLT cases. Technical complications were more abundant after LDLT than after DDLT. Infections and biliary and vascular complications were the

most common complications after LDLT. These complications may especially occur in the first 20 cases, emphasizing the role of the learning curve.

- Most A2ALL results were in concordance to other important published data from non-A2ALL centers. Similar rates of mortality were found between A2ALL and non-A2ALL centers, with older recipient age, HCC diagnosis, cold ischemia time, higher serum creatinine, and in-patient or ICU hospitalization demonstrated as significant predictors of mortality.
- Long-term outcomes demonstrated a significant and sustained survival benefit compared with DDLT. Additionally, contrary to DDLT, the survival benefit of LDLT was also seen for those with MELD less than 15.
- LDLT has an important benefit for patients with acute liver failure, without compromising donor safety.
- Similar results after LDLT and DDLT were demonstrated in patients with HCV infection and, with the anti-HCV therapy available today, LDLT can be performed with better timing of the transplant compared with DDLT.
- Despite initial reports of higher HCC recurrence rate after LDLT, similar HCC recurrence rates were seen in the MELD era when adjusted for tumor burden.
- Lower rates of acute cellular rejection can be found after LDLT in biologically related donor and recipient.
- EAD-LDLT has been internationally defined by the A2ALL criteria as the presence of jaundice (bilirubin >10 mg/dL on day 7) or coagulopathy (INR >1.6 on day 7), and is associated with a significantly higher risk of graft loss.
- There is a significant incidence of donor complications that must be recognized. Infections and biliary complications were the most common donor complications, but most are mild (Clavien grade 1 and 2) and resolved by 1 year postdonation. Aborted hepatectomies and severe complications (Clavien grade 3 and 4) were also described.
- Long-term postdonation changes included low platelet count (up to 10% of donors), as well as rare (2%–8%) psychosocial and financial problems. Most the donors did not regret undergoing the donation.

ACKNOWLEDGMENTS

The A2ALL Study centers included Northwestern University, Chicago, IL; University of California, Los Angeles, CA; University of California, San Francisco, CA; University of Colorado Health Sciences Center, Denver, CO; University of North Carolina, Chapel Hill, NC; Department of Surgery, Columbia Presbyterian Medical Center, New York, NY; University of Pennsylvania, Philadelphia, PA; Department of Internal Medicine, University of Virginia, Charlottesville, VA; Virginia Commonwealth University, Richmond, VA; Lahey Hospital and Medical Center, Burlington, MA; University of Pittsburgh Medical Center, Pittsburgh, PA; Northwestern University, Chicago, IL; University of Toronto, Toronto, ON, Canada.

The Data Coordinating Center was University of Michigan, Ann Arbor, MI; Arbor Research Collaborative for Health, Ann Arbor, MI.

The Epidemiology and Clinical Trials Branch, Division of Digestive Diseases and Nutrition, National Institute of Diabetes and Digestive and Kidney Diseases, National Institutes of Health, Bethesda, MD were integral to the study.

REFERENCES

1. Wachs ME, Bak TE, Karrer FM, et al. Adult living donor liver transplantation using a right hepatic lobe. Transplantation 1998;66(10):1313–6.

2. Gillespie BW, Merion RM, Ortiz-Rios E, et al. Database comparison of the adult-to-adult living donor liver transplantation cohort study (A2ALL) and the SRTR U.S. Transplant Registry. Am J Transplant 2010;10(7):1621–33.
3. Olthoff KM, Merion RM, Ghobrial RM, et al. Outcomes of 385 adult-to-adult living donor liver transplant recipients: a report from the A2ALL consortium. Ann Surg 2005;242(3):314–23 [discussion: 323–5].
4. Berg CL, Gillespie BW, Merion RM, et al. Improvement in survival associated with adult-to-adult living donor liver transplantation. Gastroenterology 2007;133(6):1806–13.
5. Olthoff KM, Abecassis MM, Emond JC, et al. Outcomes of adult living donor liver transplantation: comparison of the Adult-To-Adult Living Donor Liver Transplantation Cohort Study and the national experience. Liver Transpl 2011;17(7):789–97.
6. Olthoff KM, Smith AR, Abecassis M, et al. Defining long-term outcomes with living donor liver transplantation in North America. Ann Surg 2015;262(3):465–75 [discussion: 473–5].
7. Hoehn RS, Wilson GC, Wima K, et al. Comparing living donor and deceased donor liver transplantation: a matched national analysis from 2007 to 2012. Liver Transpl 2014;20(11):1347–55.
8. Goldberg DS, French B, Abt PL, et al. Superior survival using living donors and donor-recipient matching using a novel living donor risk index. Hepatology 2014;60(5):1717–26.
9. Merion RM, Schaubel DE, Dykstra DM, et al. The survival benefit of liver transplantation. Am J Transplant 2005;5(2):307–13.
10. Campsen J, Blei AT, Emond JC, et al. Outcomes of living donor liver transplantation for acute liver failure: the Adult-To-Adult Living Donor Liver Transplantation Cohort Study. Liver Transpl 2008;14(9):1273–80.
11. Freise CE, Gillespie BW, Koffron AJ, et al. Recipient morbidity after living and deceased donor liver transplantation: findings from the A2ALL retrospective cohort study. Am J Transplant 2008;8(12):2569–79.
12. Ghobrial RM, Freise CE, Trotter JF, et al. Donor morbidity after living donation for liver transplantation. Gastroenterology 2008;135(2):468–76.
13. Kim TS, Kim JM, Kwon CHD, et al. Prognostic factors predicting poor outcome in living-donor liver transplantation for fulminant hepatic failure. Transplant Proc 2017;49(5):1118–22.
14. Choudhary NS, Saigal S, Saraf N, et al. Good outcome of living donor liver transplantation in drug-induced acute liver failure: a single-center experience. Clin Transplant 2017;31(3):e12907.
15. Goldaracena N, Spetzler VN, Marquez M, et al. Live donor liver transplantation: a valid alternative for critically ill patients suffering from acute liver failure. Am J Transplant 2015;15(6):1591–7.
16. Maluf DG, Stravitz RT, Cotterell AH, et al. Adult living donor versus deceased donor liver transplantation: a 6-year single center experience. Am J Transplant 2005;5(1):149–56.
17. Thuluvath PJ, Yoo HY. Graft and patient survival after adult live donor liver transplantation compared to a matched cohort who received a deceased donor transplantation. Liver Transpl 2004;10(10):1263–8.
18. Terrault NA, Shiffman ML, Lok AS, et al. Outcomes in hepatitis C virus-infected recipients of living donor vs. deceased donor liver transplantation. Liver Transpl 2007;13(1):122–9.

19. Terrault NA, Stravitz RT, Lok AS, et al. Hepatitis C disease severity in living versus deceased donor liver transplant recipients: an extended observation study. Hepatology 2014;59(4):1311–9.

20. Everson GT, Hoefs JC, Niemann CU, et al. Functional elements associated with hepatic regeneration in living donors after right hepatic lobectomy. Liver Transpl 2013;19(3):292–304.

21. Fisher RA, Kulik LM, Freise CE, et al. Hepatocellular carcinoma recurrence and death following living and deceased donor liver transplantation. Am J Transplant 2007;7(6):1601–8.

22. Kulik L, Abecassis M. Living donor liver transplantation for hepatocellular carcinoma. Gastroenterology 2004;127(5 Suppl 1):S277–82.

23. Kulik LM, Fisher RA, Rodrigo DR, et al. Outcomes of living and deceased donor liver transplant recipients with hepatocellular carcinoma: results of the A2ALL cohort. Am J Transplant 2012;12(11):2997–3007.

24. Hong SK, Lee KW, Kim HS, et al. Living donor liver transplantation for hepatocellular carcinoma in Seoul National University. Hepatobiliary Surg Nutr 2016;5(6):453–60.

25. Park MS, Lee KW, Kim H, et al. Primary living-donor liver transplantation is not the optimal treatment choice in patients with early hepatocellular carcinoma with poor tumor biology. Transplant Proc 2017;49(5):1103–8.

26. Marcos A. Right-lobe living donor liver transplantation. Liver Transpl 2000;6(6 Suppl 2):S59–63.

27. Samstein B, Smith AR, Freise CE, et al. Complications and their resolution in recipients of deceased and living donor liver transplants: findings from the A2ALL cohort study. Am J Transplant 2016;16(2):594–602.

28. El-Meteini M, Hamza A, Abdalaal A, et al. Biliary complications including single-donor mortality: experience of 207 adult-to-adult living donor liver transplantations with right liver grafts. HPB (Oxford) 2010;12(2):109–14.

29. Kohler S, Pascher A, Mittler J, et al. Management of biliary complications following living donor liver transplantation–a single center experience. Langenbecks Arch Surg 2009;394(6):1025–31.

30. Soin AS, Kumaran V, Rastogi AN, et al. Evolution of a reliable biliary reconstructive technique in 400 consecutive living donor liver transplants. J Am Coll Surg 2010;211(1):24–32.

31. Olthoff KM, Emond JC, Shearon TH, et al. Liver regeneration after living donor transplantation: Adult-To-Adult Living Donor Liver Transplantation Cohort Study. Liver Transpl 2015;21(1):79–88.

32. Pomposelli JJ, Goodrich NP, Emond JC, et al. Patterns of early allograft dysfunction in adult live donor liver transplantation: the A2ALL experience. Transplantation 2016;100(7):1490–9.

33. Pomfret EA, Pomposelli JJ, Gordon FD, et al. Liver regeneration and surgical outcome in donors of right-lobe liver grafts. Transplantation 2003;76(1):5–10.

34. Gruttadauria S, Parikh V, Pagano D, et al. Early regeneration of the remnant liver volume after right hepatectomy for living donation: a multiple regression analysis. Liver Transpl 2012;18(8):907–13.

35. Kim SJ, Na GH, Choi HJ, et al. Effect of donor right hepatectomy on splenic volume and platelet count for living donor liver transplantation. J Gastrointest Surg 2013;17(9):1576–83.

36. Emond JC, Fisher RA, Everson G, et al. Changes in liver and spleen volumes after living liver donation: a report from the Adult-To-Adult Living Donor Liver Transplantation Cohort Study (A2ALL). Liver Transpl 2015;21(2):151–61.

37. Liu LU, Bodian CA, Gondolesi GE, et al. Marked differences in acute cellular rejection rates between living-donor and deceased-donor liver transplant recipients. Transplantation 2005;80(8):1072–80.
38. Shaked A, Ghobrial RM, Merion RM, et al. Incidence and severity of acute cellular rejection in recipients undergoing adult living donor or deceased donor liver transplantation. Am J Transplant 2009;9(2):301–8.
39. Levitsky J, Goldberg D, Smith AR, et al. Acute rejection increases risk of graft failure and death in recent liver transplant recipients. Clin Gastroenterol Hepatol 2017;15(4):584–93.e2.
40. Charlton M, Seaberg E. Impact of immunosuppression and acute rejection on recurrence of hepatitis C: results of the National Institute of Diabetes and digestive and kidney diseases liver transplantation database. Liver Transpl Surg 1999; 5(4 Suppl 1):S107–14.
41. Wiesner RH, Goldstein RM, Donovan JP, et al. The impact of cyclosporine dose and level on acute rejection and patient and graft survival in liver transplant recipients. Liver Transpl Surg 1998;4(1):34–41.
42. Levitsky J, Kaneku H, Jie C, et al. Donor-specific HLA antibodies in living versus deceased donor liver transplant recipients. Am J Transplant 2016;16(8):2437–44.
43. Northup PG, Abecassis MM, Englesbe MJ, et al. Addition of adult-to-adult living donation to liver transplant programs improves survival but at an increased cost. Liver Transpl 2009;15(2):148–62.
44. Merion RM, Shearon TH, Berg CL, et al. Hospitalization rates before and after adult-to-adult living donor or deceased donor liver transplantation. Ann Surg 2010;251(3):542–9.
45. Valentín-Gamazo C, Malagó M, Karliova M, et al. Experience after the evaluation of 700 potential donors for living donor liver transplantation in a single center. Liver Transpl 2004;10(9):1087–96.
46. Dirican A, Baskiran A, Dogan M, et al. Evaluation of potential donors in living donor liver transplantation. Transplant Proc 2015;47(5):1315–8.
47. Trotter JF, Wisniewski KA, Terrault NA, et al. Outcomes of donor evaluation in adult-to-adult living donor liver transplantation. Hepatology 2007;46(5):1476–84.
48. Freeman J, Emond J, Gillespie BW, et al. Computerized assessment of competence-related abilities in living liver donors: the Adult-To-Adult Living Donor Liver Transplantation Cohort Study. Clin Transplant 2013;27(4):633–45.
49. Abecassis MM, Fisher RA, Olthoff KM, et al. Complications of living donor hepatic lobectomy–a comprehensive report. Am J Transplant 2012;12(5):1208–17.
50. Cheah YL, Simpson MA, Pomposelli JJ, et al. Incidence of death and potentially life-threatening near-miss events in living donor hepatic lobectomy: a world-wide survey. Liver Transpl 2013;19(5):499–506.
51. DuBay DA, Holtzman S, Adcock L, et al. Adult right-lobe living liver donors: quality of life, attitudes and predictors of donor outcomes. Am J Transplant 2009;9(5): 1169–78.
52. Miyagi S, Kawagishi N, Fujimori K, et al. Risks of donation and quality of donors' life after living donor liver transplantation. Transpl Int 2005;18(1):47–51.
53. Dew MA, Zuckoff A, DiMartini AF, et al. Prevention of poor psychosocial outcomes in living organ donors: from description to theory-driven intervention development and initial feasibility testing. Prog Transplant 2012;22(3):280–92 [quiz: 293].
54. Brown RS, Smith AR, Dew MA, et al. Predictors of donor follow-up after living donor liver transplantation. Liver Transpl 2014;20(8):967–76.

55. Trotter JF, Gillespie BW, Terrault NA, et al. Laboratory test results after living liver donation in the Adult-To-Adult Living Donor Liver Transplantation Cohort Study. Liver Transpl 2011;17(4):409–17.
56. Trotter JF, Hill-Callahan MM, Gillespie BW, et al. Severe psychiatric problems in right hepatic lobe donors for living donor liver transplantation. Transplantation 2007;83(11):1506–8.
57. Dew MA, DiMartini AF, Ladner DP, et al. Psychosocial outcomes 3 to 10 years after donation in the adult to adult living donor liver transplantation cohort study. Transplantation 2016;100(6):1257–69.
58. Butt Z, Dew MA, Liu Q, et al. Psychological outcomes of living liver donors from a multicenter prospective study: results from the Adult-To-Adult Living Donor Liver Transplantation Cohort Study2 (A2ALL-2). Am J Transplant 2017;17(5):1267–77.
59. DiMartini A, Dew MA, Liu Q, et al. Social and financial outcomes of living liver donation: a prospective investigation within the Adult-To-Adult Living Donor Liver Transplantation Cohort study 2 (A2ALL-2). Am J Transplant 2017;17(4):1081–96.
60. Reimer J, Rensing A, Haasen C, et al. The impact of living-related kidney transplantation on the donor's life. Transplantation 2006;81(9):1268–73.
61. DiMartini AF, Dew MA, Butt Z, et al. Patterns and predictors of sexual function after liver donation: the Adult-To-Adult Living Donor Liver Transplantation Cohort Study. Liver Transpl 2015;21(5):670–82.

Modern Management of Acute Liver Failure

Ruben Khan, MD, Sean Koppe, MD*

KEYWORDS

- Liver transplant • Acute liver failure • MELD

KEY POINTS

- Acute liver failure causes a systemic response leading to multiorgan failure that requires supportive care in the critical care setting.
- N-Acetylcysteine is beneficial for acetaminophen-induced acute liver failure and may provide a survival benefit in nonacetaminophen causes when administered before the onset of advanced encephalopathy.
- Progressive encephalopathy and intracranial hypertension continue to be the most important factors to prognosticate survival and must be avoided or reduced as much as possible.
- Many prognostic tools are available, but the decision to pursue transplantation should not be based on a single tool, but rather with a multifactorial approach.

INTRODUCTION

Acute liver failure (ALF) is a rare disease, but when it occurs, it can be life-threatening. The most widely accepted definition of ALF is an abnormal International Normalized Ratio (INR) of greater than or equal to 1.5 and any degree of encephalopathy in a patient without preexisting underlying chronic liver disease.[1] Based on the American Association for the Study of Liver Diseases guidelines, the timeframe between the onset of acute symptoms should be within 26 weeks to be considered acute rather than chronic liver failure.[2] Some exceptions to the definition of ALF are patients with Wilson disease, acute presentation of autoimmune hepatitis (AIH) or Budd-Chiari syndrome, which can all present with ALF even if there is some degree of underlying chronic liver disease. These patients are treated as having ALF rather than acute-on-chronic liver failure.[2]

Although there are various guidelines to help clinicians with the management of ALF, there can be wide variation in clinical practice.[3] This is partly due to a lack of

Disclosure: The authors have nothing to disclose.
Department of Gastroenterology and Hepatology, University of Illinois at Chicago, 840 South Wood Street, CSB Suite 718E (MC 716), Chicago, IL 60612, USA
* Corresponding author.
E-mail address: skoppe1@uic.edu

randomized, controlled trials providing firm data on particular management strategies owing to the rarity of the disease. As critical care medicine and access to emergency liver transplantation have improved over the years, it becomes increasingly important to understand how to improve survival in patients presenting with ALF. In this article, we discuss the current management strategies for ALF.

DISCUSSION
Etiology of Acute Liver Failure

The etiology of ALF plays into the decision-making process and treatment of ALF. Depending on the etiology of ALF, patients may or may not be candidates for liver transplantation.[1,4] The epidemiologic etiologies of ALF vary depending on the geographic region, with viral hepatitis being the most common causes in the developing world, whereas drug-induced liver injury, specifically acetaminophen toxicity, is the most common etiology in the United States.[2,4] Multiple medications have been associated with ALF and a thorough history of any medication use as well as herbal or supplement use must be assessed at the time of admission[2] (**Box 1**).

Certain conditions preclude emergency listing for transplant, and include malignant infiltration of the liver, usually from lymphoma, extensive metastases, or acute ischemic injury and hypoxic hepatitis from cardiovascular or respiratory system disorders.[1] In patients presenting with Budd-Chiari syndrome, malignancy should be investigated before listing for liver transplantation; however, frequently Budd-Chiari syndrome may be related to an underlying myeloproliferative disorder and this is not necessarily a contraindication to liver transplant.[5] Relative contraindications for emergency liver transplantation include those systemic diseases that can cause secondary liver failure, including hemophagocytic lymphohistiocytosis or infectious processes such as malaria, dengue, and rickettsial disease, or certain toxin ingestions causing multiorgan failure.[1,6,7]

ALF has been classified in 3 well-known systems: the O'Grady, Bernuau, and Japanese systems.[8–10] These systems can help to identify potential causes of ALF given the timing of injury, but these systems may not be particularly helpful, because the different varieties of ALF, namely, hyperacute, acute, or subacute, are not typically used for prognostication.[1]

DIAGNOSTIC STUDIES

Initial diagnostic testing for all patients involves blood testing for specific etiologies of ALF and blood work to assess the severity of the condition. Initial evaluation typically includes:

Hepatitis A immunoglobulin (Ig)M
Hepatitis B core IgM
Hepatitis B surface antigen
Hepatitis C antibody
Hepatitis C virus RNA
Herpes simplex virus IgM
Human immunodeficiency virus antibody
Antinuclear antibody
Anti–smooth muscle antibody
IgG levels
Lipase/amylase (for complications)
Toxicology screen

Box 1
Medications and substances associated with acute liver failure

Antituberculosis drugs

- Isoniazid
- Rifampin
- Pyrazinamide

Antibiotics

- Trimethoprim-sulfamethoxazole
- Amoxicillin/amoxicillin-clavulanate
- Nitrofurantoin
- Ciprofloxacin
- Doxycycline
- Cephalosporins
- Dapsone

Antifungal agents

- Terbinafine
- Itraconazole
- Ketoconazole

Antiretroviral

- Didanosine
- Efavirenz
- Abacavir

Other

- Statins
- Amiodarone
- Sulfasalazine
- Methyldopa
- Labetalol
- Trazadone

Antiepileptics

- Phenytoin
- Valproic acid
- Carbamazepine

Antimetabolites and enzyme inhibitors

- Propylthiouracil
- Disulfiram
- Allopurinol

Nonsteroidal antiinflammatory drugs

- Etodolac
- Diclofenac

Herbals/substances

- Kava Kava
- Herbalife
- Hydroxycut
- Ma Huang
- Black cohosh
- Comfrey
- Greater celandine
- Germander
- Cocaine
- Ecstasy (MDMA)
- Amanita mushrooms

Data from Wendon J, Cordoba J, Dhawan A, et al. EASL clinical practical guidelines on the management of acute (fulminant) liver failure. J Hepatol 2017;66(5):1047–81.

Alcohol level
Acetaminophen level
Blood type and screen
Complete blood count
Liver panel
Basic metabolic panel
Phosphorous level
Prothrombin/INR
Factor V level
Arterial lactate
Arterial blood gas
Arterial ammonia level
Pregnancy test (females)

Specific diagnostic testing is recommended for certain conditions:
Immunosuppressed patients
    Varicella zoster virus polymerase chain reaction
    Cytomegalovirus polymerase chain reaction
    Epstein-Barr virus polymerase chain reaction
    Hepatitis E IgM (pregnancy)
    Hepatitis D antibody (hepatitis B positive)
    Ceruloplasmin/copper levels (Wilson disease)

Given the rarity of Wilson's disease, it is no longer clinically useful to routinely check for Wilson's disease unless clinical suspicion is elevated for the disorder owing to frequent false-positive or indeterminate results in the setting of ALF. Additionally, routine testing for herpes simplex virus is recommended. Albeit rare, if herpes simplex virus is the cause for ALF, some case reports have shown that patients have better outcomes with treatment compared with no treatment. Furthermore, there is little downside to acyclovir treatment if patients are found to be herpes simplex virus positive.[11]

Other diagnostic studies routinely recommended include some type of baseline abdominal imaging, usually an ultrasound examination with dopplers.

Cross-sectional imaging is not necessary and often uses intravenous contrast media, which may play into further renal failure given the already hypoperfused renal system in ALF. Liver biopsy must be assessed case by case and is not recommended routinely.[11] For the majority of cases, history along with noninvasive testing is enough to give a probable cause for ALF and liver biopsy may not add further information or change management. However, if there is concern for underlying chronic disease, malignant infiltration, AIH, or ALF of unclear etiology, liver biopsy can be pursued with care and attention to coagulation parameters.[2]

CARDIOVASCULAR MANAGEMENT

Because patients with ALF can deteriorate rapidly, appropriate initial treatment is crucial to the prognosis of the patient. Without appropriate resuscitative efforts and appreciation of early onset ALF, patients are at a much greater risk of multiorgan failure and death.[12,13] The initial management should focus on volume resuscitation and preserving organ perfusion.[14,15] Additionally, echocardiography is obtained routinely to rule out cardiogenic shock, especially in the setting of hypotension.

For patients who are hypotensive and not fluid responsive, norepinephrine is the initial pressor of choice followed by vasopressin.[16] It should be noted, however, that vasopressin has been suggested to be detrimental with regard to increasing intracranial pressure (ICP), but more recent studies have not reproduced this finding.[1]

ACETAMINOPHEN-INDUCED LIVER FAILURE

In the United States, acetaminophen is the most common cause of ALF, comprising approximately 50% of ALF cases. Although acetaminophen-induced ALF is often thought of due to a single large dose, the risk of ALF is even higher with substantial ingestion over days and often accidental rather than intentional. Furthermore, patients with a single large intentional dose are more likely to present for medical care earlier compared with those patients with staggered acetaminophen use.[17] Additionally, those with baseline depleted glutathione reserves, such as patients with alcohol dependence or malnutrition, have an increased sensitivity to acetaminophen overdose.[18,19]

The early identification of acetaminophen overdose remains crucial to the treatment and prevention of ALF requiring transplantation. Patients who present with acetaminophen toxicity will usually have a marked transaminitis with relatively low bilirubin and very elevated INR.[20] Patients with acetaminophen-induced ALF who do not meet criteria for transplantation generally have a good prognosis as long as medical care is received in an appropriate timeframe.

N-ACETYLCYSTEINE

N-Acetylcysteine (NAC) remains the mainstay of early treatment in acetaminophen overdose before or after ALF. NAC remains the only antidote studied in a randomized controlled trial which improves spontaneous survival in the setting of ALF.[14] The clear benefit of NAC in acetaminophen overdose is to provide the precursor for glutathione synthesis to combine and neutralize the toxic metabolite of acetaminophen in the liver.

NAC has also been used for non–acetaminophen-induced ALF given the antioxidant and vasodilatory effects of NAC. Small studies have demonstrated improvement of oxygen consumption and increased nitric oxide levels, leading to vasodilation and increased renal perfusion. NAC has also been shown to have anti-inflammatory properties via nuclear factor-κB, which may also serve in reducing the amount of immune-mediated injury in all cases of ALF.[21] Owing to these antiinflammatory properties, however, NAC is not recommended for use for more than 5 days owing to functional immunosuppression and an increased risk for nosocomial infections.[22,23]

NAC has been shown in a randomized, controlled trial to improve transplant-free survival in patients with non–acetaminophen-induced ALF with early stage encephalopathy (grades I-II).[24] Given the general safety profile of NAC and rarity side effects, in the acute setting when the etiology of ALF is unclear, NAC has very little downside while medical teams are awaiting laboratory and imaging studies to return. In clinical practice, NAC is often used in the initial stages for all suspected cases of drug-induced liver injury as well as for other etiologies of ALF.[1–4,21]

MUSHROOM-INDUCED ACUTE LIVER FAILURE

Mushroom poisoning, most commonly by the *Aminata* species, can be a rapidly fatal cause of ALF. In the United States, there have been outbreaks in California, but cases have been reported throughout the entire country. Patients often present with multiorgan failure before liver failure as well as prominent gastrointestinal complaints. In 1 study, the total bilirubin and activated partial thromboplastin time had a correlation with prediction of survival and need for liver transplantation.[25] These criteria for transplantation of those patients with mushroom poisoning may aid the already available validated prognostic scoring systems for ALF. Intravenous silibinin, a milk thistle product, has been shown in observational studies to reduce mortality in mushroom poisoning.[26] It is available already in Europe and is being investigated in a clinical trial in the United States; it is available on an emergent basis and free of charge for patients enrolled in the study.

PREGNANCY AND ACUTE LIVER FAILURE

There are 2 liver-related emergencies that occur during the third trimester of pregnancy: hemolysis, elevated liver enzymes, and low platelets (HELLP) syndrome and acute fatty liver of pregnancy. HELLP can seem to be similar to other hemolytic disease, so these must be worked up to differentiate the etiology.[27] In acute fatty liver of pregnancy, transaminases are relatively low and there is extensive steatosis of the liver. Prompt delivery is the primary treatment in both these syndromes, but rarely, emergency liver transplantation is needed. Additionally, when a pregnant patient presents with ALF, hepatitis E should also be routinely checked.[1,2,11,15]

STEROIDS AND AUTOIMMUNE HEPATITIS

Steroids are used for a wide variety of conditions causing increased ICP such as brain masses or infections; however, in ALF steroids are not routinely recommended owing to suppression of the already relatively suppressed immune system and because there is no survival benefit in patients with ALF. Stress dose steroids may assist in reducing vasopressor requirements, but steroids have not shown a mortality benefit for ALF.[1]

An exception to steroids comes with documented AIH with either biopsy-proven AIH or biomarkers with clinical presentation consistent with AIH. In cases when there is a high suspicion of AIH, but biomarkers are negative, a liver biopsy may be warranted to confirm the diagnosis.[2,28] If AIH is the cause of ALF, steroids are recommended with close attention to sepsis. Steroid use, however, should not delay listing for transplantation.[29]

ANTIBIOTICS AND ANTIFUNGALS

Given the severe immune system disturbance and associated volume depletion in ALF, there is often worry for sepsis. Infection, however, more often occurs later in hospitalization and is not typically part of the presenting symptoms of ALF. Multiple guidelines do not recommend the prophylactic use of antibiotics or antifungals upon admission.[1,2,11] However, in clinical practice, if there is any persistent hypotension or need for vasopressors, or if encephalopathy is worsening, antibiotics and antifungals are commonly used given the severity of disease.[4]

ENCEPHALOPATHY

Encephalopathy is of critical concern and part of the definition of ALF. Encephalopathy is usually multifactorial, related to hypotension, sepsis, and ammonia buildup from the failing liver itself and progressive encephalopathy has a poor prognosis.[15] Even low-grade encephalopathy can suggest a poor prognosis, especially if patients present in a subacute manner. Additionally, high-grade encephalopathy and hyperammonemia, usually sustained arterial levels of more than 150 to 200 μmol/L, can lead to increased intracranial hypertension, which has its own set of complications and treatment.[30] Ammonia is converted to glutamine after passing the blood–brain barrier and contributes to cerebral edema and altered cerebral function. Thus, hyperammonemia is linked directly to cerebral edema and intracranial hypertension.[14]

The use of lactulose and rifaximin has clear benefits in chronic liver disease to decrease the chance of hepatic encephalopathy. However, there is no clear evidence for their use in ALF.[1] In patients with ALF, they may have an ongoing ileus and thus, lactulose may contribute to abdominal bloating and distension. Furthermore, should a patient need liver transplantation, there is some theoretic concern that the bloating effect of lactulose could make the surgery technically more difficult.[2,15] That being said, owing to the serious complications of progressive or high-grade encephalopathy, lactulose and rifaximin are commonly used to reduce hyperammonemia and decrease the risk of intracranial hypertension if able to be tolerated.[31] If it is deemed too risky to use lactulose given issues with ileus, or if hyperammonemia is refractory, renal replacement therapy (RRT) can be used to reduce ammonia levels.[32]

INTRACRANIAL HYPERTENSION AND PRESSURE MONITORING

Intracranial hypertension is a feared complication of ALF and is multifactorial in nature. Intracranial hypertension can lead to irreversible brainstem herniation and death.[33,34] There is wide variety with regard to ICP monitoring and the treatment of increased ICP. Direct measurement with ICP monitoring has its own risks, particularly intracranial hemorrhage, especially given the coagulation abnormalities in ALF. Epidural catheters have fewer complications compared with subdural or intraparenchymal locations, but there is increased variability in the readings of these less invasive epidural monitors compared with the intraparenchymal and subdural space.[35] The rate of elevated ICP is so high in grade III and IV encephalopathy, reaching approximately 80% to 95%, that the risks of introducing an intracranial monitor may outweigh the benefit. Thus, many practitioners assume an increased ICP and treat the patient accordingly in grade III and IV encephalopathy. There are no randomized, controlled trials demonstrating overall survival benefit with ICP monitoring; there are only some case reports suggesting that ICP monitoring may extend the survival time.[36] Noninvasive techniques to estimate ICP include measuring flow and resistance of the middle cerebral artery via doppler imaging. These techniques, however, demonstrate interassay and intraassay variability.[37] Some have also tried to measure optic nerve sheath diameter as a proxy for ICP measurement with varied success.[38]

Patients at higher risk for intracranial hypertension are those with a shorter symptom-to-encephalopathy interval, younger age, renal impairment, sustained arterial ammonia of greater than 150 to 200 μmol/L, need for vasopressors, and higher grades of encephalopathy.[8,39] Despite the lack of evidence to use ICP monitoring, some centers will use ICP monitoring if there is evidence of papilledema, need for RRT, or progressive encephalopathy, but overall ICP monitoring is used in a minority of cases.[3] Should ICP monitoring be pursued, the target ICP should be less than 20 to 25 mm Hg with a goal cerebral perfusion pressure of 50 to 70 mm Hg. Treatments to decrease an elevated ICP include brief periods of hyperventilation (transient benefit) and either mannitol or hypertonic saline.[1,2] Although barbiturates are in the guidelines as a potential treatment for severe refractory elevated ICP, these agents are rarely used because of the sedative effects contributing to worsened encephalopathy.

RENAL REPLACEMENT THERAPY

In addition to the common indications for RRT, there are some specific conditions in which RRT may be considered in ALF. Refractory hyperammonemia, progressive encephalopathy, or evidence of intracranial hypertension are situations to consider RRT, even if there are no other renal-specific indications. The renal-specific indications for RRT remain hyperkalemia, refractory metabolic acidosis, volume overload, or uremia.[1] Many patients who present with ALF, regardless of hyperammonemia or elevated ICP, will require RRT regardless, owing to the multiorgan failure caused by liver dysfunction.[15]

In contrast, if RRT is needed for reasons other than intracranial hypertension, adequate sodium levels should be maintained because hyponatremia, specifically sodium of less than 140 mmol/L, can worsen intracranial hypertension.[14] Additionally, hyponatremia has been shown to independently have increased mortality in ALF patients. Thus, care must be taken by the nephrologist to adjust the dialysate baths to maintain adequate serum sodium levels and appropriate serum osmolarity.[40] Care must also be taken when placing central venous access in these patients for RRT given the coagulopathy seen in patients with ALF.

COAGULOPATHY

In addition to the presence of encephalopathy, the other key component of the definition of ALF is an alteration in coagulopathy, in particular, an INR of greater than or equal to 1.5. Although patients with ALF may present with thrombocytopenia and an elevated INR, typically ALF patients do not have spontaneous bleeding complications.[41] In the American Association for the Study of Liver Diseases guidelines, the routine administration of vitamin K is recommended to address any underlying nutritional deficiency that may be contributing to an elevated INR.[2] Given the importance of the INR as an assessment of the liver function and given the potential risk of transfusions, the routine use of coagulation factors to correct the INR is not recommended unless there is an invasive procedure planned.[1,4] Additionally, given the proinflammatory state of patients with ALF, there may be some risk for blood clots, especially portal vein thrombus.

THERAPEUTIC HYPOTHERMIA

Therapeutic hypothermia has been used in many life-threatening conditions to slow metabolism and decrease oxygen consumption of tissues. A reduction in body temperature can also decrease the cerebral ammonia concentration, helping reduce encephalopathy and ICP. This is partly due to the decreased cerebral blood flow in hypothermic conditions, which allows for less delivery of ammonia to the brain.[42,43]

Therapeutic hypothermia may lead to decreased inflammation of the liver, but in turn, may also lead to decreased regeneration of the liver.[44] There are no good prospective studies to suggest the routine use of therapeutic hypothermia and observational studies also fail to demonstrate any clear benefit of hypothermia.[45,46]

LIVER ASSIST DEVICES

There is much unknown about newly designed liver assisted devices and plasma exchange in ALF, yet some rare centers are using these methods. In ALF, there are circulating cytokines causing a diffuse systemic inflammatory response, which contributes to many of the hemodynamic changes. Plasma exchange has been used to try to clear these cytokines and reduce the inflammatory response.[47,48] There are small case series and case studies to demonstrate a good survival rate, but given the rarity of disease and rarity of use, plasma exchange is not routinely recommended unless in a study setting.

Additionally, there has been recent attention paid to extracorporeal liver assist devices in ALF. These support systems are designed to allow the liver more time for spontaneous recovery and either avoid liver transplantation or act as a bridge to transplantation.[1,2] Thus far, there has been mixed data regarding survival and mortality benefit with these devices, which have not been convincing enough to recommend widespread use. Additionally, these extracorporeal systems are highly demanding of resources and may have significant potential toxicities.[11,49]

Hepatocyte transplantation is another method designed to delay transplantation or allow enough time for spontaneous recovery. Tissue is obtained from donor liver not used for transplantation, which already preselects hepatocytes that would provide marginal rather than excellent graft tissue. These cells are preserved in NAC or cryopreserved for emergency use. Most data for hepatocyte transplantation are for inborn metabolic disorders of the liver, and there has not been widespread evidence of their benefit in ALF yet.[50]

PROGNOSTIC BIOMARKERS

The etiology of ALF is of important prognostic significance. Patients who do poorly are those with an idiosyncratic drug injury, seronegative hepatitis, autoimmune hepatitis, mushroom poisoning, Wilson disease, Budd-Chiari syndrome, or ALF of unknown cause. The most used standard biomarkers thus far are lactate and pH levels, which are nonspecific, but can help to determine the severity of illness.[51] Additionally, the INR is used to prognosticate mortality and severity of disease. Age and duration of time between the onset of illness and the onset of encephalopathy have been studied as independent prognostic indicators in ALF, but these factors did not affect mortality or outcome. Currently, there are few biomarkers that may help to prognosticate the severity of ALF patients. Newer potential biomarkers continue to be studied. Some of the biomarkers which may have some prognostic value include:

- Phosphate: higher levels indicate poor prognosis[52];
- AFP ratio: AFP levels on day 3 divided by AFP levels on day 1 of greater than 1 indicate improved survival rates than AFP ratio less than 1[53]; and
- Factor V levels: lower levels, particularly levels less than 10%, indicate poor prognosis and need for liver transplantation.[54]

CRITERIA FOR EMERGENCY LIVER TRANSPLANTATION

There are good validated scoring systems that can assist in the decision of whether to pursue liver transplantation or not. The Model for End-stage Liver disease (MELD) score is used more often compared with the traditional King's College Hospital (KCH) Criteria or the Clichy Criteria, which are more often used in Europe.[11] Several studies have demonstrated that a MELD score of greater than 30.5 has a high positive predictive value for the need of emergency liver transplantation. All these scoring systems have fairly good (>70%) positive predictive values, but in further studies, the KCH Criteria tend to have a slightly higher accuracy in predicting outcome compared with the Clichy criteria or the MELD score (**Box 2**), but generally lower sensitivity.[11,55]

There are other scoring systems that have been developed recently and are being studied currently, but these have not yet been validated yet. One is the Sequential Organ Failure Assessment score, which was not initially designed for ALF, but has recently been applied to patients with cirrhosis. A prognostic system from the Acute Liver Failure Study Group includes coma grade, INR, serum phosphate, bilirubin, and a new marker of apoptosis known as M30, which is elevated in ALF. In a small study, this system outperformed both the MELD and KCH Criteria in predicting outcome, but it has not been widely validated yet.[56] Additionally, M30 levels are not

---

Box 2
Criteria for emergency liver transplantation

MELD/MELD-Na greater than 30.5 for emergency liver transplantation
- Creatinine
- Bilirubin
- INR
- Sodium

King's College Criteria (acetaminophen induced)
- Arterial lactate >3 mmol/L after early fluid resuscitation
- Arterial pH <7.3 after resuscitation and it has been >24 hours after ingestion
- List for transplant if all 3 occur within a 24-hour period:
  ○ Presence of grade III to IV encephalopathy
  ○ INR >6.5
  ○ Creatinine >3.4 mg/dL

King's College Criteria (NAI-ALF)
- List for transplant if INR >6.5 and any grade of encephalopathy is present or any 3 of the following plus encephalopathy:
  ○ Age <10 or >40 years
  ○ Jaundice for >7 days before encephalopathy
  ○ INR >3.5
  ○ Bilirubin >17 mg/dL
  ○ Unfavorable etiology such as Wilson Disease, DILI, seronegative hepatitis

Clichy criteria
- Confusion or encephalopathy grades III or IV
- Factor V <20% of normal is <30 years old or Factor V <30% of normal if age >30 years old

Abbreviations: DILI, drug-induced liver injury; INR, International Normalized Ratio; MELD, Model for End-stage Liver Disease; MELD-Na, Model for End-stage Liver Disease with serum sodium; NAI-ALF, non–acetaminophen-induced acute liver failure.
Data from Wendon J, Cordoba J, Dhawan A, et al. EASL Clinical practical guidelines on the management of acute (fulminant) liver failure. J Hepatol 2017;66(5);1047–81; and Lee WM, Larson AM, Stravitz RT. Introduction to the revised American Association for the study of liver diseases position paper on acute liver failure 2011. Hepatology 2012;55(3):965–7.

clinically available at all laboratories, which limits its use. As good as the scoring systems have become, reliance completely on these guidelines is still not recommended because the entire clinical context needs to be reviewed in make the decision of whether to pursue liver transplantation.

SUMMARY

ALF continues to be a rare but life-threatening disease requiring specialized care. As we gain more experience over the years in treating this subset of patients, survival without the need for emergency transplantation is also improving. ALF care remains an ever-changing field that will continue to progress. Furthermore, classification systems continue to evolve and potential biomarkers continue to be investigated, which may help to refine our understanding of which patients need transplantation versus which will recover.

REFERENCES

1. European Association for the Study of the Liver, Wendon J, Cordoba J, Dhawan A, et al. EASL clinical practical guidelines on the management of acute (fulminant) liver failure. J Hepatol 2017;66(5):1047–81.
2. Lee WM, Larson AM, Stravitz RT. Introduction to the revised American Association for the Study of Liver Diseases Position Paper on acute liver failure 2011. Hepatology 2012;55:965–7.
3. Rabinowich L, Wendon J, Bernal W, et al. Clinical management of acute liver failure: results of an international multi-center survey. World J Gastroenterol 2016; 22(33):7595–603.
4. Bernal W, Auzinger G, Dhawan A, et al. Acute liver failure. Lancet 2010;376: 190–201.
5. Parekh J, Matei VM, Canas-Coto A, et al, Acute Liver Failure Study Group. Budd-Chiari syndrome causing acute liver failure: a multicenter case series. Liver Transpl 2017;23(2):135–42.
6. Price B, Lines J, Lewis D, et al. Haemophagocytic lymphohistiocytosis: a fulminant syndrome associated with multiorgan failure and high mortality that frequently masquerades as sepsis and shock. S Afr Med J 2014;104:401–6.
7. Anand AC, Garg HK. Approach to clinical syndrome of jaundice and encephalopathy in tropics. J Clin Exp Hepatol 2015;5:S116–30.
8. O'Grady JG, Schalm SW, Williams R. Acute liver failure: redefining the syndromes. Lancet 1993;342:273–5.
9. Bernuau J, Rueff B, Benhamou JP. Fulminant and subfulminant liver failure: definitions and causes. Semin Liver Dis 1986;6:97–106.
10. Mochida S, Nakayama N, Matsui A, et al. Re-evaluation of the guideline published by the acute liver failure study group of Japan in 1996 to determine the indications of liver transplantation in patients with fulminant hepatitis. Hepatol Res 2008;38:970–9.
11. Flamm SL, Yang Y, Singh S, et al, AGA Institute Clinical Guidelines Committee. American Gastroenterological Association Institute guidelines for the diagnosis and management of acute liver failure. Gastroenterology 2017;152:644–7.
12. Vaquero J, Polson J, Chung C, et al. Infection and the progression of hepatic encephalopathy in acute liver failure. Gastroenterology 2003;125:755–64.
13. Karvellas CJ, Pink F, McPhail M, et al. Predictors of bacteraemia and mortality in patients with acute liver failure. Intensive Care Med 2009;35:1390–6.

14. McPhail MJ, Kriese S, Heneghan MA. Current management of acute liver failure. Curr Opin Gastroenterol 2015;31(3):209–14.
15. Bernal W, Wendon J. Acute liver failure. N Engl J Med 2013;369:2525–34.
16. Eefsen M, Dethloff T, Frederiksen H-J, et al. Comparison of terlipressin and noradrenalin on cerebral perfusion, intracranial pressure and cerebral extracellular concentrations of lactate and pyruvate in patients with acute liver failure in need of inotropic support. J Hepatol 2007;47:381–6.
17. Craig DG, Bates CM, Davidson JS, et al. Staggered overdose pattern and delay to hospital presentation are associated with adverse outcomes following paracetamol-induced hepatotoxicity. Br J Clin Pharmacol 2012;73:285–94.
18. Craig DG, Reid TW, Martin KG, et al. The systemic inflammatory response syndrome and sequential organ failure assessment scores are effective triage markers following paracetamol (acetaminophen) overdose. Aliment Pharmacol Ther 2011;34:219–28.
19. Myers RP, Shaheen AAM, Li B, et al. Impact of liver disease, alcohol abuse, and unintentional ingestions on the outcomes of acetaminophen overdose. Clin Gastroenterol Hepatol 2008;6:918–25.
20. Zimmerman JH, Maddrey WC. Acetaminophen (paracetamol) hepatotoxicity with regular intake of alcohol: analysis of instances of therapeutic misadventure. Hepatology 1995;22:767–73.
21. Sales I, Dzierba AL, Smithburger PL, et al. Use of acetylcysteine for non-acetaminophen-induced acute liver failure. Ann Hepatol 2013;12(1):6–10.
22. Stravitz RT, Sanyal AJ, Reisch J, et al, Acute Liver Failure Study Group. Effects of N-acetylcysteine on cytokines in non-acetaminophen acute liver failure: potential mechanism of improvement in transplant-free survival. Liver Int 2013;33:1324–31.
23. Kim DY, Jun JH, Lee HL, et al. N-acetylcysteine prevents LPS-induced pro-inflammatory cytokines and MMP2 production in gingival fibroblasts. Arch Pharm Res 2007;30:1283–92.
24. Lee WM, Hynan LS, Rossaro L, et al, Acute Liver Failure Study Group. Intravenous N-acetylcysteine improves transplant-free survival in early stage non-acetaminophen acute liver failure. Gastroenterology 2009;137(3):856–64.
25. Kim T, Lee D, Lee JH, et al. Predictors of poor outcomes in patients with wild mushroom-induced acute liver injury. World J Gastroenterol 2017;23(7):1262–7.
26. Hruby K, Csomos G, Fuhrmann M, et al. Chemotherapy of Aminata phalloides poisoning with intravenous silibinin. Hum Toxicol 1983;2:183–95.
27. Westbrook RH, Yeoman AD, Joshi D, et al. Outcomes of severe pregnancy-related liver disease: refining the role of transplantation. Am J Transplant 2010;10:2520–6.
28. Stravitz RT, Lefkowitch JH, Fontana RJ, et al, Acute Liver Failure Study Group. Autoimmune acute liver failure: proposed clinical and histological criteria. Hepatology 2011;53:517–26.
29. Viruet EJ, Torres EA. Steroid therapy in fulminant hepatic failure secondary to autoimmune hepatitis. P R Health Sci J 1998;17:297–300.
30. Clemmesen JO, Larsen FS, Kondrup J, et al. Cerebral herniation in patients with acute liver failure is correlated with arterial ammonia concentration. Hepatology 1999;29:648–53.
31. Kumar R, Shalimar, Sharma H, et al. Persistent hyperammonemia is associated with complications and poor outcomes in patients with acute liver failure. Clin Gastroenterol Hepatol 2012;10:925–31.
32. Slack AJ, Aunzinger G, Willar C, et al. Ammonia clearance with haemofiltration in adults with liver disease. Liver Int 2014;34:42–8.

33. Ware AJ, D'Agostino AN, Combes B. Cerebral edema: a major complication of massive hepatic necrosis. Gastroenterology 1971;61:877–84.
34. O'Brien CJ, Wise RJS, O'Grady JG, et al. Neurological sequelae in patients recovered from fulminant hepatic failure. Gut 1987;28:93–5.
35. Blei AT, Olafsson S, Webster S, et al. Complications of intracranial pressure monitoring in fulminant hepatic failure. Lancet 1993;341:157–8.
36. Fortea JI, Banares R, Vaquero J. Intracranial pressure in acute liver failure: to bolt or not to bolt-that is the question. Crit Care Med 2014;42(5):1304–5.
37. Larsen FS, Strauss G, Moller K, et al. Regional cerebral blood flow autoregulation in patients with fulminant hepatic failure. Liver Transpl 2000;6:795–800.
38. Krishnamoorthy V, Beckmann K, Mueller M, et al. Perioperative estimation of the intracranial pressure using the optic nerve sheath diameter during liver transplantation. Liver Transpl 2013;19(3):246–9.
39. Bernal W, Hall C, Karvellas CJ, et al. Arterial ammonia and clinical risk factors for encephalopathy and intracranial hypertension in acute liver failure. Hepatology 2007;46:1844–52.
40. Bagshaw SM, Bellomo R, Devarajan P, et al. Review article: renal support in critical illness. Can J Anaesth 2010;57:999–1013.
41. Habib M, Roberts LN, Patel RK, et al. Evidence of rebalanced coagulation in acute liver injury and acute liver failure as measured by thrombin generation. Liver Int 2014;34:672–8.
42. Chatauret N, Rose C, Therien G, et al. Mild hypothermia prevents cerebral edema and CSF lactate accumulation in acute liver failure. Metab Brain Dis 2001;16: 95–102.
43. Rose C, Michalak A, Pannunzio M, et al. Mild hypothermia delays the onset of coma and prevents brain edema and extracellular brain glutamate accumulation in rats with acute liver failure. Hepatology 2000;31:872–7.
44. Vaquero J. Therapeutic hypothermia in the management of acute liver failure. Neurochem Int 2012;60(7):723–35.
45. Bernal W, Murphy N, Brown S, et al. A multicentre randomized controlled trial of moderate hypothermia to prevent intracranial hypertension in acute liver failure. J Hepatol 2016;65(2):273–9.
46. Karvellas CJ, Todd Stravitz R, Battenhouse H, et al, US Acute Liver Failure Study Group. Therapeutic hypothermia in acute liver failure: a multicenter retrospective cohort analysis. Liver Transpl 2015;21(1):4–12.
47. Bernsmeier C, Antionades CG, Wendon J. What's new in acute liver failure? Intensive Care Med 2014;40:1545–8.
48. Larsen FS, Schmidt LE, Bernsmeier C, et al. High-volume plasma exchange in patients with acute liver failure: an open randomised controlled trial. J Hepatol 2016;64:69–78.
49. Struecker B, Raschzok N, Sauer IM. Liver support strategies: cutting-edge technologies. Nat Rev Gastroenterol Hepatol 2014;11:166–76.
50. Hughes RD, Mitry RR, Dhawan A. Current status of hepatocyte transplantation. Transplantation 2012;93:342–7.
51. Hadem J, Stiefel P, Bahr MJ, et al. Prognostic implications of lactate, bilirubin, and etiology in German patients with acute liver failure. Clin Gastroenterol Hepatol 2008;6:339–45.
52. Baquerizo A, Anselmo D, Shackleton C, et al. Phosphorus as an early predictive factor in patients with acute liver failure. Transplantation 2003;75(12):2007–14.
53. Schiodt F, Ostapowicz G, Murray N, et al. Alpha-fetoprotein and prognosis in acute liver failure. Liver Transpl 2006;12(12):1776–81.

54. Izume I, Langley PG, Wendon J, et al. Coagulation factor V levels as a prognostic indicator in fulminant hepatic failure. Hepatology 1996;23(6):1507–11.
55. McPhail MJ, Farne H, Senvar N, et al. Ability of King's College criteria and model for end-stage liver disease scores to predict mortality of patients with acute liver failure: a meta-analysis. Clin Gastroenterol Hepatol 2016;14(4):516–25.
56. Cholongitas E, Theocharidou E, Vasianopoulou P, et al. Comparison of the sequential organ failure assessment score with the King's College Hospital criteria and the model for end-stage liver disease score for the prognosis of acetaminophen-induced acute liver failure. Liver Transpl 2012;18:405–12.

Intestinal Failure and Rehabilitation

Alan L. Buchman, MD, MSPH

KEYWORDS

- Intestinal failure • Intestinal rehabilitation • Short bowel syndrome
- Home parenteral nutrition • Intestinal adaptation

KEY POINTS

- Following a massive enterectomy, the intestine hypertrophies over time and segmental absorption improves.
- Medication malabsorption occurs in patients with intestinal failure.
- Diarrhea control in patients with intestinal failure may involve the use of several medications at unconventional dose.
- Development of hyperphagia and a high complex carbohydrate diet is critically important in patients with residual colon on continuity with small bowel, but has little role in patients with a jejunostomy.
- Teduglutide, a GLP-2 analog, may be useful to enhance intestinal adaptation, enhance nutrient and fluid absorption, and help wean patients from parenteral nutrition when conventional methods have been unsuccessful.

INTRODUCTION TO INTESTINAL FAILURE

Intestinal failure has been defined as a condition that "results from obstruction, dysmotility, surgical resection, congenital defect, or disease-associated loss of absorption and is characterized by the inability to maintain protein-energy, fluid, electrolyte, or micronutrient balance."[1] Not all patients who have undergone intestinal resection, or even have developed short bowel syndrome (SBS) will develop intestinal failure and, of course, there are causes for intestinal failure other than SBS. This article addresses the management of those patients with SBS and intestinal failure, a group that has been defined as "type 2," referring to those patients who may require intravenous nutrition and/or fluid and electrolyte supplementation for a period of weeks to months, or "type 3" wherein intestinal failure may require years to reverse, if at all.[2] SBS may develop as a consequence of mesenteric thrombosis (venous or arterial), mesenteric embolism (arterial), resections for Crohn disease, volvulus,

Disclosure: The author has nothing to disclose.
Department of Surgery, Intestinal Rehabilitation and Transplant Center, University of Illinois at Chicago, Health Care Services Corporation, 959 Oak Drive, Glencoe, IL 60022, USA
E-mail address: buchman@uic.edu

intussusception, polyposis, aganglionosis, radiation enteritis, necrotizing enterocolitis, trauma, or surgical misadventures. SBS also may be congenital in the form of jejunal or ileal atresia, gastroschisis, or omphalocele.

Normally in adults, intestinal length varies between approximately 275 and 850 cm.[3] In general, intestinal failure results when there is less than 35 cm of residual small bowel with a jejunoileal anastomosis when the colon is intact and in continuity; less than 60 cm with a jejunocolonic anastomosis and an intact colon; or less than 115 cm when there is an end-jejunostomy. From an energy-absorptive perspective, approximately half of the colon is roughly equivalent to 50 cm of small intestine. This article focuses on the adult, although applicable data from children are cited and described. Children have all the same issues as adults, but also some unique issues that are important in adaptation and weaning of parenteral nutrition (PN), such as different macronutrient and micronutrient requirements, and food aversion if they have received PN since birth or a very early age, which is not be discussed here.

INTESTINAL REHABILITATION AND ADAPTATION

Intestinal rehabilitation is defined as the restoration of lost intestinal function. Specifically, that refers to increased macronutrient and micronutrient as well as fluid absorption. This process begins immediately following an intestinal resection and is mediated by various interactive factors, including presence or absence of an ileocecal valve, comorbid conditions, age, blood flow, dietary elements, gastrointestinal secretions, cytokines, and hormone/growth factors.[4] The intestine increases slightly in length, but more importantly increases in overall surface area via longer villi (and increased crypt depth), likely resulting in more efficient absorption per square centimeter.[5–8] This process is thought to take up to 1 to 2 years in humans, although there are few instructive data.[3,9,10] There are isolated experiences of patients gaining weight while on PN and being weaned after many years. Minimal, if any adaptation occurs in patients with an end-jejunostomy.[4] One series of 28 children with less than 20 cm of small bowel showed that nearly half were able to become nutritional independent within 2 years, although those with an intact colon in continuity were more likely to achieve nutritional autonomy.[11] In general, in adults, intestinal adaptation will be suboptimal in those with less than 75 to 100 cm of healthy residual small bowel.[9,12] Most macronutrients are absorbed within the initial 100 to 150 cm of jejunum.[13] If residual colon remains in continuity with the small bowel, unabsorbed carbohydrates may be salvaged by colonic bacteria and fermented to short-chain fatty acids (SCFAs), an energy source.[14] Therefore, less small residual small bowel is required in the presence of colon. Patients with radiation enteritis, an increasingly greater percentage of the population of patients with intestinal failure, generally have blunted adaptation, although an observational study from France has suggested upward of as many as two-thirds may be successfully weaned from PN.[15] The degree to which the intestine "adapts" and PN can be weaned may be highly individualized, although a plasma citrulline concentration of less than 20 μmol/L predicted the presence of permanent intestinal failure in a study of 57 patients (sensitivity 92%; specificity 90%).[16,17]

PARENTERAL NUTRITION

The first step in intestinal rehabilitation is to determine the patient's fluid and macronutritional and micronutritional requirements to avoid the provision of excessive amounts. In general, fluid requirements for adults average approximately 35 mL/kg body weight, although slightly less if age is >60 years.[18] Diseases such as renal failure, cirrhosis, or congestive heart failure obviously lead to decreased requirements.

Diarrhea, very significant sweating, and fever increase fluid requirements. Sodium and potassium are generally provided at a dosage of 1.0 to 1.5 mmol/kg per day; magnesium at 0.1 to 0.2 mmol/kg per day, calcium at 0.1 to 0.15 mmol/kg per day, chloride (as sodium or potassium) at 1.0 to 1.5 mmol/kg per day, and phosphate (as potassium or sodium) at 0.3 to 0.5 mmol/kg per day[18] disease states may alter these doses. It must be noted that magnesium deficiency can precipitate calcium deficiency because of impaired parathyroid hormone release[19]; this may occur in spite of normal serum magnesium concentration and therefore a 24-hour urine magnesium must be measured.[20] Magnesium deficiency can be challenging to correct using the oral route, as it is a cathartic.

Acid/base status should be optimized using chloride or acetate salts (bicarbonate is not compatible with PN) as appropriate. Metabolic acidosis with an increased anion gap may also develop as a result of colonic bacterial fermentation of nonabsorbed carbohydrate (often by *Clostridium perfringens* and *Streptococcus bovis*), with a resultant production of D-lactic acid. These bacteria may proliferate in the acidic environment created by the production of SCFAs from carbohydrate salvage. D-lactic acidosis also may develop in cases of thiamine deficiency.[21] Clinical manifestations include ataxia, dysarthria, and encephalopathy. The typically measured L-lactate will be normal and D-lactate must be specifically requested. Treatment is by a reduction of "refined" dietary carbohydrate. Oral antibiotic therapy (metronidazole, neomycin, vancomycin) has been used, but it is unclear whether this is necessary.

Parenteral energy is typically supplied by a mixture of dextrose monohydrate and lipid emulsion at a level of 20 to 35 kcal/kg per day depending on oral intake, weight gain/loss, fever/inflammation, and/or tumor burden. Lipid typically provides 15% to 30% of energy needs, although a minimum of 4% of energy intake should be from linoleic fatty acid to prevent development of essential fatty acid deficiency. In general, lipid emulsion intake should generally not exceed 1 g/kg per day due to an association with intestinal failure–associated liver disease (IFALD).[22] Protein is supplied as a balanced free amino acid solution at a typical dosage of 0.8 to 1.0 g/kg per day, modified on the basis of disease state (as low as 0.4 g/kg per day for impending renal failure or as high as 1 g/kg for patients with concomitant head injury or major burn). A recent study has noted, however, that the intravenously infused amino acids may not be equivalent to dietary protein and may in fact provide as much as 17% less protein substrate.[23] Water-soluble and fat-soluble vitamins are added to the PN solution, as are the trace elements copper, zinc, and selenium. The use of other trace elements, such as chromium, remains controversial.[24] Although obviously there is significant malabsorption, but oral intake of macronutrients and micronutrients must also be considered. It goes without saying that provision of PN at home (HPN) should be provided via a single-lumen tunneled, cuffed catheter or implanted port, without other medications without PN being infused and no blood being drawn from the catheter to reduce the risk of infection, which obviously would complicate the intestinal rehabilitation process.[25]

The next step in the process is to provide for formal teaching of the patient and/or caregiver in the management of HPN and the overall strategy of intestinal rehabilitation. This includes assessment of the patient and caregivers' cognitive and physical capabilities, as well as an assessment of the home environment and related social and economic factors. For example, as the patient is encouraged to develop hyperphagia, where hyperphagia is defined as the spontaneous intake of more than 1.5 times their individual resting energy expenditure,[26] it must be certain there are financial resources to cover the increased grocery bill. Total nutrient absorption is a function of the amount of intake, as well as the percentage of intake absorbed. Although this article is focused on the actual intestinal adaptation/rehabilitation process, it is critical that patient/caregiver teaching also include specific instruction on appropriate catheter care, prevention, and recognition of complications such as catheter occlusion, pump issues, storage of PN solutions and their preparation for infusion, and ostomy care if one is present. Indeed, referral to a team specialized in this patient group and approach to their care is highly recommended.[18] The patient should be encouraged to join a patient support group, such as the Oley Foundation (www.Oley.org).[27] There is a suggestion that the catheter infection rate may decrease, quality of life improves, and there is less depression among those who have joined such support groups.[28,29]

MEDICAL THERAPY AND CONTROL OF DIARRHEA

Small bowel resection is often associated with the development of hypergastrinemia, which in turn may result in increased fluid loss from the digestive tract. In addition, the low-pH environment may lead to a denaturing of bile salts as well as pancreatic enzymes, further compromising digestion.[30] Therefore, proton pump inhibitors (PPI) should be used. Given that oral medication absorption, much like nutrients, is usually impaired, intravenous use is prepared with consideration given to adding it to the PN solution, followed by enhanced oral dosing (to account for malabsorption) at the end of the nightly PN infusion.[31,32] The optimal duration of PPI therapy is unknown, but should be continued for approximately 6 months; possibly longer in select cases.

Antimotility medications are also critical to slow intestinal transit, potentially improve absorption by increasing nutrient/enterocyte contact time, and decreasing diarrheal fluid losses.[33–37] These include loperamide hydrochloride (Imodium), diphenoxylate/atropine (Lomotil), tincture of opium, and codeine phosphate. Very little loperamide is absorbed and therefore it has few, if any, central nervous system effects. Doses are shown in **Table 1**. Fecal output can be expected to decrease by 15% to 30% or more. Overzealous use of antidiarrheal medication also is to be avoided to avoid development of abdominal cramping and bloating; the goal is not intestinal stasis! In addition, these medications should be avoided in cases of chronic intestinal pseudo-obstruction syndrome. Clonidine, an $\alpha 2$-adrenergic receptor agonist, antihypertensive agent, enhances colonic chloride absorption and may be useful in patients with an intact colon,[38] unlike the other medications (not octreotide).

Bile acid sequestering agents, such as cholestyramine, should *not* be used in patients with SBS; investigation has shown no improvement in diarrhea if >100 cm of ileum has been resected, and/or steatorrhea is >20 g/d.[39] In addition, these medications may bind other medications and fat-soluble vitamins.

Octreotide is a long-acting analog of the peptide hormone somatostatin. It increases gastrointestinal transit time and reduces gastrointestinal secretions,

Table 1		
Recommended medication doses for the control of diarrhea		
Medication	**Dose**	**Frequency**
Loperamide hydrochloride	4 mg (up to 12–24 mg)	3–4 times daily
Diphenoxylate/atropine	2 mg (up to 4–8 mg)	3–4 times daily
Tincture of opium	0.3–1.0 mL	3–4 times daily
Codeine phosphate	40 mg (up to 80–160 mg)	3–4 times daily
Clonidine hydrochloride	0.3 mg	One patch weekly
Octreotide	100 µg	3 times daily (subcutaneous)

particularly those pancreatic in origin, through an as-yet unidentified mechanism, and may be useful for effecting substantial reductions in jejunostomy output.[40] However, it also reduces splanchnic protein synthesis and mucosal blood flow, which may compromise intestinal adaptation.[40–44] Because it slows biliary tract motility as well, there is an increased risk for the development of cholelithiasis in a group of patients already at increased risk.[45,46]

Routine antibiotic use to treat presumed "bacterial overgrowth" is not warranted, and possibly even contraindicated. It is to be noted that the standard breath hydrogen tests are useless in patients with SBS, as the early hydrogen peak simply reflects rapid transit. In fact, given the substantial bacterial production of folate, vitamin K, and SCFAs, such therapy has the potential to be harmful.[27] However, those patients with segmental dilated loops of small intestine, in which motility is impaired, may benefit from occasional antibiotic treatment, although this approach is temporizing only and consideration should be given for a definitive procedure, such as serial transverse enteroplasty (STEP).[47]

DIETARY MANAGEMENT OF INTESTINAL FAILURE

Dietary management includes oral fluid ingestion in addition to traditional food. As such, fluid management is an integral part of dietary management in patients with intestinal failure. Urine output should be at least 1000 mL per 24 hours and should be measured at home by patients. If urine volume is less, parenteral fluid provision should be increased, although there have been no studies on the optimal volume, and parenteral fluid volume is not perfectly correlated with urine output.

Oral rehydration solution (ORS) is useful to improve hydration and to decrease parenteral fluid requirements.[48] Such solutions operate on the principle that sodium and glucose are co-transported into the enterocyte, and water follows as a result of solvent drag.[49] Stomal sodium loss in effluent is approximately 90 to 100 mmol/L, and therefore such patients often secrete more sodium than they consume orally.[50,51] Therefore, ORS should ideally contain 100 mmol/L of sodium. This may make long-term patient compliance a challenge. Nevertheless, patients should be encouraged to drink ORS when thirsty instead of drinking low-sodium, hyperosmolar compounds or plain water, which may enhance sodium losses.[52] There are a number of "just add water" and ready-to-use commercial products available, although the least expensive is the World Health Organization formula, which can be easily made at home by dissolving 2.6 g table salt, 1.5 g potassium chloride ("salt substitute"), 2.5 g baking soda, and 20 g table sugar into 1 L of tap water.[53] It should be noted that most of the commercially available formulas contain less than the optimal amount of sodium. Some evidence suggests that hypotonic solutions (eg, 160 mOsmol/kg) may have greater efficacy than isotonic solutions because of a decreased intraluminal duodeno-jejunal fluid flow rate, but such solutions have not been thoroughly investigated in patients with SBS or intestinal failure.[54] For patients with residual colon in continuity with small bowel, ORS is not as critical if there is sufficient dietary sodium consumption; the colon absorbs sodium and water against a steep electrochemical gradient.[55] In addition, because ileal fluid absorption is not affected by the presence of glucose, the use of ORS is not critical in patients who have had most of the jejunum resected.[56]

Induction of hyperphagia, as previously described, is the most critical part of the prescribed diet, regardless of its composition. Most macronutrients (carbohydrates, protein, fat) are absorbed within the first 100 to 150 cm of jejunum.[57] Given that it is the very rare patient only with intestinal failure who is missing their duodenum and proximal jejunum, a lactose-containing diet can be provided. This is a vital source of calcium. Two studies have shown that a diet that contained 20 g/d (a glass of milk) of lactose did not increase diarrhea, flatulence, or breath hydrogen production in patients with SBS.[58,59]

Because nitrogen is the macronutrient whose absorption is least affected in SBS due to its proximal absorption,[57] the use of peptide-based formula likely has little merit. This concept is supported by 2 small clinical trials.[60,61] Nitrogen absorption may be modestly enhanced, however, in patients with short residual bowel ending in a jejunostomy, related to the extreme loss of absorptive surface area.[62]

As mentioned earlier, in patients with SBS, the colon becomes and important digestive organ. Soluble fiber and resistant starch pass through undigested and unabsorbed into the colon where they are undergo bacterial-catalyzed fermentation to the SCFAs butyrate, propionate, and acetate, the preferred fuel for colonocytes.[63,64] Different carbohydrates will be fermented to different ratios of these SCFAs. Approximately 75 mmol of SCFA are produced from 10 g of unabsorbed carbohydrate.[65] Patients with SBS, but their entire colon remaining, and in continuity with the residual small bowel, in one study were able to reduce their fecal energy loss by 310 to 740 kcal/d (1.3–3.1 MJ/d) when they consumed a diet that consisted of 60% carbohydrates.[14] The SCFAs also stimulate water absorption by the colonocyte and hypothetically could result in decreased diarrhea, although this has not been observed clinically, as there are many factors that come into play with regard to diarrhea in these patients. The colon, or more likely, the colonic microbiome may also "adapt" after resection, and colonic fermentation may increase further.[66]

Besides the potential of carbohydrate restriction in the rare patient with colon in continuity who develops D-lactic acidosis, the only other dietary constituent that may require restriction is oxalate.[3] Patients with colon in situ and in continuity with the small intestine are at risk for development of hyperoxaluria and calcium oxalate kidney stones.[67] Hyperoxaluria develops because the calcium that normally binds dietary oxalate, binds fatty acids instead in the presence of significant fat malabsorption. Thereby, uncomplexed dietary oxalate basses into the colon where it is absorbed, and the absorbed oxalate accumulates in the renal tubules. Such patients should receive instructions and written information on a low-oxalate diet. Oral calcium supplementation also may be of benefit, as the calcium will bind some of the oxalate so that it is excreted in the stool; decreasing dietary fat intake also may be useful. Of note is that vitamin C may degrade to oxalate when exposed to light.[68] Therefore, not just patients with colon in continuity may be at risk for development of hyperoxaluria.[69]

With regard to lipid, it is not clear whether a high-fat or low-fat diet is advantageous. On the one hand, fat is the most energy-dense macronutrient, but it also delays gastric emptying and may be associated with early satiety. In addition, limited data from patients with a jejunostomy suggest a high-fat diet leads to increased fecal loss of the divalent cations calcium, magnesium, zinc, and copper,[70] yet murine studies suggest a high-fat diet may be beneficial for intestinal adaptation, although this has not been studied in humans.[71] Medium-chain triglyceride (C8–C10; 8.3 kcal/g) does not supply essential fatty acids, but is an energy source that may be absorbed directly into the portal circulation(even in the stomach and colon) unlike long-chain fats that require digestion, although for all practical purposes the amount of energy supplied by a maximal tolerable dose is small.

PHARMACOLOGIC ENHANCEMENT OF INTESTINAL ADAPTATION

Two medications are approved by the Food and Drug Administration for the treatment of SBS with intestinal failure. These include growth hormone (Zorbtive; EMD Serono,

Rockland, MA) as well as growth hormone manufactured by others (Pfizer, Eli Lilly, Novo Nordisk, and Sandoz) with glutamine, and teduglutide (Gattex; Shire, Zug, Switzerland).

There are few data on the effect of growth hormone with and without glutamine (oral or intravenous) on the human intestine, and the data that exist suggest they have no effect.[72] However, the growth hormone stimulates tubular reabsorption of sodium from the renal tubule and this may be very useful for the conservation of fluid.[73] Indeed, the use of growth hormone (0.1 mg/kg per day subcutaneous [SQ]) has allowed PN to be decreased.[74] This study was confounded, however, by the fact there was no true placebo, diets were also provided with ORS and a high complex carbohydrate diet, and in many cases, antidiarrheal medication. Other studies though have shown no improvement in electrolyte or nutrient absorption,[75] or more modest improvements in absorption.[76] Nevertheless, this medication may be useful in some patients. Side effects that have been recognized in patients with SBS/intestinal failure include edema and anasarca from excess fluid retention and carpal tunnel syndrome.

Teduglutide is an analog of a naturally occurring hormone GLP-2 (secreted from L cells in the ileum and possibly right colon) where a glycine residue is substituted for an alanine at position 2 of the native hormone. This renders the molecule partially resistant to degradation by dipeptidyl-peptidase and prolongs its half-life. GLP-2 decreases gastrointestinal motility, although that has not been observed in all studies,[77–79] and stimulates splanchnic blood flow.[80,81] Teduglutide (0.5 mg/kg per day SQ) promotes mucosal hyperplasia and results in enhanced fluid and nutrient absorption.[82] This has resulted in the ability to decrease HPN by 1 to 2 days per week, and in some cases in which PN is low volume, to discontinue HPN.[83] In this study, approximately 65% of patients responded to the therapy, although the factors that predict efficacy of teduglutide are not well delineated. Attempted PN weaning can begin after 2 to 4 weeks of therapy. If a response to therapy is achieved, teduglutide must be continued lifelong, as the mucosa regresses toward baseline once it has been discontinued.[82] It is likely those patients with the least native GLP-2 production, namely those with ileal and right colon resections, are the most likely to benefit, and preliminary data support that theory.[84] More recent preliminary data suggested that although GLP-2 appears to have greater intestinalotropic effects when compared with GLP-1, there may be an additive effect from combination therapy, possibly due to the inhibitory effects of GLP-1 on gastric emptying.[85] However, one does not want to trade off early satiety and decrease hyperphagia for increased nutrient and fluid absorption. There are no currently published data on the use of combination therapy with growth hormone and teduglutide.

WEANING PARENTERAL NUTRITION

A retrospective European study found the likelihood of weaning patients from HPN successfully was approximately 6% if not accomplished within the first 2 years of starting HPN.[9] It must be recognized that the provision of one's complete energy needs parenterally does not stimulate hunger and, therefore, PN must be decreased to stimulate appetite. Paradoxically, PN often is not reduced because the patient has a poor appetite without recognition of the role PN plays. In fact, studies have suggested intravenous lipids delay gastric emptying,[86] which may result in early satiety and confound efforts to induce permanent hyperphagia. This finding was not observed in all studies, however.[87] In addition, intravenous amino acid infusion has been shown to reduce oral intake in some,[88,89] but not all studies.[90] Recall that the induction of hyperphagia is important to account for the decreased nutrient absorption found with

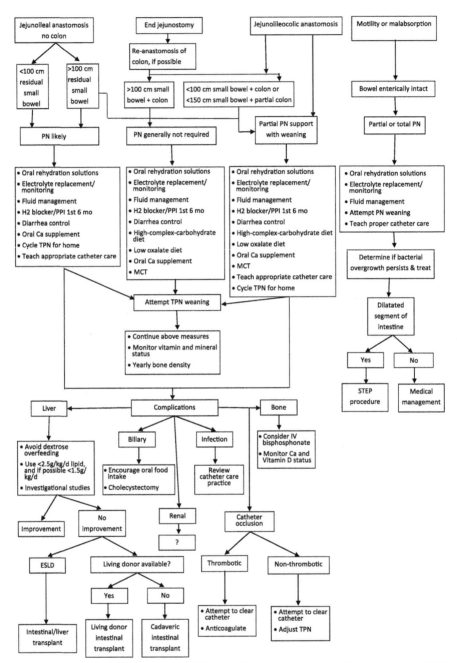

Fig. 1. Intestinal failure flowchart. ESLD, end-stage liver disease; IV, intravenous; MCT, medium-chain tryglyceride; PPI, proton pump inhibitor; TPN, total parenteral nutrition.

intestinal failure. Therefore, the first step in the weaning of PN is to reduce the PN and stimulate hunger. Lipids should be discontinued first, given the aforementioned effects on gastric emptying, as PN is reduced by increments of 10% to 20% on a daily basis. Urine output should be measured and should be consistently at least 1000 mL per

24 hours. Patients need to be instructed to keep a log of their urine outputs and call in with the results; the urine need not be saved. Once the daily PN volume has decreased to less than 1.5 L/d, 1 night may be eliminated, followed by a second night, and so on. Twenty-four-hour or 48-hour urine volume measurements should be made on off-PN nights, or include an off-PN night if a 48-hour measurement. Once PN is down to 3 nights a week at less than 1.5 L/night, the PN can be discontinued. Typically, 1 week elapses between changes.

It must be recognized that as the frequency of PN is decreased, the frequency during which micronutrients are infused also decreases. Therefore, vitamin status must be monitored. This may involve measurement of the vitamin (not immediately after PN has been completed from the infusion catheter!) or vitamin metabolites where appropriate. Trace metal status also will require monitoring, although there is some controversy as to effectively and appropriately determine trace metal status.

SUMMARY

The rendering of proper care for the patient with intestinal failure requires the provider to have a functional understanding of digestion and absorption, nutrient requirements, and intestinal adaptation. Inherent in those concepts are that not only is nutritional absorption compromised, but medication absorption is as well. The principles of the management of HPN must be mastered and then proper and controlled weaning of PN may be commenced by use of dietary and pharmacologic means with appropriate clinical outcome measures followed. The most important aspects of care include the development of hyperphagia, appropriate oral fluid intake, and appropriate pharmacologic control of diarrhea, which may involve higher or even much higher doses of medication than used in other patient groups. Teduglutide, a GLP-2 analog, may also be used not in place of, but in addition to proper conservative management, as outlined in this article. For those patients with dilated loops of small intestine in which bacterial overgrowth becomes a problem, the STEP is an excellent alternative in experienced centers. Intestinal transplantation is not currently a replacement for HPN, but rather, is a potential alternative to death for those patients who have developed what could become life-threatening complications of SBS, namely IFALD, true loss of venous access (although access must be reserved for a transplant), or the rare cases of true "refractory" dehydration. This complicated management requires a team experienced in both the medical and the surgical management of intestinal failure. An algorithm for the management of patients with intestinal failure is depicted in **Fig. 1**.

REFERENCES

1. O'Keefe SJ, Buchman AL, Fishbein TM, et al. Short bowel syndrome and intestinal failure: consensus definitions and overview. Clin Gastroenterol Hepatol 2006; 4:6–10.
2. Pironi L, Arends J, Baxter J, et al. ESPEN endorsed recommendations: definition and classification of intestinal failure in adults. Clin Nutr 2015;34:171–80.
3. Buchman AL, Scolapio J, Fryer J. AGA technical review on short bowel syndrome and intestinal transplantation. Gastroenterology 2003;124:1111–34.
4. Cisler JJ, Buchman AL. Intestinal adaptation in short bowel syndrome. J Investig Med 2005;53:402–13.
5. Solhaug JH, Tvete S. Adaptive changes in the small intestine following bypass operation for obesity. Scand J Gastroenterol 1978;13:401–8.
6. Doldi SB. Intestinal adaptation following jejeuno-ileal bypass. Clin Nutr 1991;10: 138–45.

7. Dowling RH, Booth CC. Functional compensation after small bowel resection in man. Lancet 1966;1:146–7.
8. Weinnstein LD, Shoemaker CP, Hersh T, et al. Enhanced intestinal absorption after small bowel resection in man. Arch Surg 1968;99:560–1.
9. Messing B, Crenn P, Beau P, et al. Long-term survival and parenteral nutrition dependence in adult patients with short bowel syndrome. Gastroenterology 1999;117:1043–50.
10. Dibb M, Soop M, Teubner A, et al. Survival and nutritional dependence of home parenteral nutrition: three decades of experience from a single referral centre. Clin Nutr 2017;36(2):570–6.
11. Infantino BJ, Mercer DF, Hobson BD, et al. Successful rehabilitation in pediatric ultrashort small bowel syndrome. J Pediatr 2013;163:1361–6.
12. Carbonnel F, Cosnes J, Chevret S, et al. The role of anatomic factors in nutritional autonomy after extensive small bowel resection. JPEN J Parenter Enteral Nutr 1996;20:275–80.
13. Ameen VZ, Powell GK, Jones LA. Quantitation of fecal carbohydrate excretion in patients with short bowel syndrome. Gastroenterology 1987;92:493–500.
14. Nordgaard I, Hansen BS, Mortensen PB. Importance of colonic support for energy absorption as small bowel failure proceeds. Lancet 1994;343:373–6.
15. Amiot A, Joly F, Lefevre JH, et al. Long-term outcome after extensive intestinal resection for chronic radiation enteritis. Dig Liver Dis 2013;45(2):110–4.
16. Crenn P, Coudray-Lucas C, Thuillier F, et al. Postabsorptive plasma citrulline concentration is a marker of absorptive enterocyte mass and intestinal failure in humans. Gastroenterology 2000;119:1496–505.
17. Picot D, Garin L, Trivin F, et al. Plasma citrulline is a marker of absorptive small bowel length in patients with transient enterostomy and acute intestinal failure. Clin Nutr 2010;29:235–42.
18. Staun M, Pironi L, Bozzetti F, et al. ESPEN guidelines on parenteral nutrition: home parenteral nutrition (HPN) in adult patients. Clin Nutr 2009;28(4):467–79.
19. Anast CS, Winnacker JL, Forte LR, et al. Impaired release of parathyroid hormone in magnesium deficiency. Clin Endocrinol Metab 1976;42:707–17.
20. Fleming CR, George L, Stoner GL, et al. The importance of urinary magnesium values in patients with gut failure. Mayo Clin Proc 1996;71:21–4.
21. Da Silva YS, Horvat CM, Dezfulian C. Thiamin deficiency as a cause of persistent hyperlactatemia in a parenteral nutrition-dependent patient. JPEN 2015;39:604–6.
22. Cavicchi M, Beau P, Crenn P, et al. Prevalence of liver disease and contributing factors in patients receiving home parenteral nutrition for permanent intestinal failure. Ann Intern Med 2000;132:525–32.
23. Hoffer LJ. How much protein do parenteral amino acid mixtures provide? Am J Clin Nutr 2011;94:1396–8.
24. Buchman AL, Howard L. Micronutrients in parenteral nutrition: too little or too much? The past, present, and recommendations for the future. Gastroenterology 2009;137:S1–6.
25. Buchman AL, Opilla M, Kwasny M, et al. Risk factors for the development of catheter-related bloodstream infections in patients receiving home parenteral nutrition. JPEN 2014;38:744–9.
26. Crenn P, Morin MC, Joly F, et al. Net digestive absorption and adaptive hyperphagia in adult short bowel patients. Gut 2004;53:1279–86.
27. Pironi L, Arends J, Bozzetti F, et al. ESPEN guidelines on chronic intestinal failure in adults. Clin Nutr 2016;35(2):247–307.

28. Smith CE. Quality of life in long term TPN patients and their family caregivers. JPEN 1993;17:501–6.

29. Smith CE, Curtas S, Werkowitch M, et al. Home parenteral nutrition: does affiliation with a national support and educational organization improve patient outcomes? JPEN 2002;26:159–63.

30. Go VL, Poley JR, Hofmann AF, et al. Disturbances in fat digestion induced by acidic jejunal pH due to gastric hypersecretion in man. Gastroenterology 1970; 58:638–46.

31. Nightingale JM, Walker ER, Farthing MJ, et al. Effect of omeprazole on intestinal output in the short bowel syndrome. Aliment Pharmacol Ther 1991;5:405–12.

32. Jeppesen PB, Staun M, Tjellesen L, et al. Effect of intravenous ranitidine and omeprazole on intestinal absorption of water, sodium, and macronutrients in patients with intestinal resection. Gut 1998;43:763–9.

33. Tytgat GN, Huibregtse K, Davevos J, et al. Effect of loperamide on fecal output and composition in well-established ileostomy and ileorectal anastomosis. Am J Dig Dis 1977;22:669–76.

34. Tygat GN. Loperamide and ileostomy output. Br Med J 1975;3:489.

35. Tytgat GN, Huibregtse K, Meuwissen SG. Loperamide in chronic diarrhea and after ileostomy: a placebo-controlled double-blind cross-over study. Arch Chir Neerl 1976;28:13–20.

36. Newton CR. Effect of codeine phosphate, Lomotil, and Isogel on ileostomy function. Gut 1978;19:377–83.

37. King RF, Norton T, Hill GL. A double-blind crossover study of the effect of loperamide hydrochloride and codeine phosphate on ileostomy output. Aust N Z J Surg 1982;52:121–4.

38. Buchman AL, Fryer J, Wallin A, et al. Clonidine reduces diarrhea and sodium loss in patients with proximal jejunostomy: a controlled study. JPEN 2006;30:487–91.

39. Hofmann AF, Poley JR. Cholestyramine treatment of diarrhea associated with ileal resection. N Engl J Med 1969;281:397–402.

40. O'Keefe SJD, Haymond MW, Bennet WM, et al. Long-acting somatostatin analogue therapy and protein metabolism in patients with jejunostomies. Gastroenterology 1994;107:379–88.

41. Niv Y, Charash B, Sperber AD, et al. Effect of octreotide on gastrostomy, duodenostomy, and cholecysostomy effluents: a physiologic study of fluid and electrolyte balance. Am J Gastroenterol 1997;92:2107–11.

42. Heuser M, Popken O, Kleiman I, et al. Detrimental effects of octreotide on intestinal microcirculation. J Surg Res 2000;92:186–92.

43. Tocchi A, Costa G, Lepre L, et al. Effects of octreotide (somatostatin analog SMS 201-995) on superior mesenteric artery blood flow in swine. An experimental study using Doppler color ultrasonography. G Chir 1999;20:9–13.

44. Sukhotnik I, Khateeb K, Krausz MM, et al. Sandostatin impairs post resection intestinal adaptation in a rat model of short bowel syndrome. Dig Dis Sci 2002;47: 2095–102.

45. Catnach SM, Anderson JV, Fairclough PD, et al. Effect of octreotide on gallstone prevalence and gallbladder motility in acromegaly. Gut 1993;34:270–3.

46. Roslyn JJ, Pitt HA, Mann LL, et al. Gallbladder disease in patients on long term parenteral nutrition. Gastroenterology 1983;84:148–54.

47. Oliveira C, de Silva N, Wales PW. Five-year outcomes after serial transverse enteroplasty in children with short bowel syndrome. J Pediatr Surg 2012;47:931–7.

48. Nightingale JM, Lennard Jones JE, Walker ER, et al. Oral salt supplements to compensate for jejunostomy losses: comparison of sodium chloride capsules,

glucose electrolyte solution, and glucose polymer electrolyte solution. Gut 1992; 33:759–61.

49. Fortran JS. Stimulation of active and passive sodium absorption by sugars in the human jejunum. J Clin Invest 1975;55:728–37.

50. Nightingale JM, Lennard-Jones JE, Walker ER, et al. Jejunal efflux in short bowel syndrome. Lancet 1990;336:765–8.

51. Langefoged K, Olgaard K. Fluid and electrolyte absorption and renin-angiotensin-aldosterone axis in patients with severe short bowel syndrome. Gastroenterology 1979;14:729–35.

52. Newton CR, Gonvers JJ, McIntyre PB, et al. Effect of different drinks on fluid and electrolyte losses from a jejunostomy. J R Soc Med 1985;78:27–34.

53. Treatment and prevention of dehydration in diarrheal diseases. Geneva: WHO; 1976.

54. Pfeiffer A, Schmidt T, Kaess H. The role of osmolality in the absorption of a nutrient solution. Aliment Pharmacol Ther 1998;12:281–6.

55. Fortran JS, Rector FC Jr, Carter NW. The mechanism of sodium absorption in the human small intestine. J Clin Invest 1968;47:884–900.

56. Davis GR, Santa Ana CA, Morawski SG, et al. Permeability characteristics of human jejunum, ileum, proximal colon, and distal colon: results of potential difference measurements and unidirectional fluxes. Gastroenterology 1982;83:844–50.

57. Borgstrom B, Dahlqvist A, Lundh G, et al. Studies of intestinal digestion and absorption in the human. J Clin Invest 1957;36:1521–36.

58. Marteau P, Mesing B, Arrigoni E, et al. Do patients with short bowel syndrome need a lactose-free diet? Nutrition 1997;13:13–6.

59. Arrigoni E, Marteau P, Briet F, et al. Tolerance and absorption of lactose from milk and yogurt during short bowel syndrome in humans. Am J Clin Nutr 1994;60: 926–9.

60. McIntyre PB, Fitchew M, Lennard-Jones JE. Patients with a high jejunostomy do not need a special diet. Gastroenterology 1986;91:25–33.

61. Levy E, Frileux P, Sandrucci S, et al. Continuous enteral nutrition during the early adaptive stage of the short bowel syndrome. Br J Surg 1988;75:549–53.

62. Cosnes J, Evard D, Beaugerie L, et al. Improvement in protein absorption with a small peptide-based diet in patients with high jejunostomy. Nutrition 1992;8: 406–11.

63. Englyst HN, Trowell H, Southgate DAT, et al. Dietary fibre and resistant starch. Am J Clin Nutr 1987;46:873–4.

64. Bond JH, Currier BE, Buchwald H, et al. Colonic conservation of malabsorbed carbohydrate. Gastroenterology 1980;78:444–7.

65. Cummings JH, Gibson GR, Mcfarlane GT. Quantitative estimates of fermentation in the hind gut of man. Acta Vet Scand Suppl 1989;86:76–82.

66. Briet F, Flourie B, Achour L, et al. Bacterial adaptation in patients with short bowel and colon in continuity. Gastroenterology 1995;109:1446–53.

67. Nightingale JM, Lennard-Jones JE, Gertner DJ, et al. Colonic preservation reduces need for parenteral therapy, increases incidence of renal stones, but does not change high prevalence of gallstones in patients with a short bowel. Gut 1992;33:1493–7.

68. Fairholm L, Saqui O, Baun M, et al. Influence of multivitamin regimen on urinary oxalate in home parenteral nutrition patients. Nutr Clin Pract 2003;18:366–9.

69. Buchman AL, Moukarzel AA, Ament ME. Excessive urinary oxalate excretion occurs in long-term TPN patients both with and without ileostomies. J Am Coll Nutr 1995;14:24–8.

70. Ovesen L, Chu R, Howard L. The influence of dietary fat on jejunostomy output in patients with severe short bowel syndrome. Am J Clin Nutr 1983;38:270–7.
71. Choi PM, Sun RC, Guo J, et al. High-fat diet enhances villus growth during the adaptation response to massive proximal small bowel resection. J Gastrointest Surg 2014;18:286–94.
72. Scolapio JS, Camilleri M, Fleming CR, et al. Effect of growth hormone, glutamine, and diet on adaptation in short-bowel syndrome: a randomized, controlled study. Gastroenterology 1997;113:1074–81.
73. Hansen TK, Moller J, Thomsen K, et al. Effects of growth hormone on renal tubular handling of sodium in healthy humans. Am J Physiol Endocrinol Metab 2001;281:E1326–32.
74. Byrne TA, Wilmore DW, Iyer K, et al. Growth hormone, glutamine, and an optimal diet reduces parenteral nutrition in patients with short bowel syndrome: a prospective, randomized, placebo-controlled, double-blind clinical trial. Ann Surg 2005;242:655–61.
75. Szkudlarek J, Jeppesen PB, Mortensen PB. Effect of high dose growth hormone with glutamine and no change in diet on intestinal absorption in short bowel patients: a randomized, double blind, crossover, placebo controlled trial. Gut 2000;47:199–205.
76. Seguy D, Vahedi K, Kapel N, et al. Low-dose growth hormone in adult home parenteral nutrition-dependent short bowel syndrome patients: a positive study. Gastroenterology 2003;124:293–302.
77. Iturrino J, Camilleri M, Acosta A, et al. Acute effects of a glucagon-like peptide 2 analogue, teduglutide, on gastrointestinal moto function and permeability in adult patients with short bowel syndrome on home parenteral nutrition. JPEN 2015;40:1089–95.
78. Nagell CF, Wettergren A, Pedersen JF, et al. Glucagon-like peptide-2 inhibits antral emptying of liquids in man, but is not as potent as glucagon-like peptide-1. Scand J Gastroenterol 2004;39:353–8.
79. Schmidt PT, Naslund E, Gryback P, et al. Peripheral administration of GLP-2 to humans has no effects on gastric emptying or satiety. Regul Pept 2003;116:21–5.
80. Hoyerup P, Hellstrom PM, Schmidt PT, et al. Glucagon-like peptide-2 stimulates mucosal microcirculation measured by laser Doppler flowmetry in end-jejunostomy short bowel syndrome patients. Regul Pept 2013;180:12–6.
81. Bremholm L, Hornum M, Andersen UB, et al. The effect of glucagon-like peptide -2 on mesenteric blood flow and cardiac parameters in end-jejunostomy short bowel patients. Regul Pept 2011;168:32–8.
82. Jeppesen PB, Sanguinetti EL, Buchman AL, et al. Teduglutide (ALX-0600), a dipeptidyl peptidase IV resistant glucagon-like peptide 2 analogue, improves intestinal function in short bowel syndrome patients. Gut 2005;54:223–31.
83. Jeppesen PB, Pertkiewicz M, Messing B, et al. Teduglutide reduces need for parenteral support among patients with short bowel syndrome with intestinal failure. Gastroenterology 2012;143:1473–81.
84. Chen K, Xie J, Tang W, et al. Predictors and characteristics of early responder to teduglutide in patients with short bowel syndrome and parenteral nutrition dependency [abstract]. Gastroenterology 2017;152:S8.
85. Madsen KB, Askov-Hansen C, Naimi RM, et al. Acute effects of continuous infusions of glucagon-like peptide (GLP-1), GLP-2 and the combination (GLP-1 + GLP-2) on intestinal absorption in short bowel syndrome patients. A placebo-controlled study. Regul Pept 2013;184:30–9.

86. Casaubon PR, Dahlstrom KA, Vargas J, et al. Intravenous fat emulsion (Intralipid) delays gastric emptying, but does not cause gastroesophageal reflux in healthy volunteers. JPEN 1989;13:246–8.
87. Welch I, Saunders K, Read NW. Effect of ileal and intravenous infusions of fat emulsions on feeding and satiety in human volunteers. Gastroenterology 1985; 89:1293–7.
88. Gielkens HA, Penning C, van dan Biggelaar A, et al. Effect of I.V. amino acids on satiety in humans. JPEN 1999;23:56–60.
89. Sriram K, Pinchcofsky G, Kaminiski MV Jr. Suppression of appetite by parenteral nutrition in humans. J Am Coll Nutr 1983;3:317–23.
90. Murray CD, le Roux CW, Gouveia C, et al. The effect of different macronutrient infusions on appetite, ghrelin, and peptide YY in parenterally fed patients. Clin Nutr 2006;25:626–33.

Adult Intestinal Transplantation

Cal S. Matsumoto, MD*, Sukanya Subramanian, MD, Thomas M. Fishbein, MD

KEYWORDS

- Adult intestinal transplantation • Intestinal transplant indications
- Intestinal transplant outcome • Virtual crossmatch

KEY POINTS

- Owing to the large lymphoid load and resultant immunologically reactive graft, intestinal transplants pose a direct challenge to the recipient's immune system.
- Intestinal transplants also indirectly challenge the recipient with the compulsory augmented immunosuppression and the inherent complications associated with the higher immunosuppressed state.
- The etiologies of intestinal failure, rehabilitative prognosis, graft type, surgical techniques, nutritional autonomy, and outcomes separate adults and children with regard to intestinal transplantation.

INTRODUCTION

Adult intestinal transplantation has evolved over the past decades from a rarely performed, immunologically hazardous therapy into a mainstream therapeutic procedure with results that today approach other solid organ transplants.[1] Owing to the large lymphoid load and resultant immunologically reactive graft, the transplanted intestine poses challenges both directly and indirectly on the recipient. Directly, it poses an immediate immunologic confrontation to the recipient immune system, and indirectly on the recipient with the compulsory augmented immunosuppression and the inherent complications associated with the higher immunosuppressed state.

Despite the commonality of the transplanted intestine allograft, adult and pediatric intestinal transplantations have differences in nearly all aspects. The etiologies of intestinal failure, intestinal rehabilitative prognosis, graft type use, surgical techniques, nutritional autonomy, and outcomes are a few of the differences that separate adults and children with regard to intestinal transplantation.

Disclosure: The authors have nothing to disclose.
Medstar Georgetown University Hospital, Medstar Georgetown Transplant Institute, 3800 Reservoir Road, Northwest, 2 PHC Building, Washington, DC 20007, USA
* Corresponding author.
E-mail address: csm5@gunet.georgetown.edu

Gastroenterol Clin N Am 47 (2018) 341–354
https://doi.org/10.1016/j.gtc.2018.01.011
0889-8553/18/© 2018 Elsevier Inc. All rights reserved.

CURRENT TRENDS IN ADULT INTESTINAL TRANSPLANTATION

Unlike in the pediatric intestinal transplant population, grafts that include the liver have increased in the adult population globally over the past several years according to the latest data published by the Intestinal Transplant Registry[2] (**Fig. 1**). Not surprisingly, pre-transplant death reported from the Organ Procurement and Transplantation Network/Scientific Registry of Transplant Recipients 2015 Annual Data Intestine Report was notably higher for those patients requiring a liver containing graft at 19.9 deaths per 100 waitlist years as compared with 2.8 deaths per 100 waitlist years for recipients with isolated intestine.[3] Thus, despite the observed overall decreased morbidity associated with parenteral nutrition, largely owing to the establishment and refinement of specialized intestinal care and intestinal rehabilitation centers, pretransplant mortality remains greatest for adult intestine candidates, at 19.6 deaths per 100 waitlist years.[3]

Adult candidates, however, have differing reasons for requiring a liver-containing graft as compared with pediatric candidates. Whereas the majority of pediatric intestinal candidates that require a liver-containing graft suffer from parenteral nutrition–associated liver disease as the basis for their liver inclusion, adult candidates who require a liver-inclusive graft have other conditions such as malignancy or primary end-stage liver disease with complicated portomesenteric thrombosis that necessitates a combined or multivisceral graft for successful liver transplantation.[4] As expected, these adult multivisceral candidates do not suffer from intestinal failure and do not fall under the traditional indications of "failure of parenteral nutrition" as an indication for intestinal transplantation. Attempts to directly compare adult and pediatric indications, surgical techniques, and outcomes cannot be done without understanding the major characteristics between the 2 populations.

Adult Intestine Transplant Volume

Overall, with the exception of 2012, the number of adult intestine transplants has remained relatively steady in the United States in the past decade, ranging from 77 to 92 adult intestine transplant cases per calendar year (median, 85 cases)[5] (**Fig. 2**). This

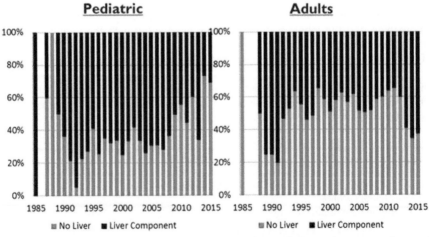

Fig. 1. International transplant registry data comparing liver inclusive grafts versus no liver graft in the adult and pediatric population. (*Courtesy of* Robert S. Venick, MD, Los Angeles, CA.)

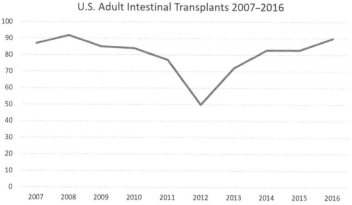

Fig. 2. United Network for Organ Sharing (UNOS) data of total number of adult (≥18 years) intestinal transplants from 2007 to 2016. (*Data from* U.S. Department of Health and Human Services. Organ procurement and transplantation network data reports. Available at: https://optn.transplant.hrsa.gov/data/view-data-reports/.)

has differed substantially with the pediatric intestinal transplant experience, which has observed a precipitous decrease in the number of intestinal transplants since 2007.[6] Much of the decrease in the number of pediatric intestinal transplants can be attributed to specialized intestinal care centers that capitalize on the increased potential that the infant pediatric gut has for adaptation, and thus rehabilitation. This condition differs from the adult patients with a short gut, who have generally maintained and sustained decades of established intestinal function before the loss of gut and, thus, harbors less potential for growth and adaptation of the remnant intestine. Prolonged parenteral nutrition exposure in the adult population, however, does account for the need for a proportion of liver-containing grafts in the adult population, and this is an area for potential improvement in decreasing the high pretransplant mortality in the adult liver–intestine transplant population. Early referral to a specialized adult intestinal transplant center and early recognition of adult recipients with intestinal failure could serve to provide the preferred option of isolated intestine transplant and subsequent withdrawal of parenteral nutrition before the development of irreversible parenteral nutrition–associated liver disease, thus, obviating the requirement for a liver-inclusive graft. Recognizing the extremely high mortality that adult patients have on the combined liver–intestine waiting list, the United Network for Organ Sharing revised allocation policy for this specific subset in 2013, allowing for a greater, nationwide pool of potential adult multivisceral donors to help mitigate the high mortality risk.[7] Current policy for adults also allocates an additional increase in their Model for End-Stage Liver Disease score equivalent to a 10% increase in risk of 3-month mortality.

Etiologies of Conditions Leading to Adult Intestinal Transplantation

Short gut syndrome remains the most common condition leading to transplant in both the adult and pediatric population, comprising approximately 60% to 65% of all transplanted cases. Conditions that lead to the short gut diagnosis, however, differ significantly between the 2 populations. Classic neonatal and infant conditions such as gastroschisis, necrotizing enterocolitis, intestinal volvulus, and jejunal ileal atresia account for the vast majority of conditions leading to short gut syndrome and transplantation in the infant and child. In the adult, mesenteric ischemia is the most common etiology of short gut syndrome followed by Crohn's disease, trauma, surgical misadventure, and volvulus.[2]

Mesenteric Infarction

Acute mesenteric infarction has a low incidence of occurrence, accounting for 0.09% to 0.20% of all acute admissions in the emergency room. The condition, however, has an accompanying mortality rate of up to 80% if not treated in a timely manner.[8] Given that there is very little collateral circulation to the small intestine, acute arterial occlusion from emboli, which accounts for approximately 50% of all cases of acute mesenteric ischemia, usually results in short gut syndrome in those patients who survive this catastrophic event.[9] Etiologies of emboli include the left ventricle from cardiac dysrhythmias, cardiac valves from endocarditis, and aortic atherosclerotic plaque, diseases which occur primarily in the adult population. Venous occlusion accounts for less than 10% of cases of mesenteric infarction and is usually associated or precipitated by a hypercoagulable state. Acute mesenteric venous hypertension leads to increased vascular resistance, bowel edema, decreased blood flow, and bowel ischemia. Mandatory thrombophilia workup and hematologic evaluation is warranted in cases of venous mesenteric thrombosis to prevent future thrombotic events, which could have a profound effect on a newly transplanted intestinal graft in the future.[8]

Crohn's Disease

Crohn's disease is the second most common etiology of short gut syndrome leading to transplantation in adults, accounting for approximately 11% of cases.[2] Common complications such as perforation, stricture, obstruction, and abscess generally lead to multiple surgical procedures over the course of time, eventually rendering the patient with intestinal failure and permanent parenteral nutrition. Nearly one-quarter of patients who recovered from a Crohn's disease–related surgery will require a subsequent surgery within 5 years and 35% within a decade.[10] Despite the general surgical teaching of avoidance of large resections in Crohn's disease complications, recurrent and refractory disease will dictate mandatory resections in life-threatening surgical emergencies. In many cases, this emergent surgery will produce more surgical complications, particularly enterocutaneous fistulae. Efforts to reestablish enteral continuity, such as stoma closure, closure of enteroatmospheric fistulas, and surgically relieving obstructions, are a few of the surgical procedures that need to be performed before establishing a diagnosis of permanent intestinal failure in patients with Crohn's disease. Newer medical treatments and advances have led to a steady decrease in initial surgery rates over the last several decades; however, since the 1980s, the rates of second surgery have not decreased.[10] Mutations of certain alleles of the *NOD2* gene have been identified as risk factors for Crohn's disease. The *NOD2* gene, which encodes for an intracellular protein that serves as a microbial sensor in macrophages, dendritic cells, and Paneth cells, if abnormal, has been identified as having a 2- to 40-fold increased risk of Crohn's disease for certain mutant alleles.[11] With regard to intestinal transplant recipients, in several independent center analyses, a higher likelihood of allograft failure has been observed in recipients with a *NOD2* mutation, some with increased failure rates as high as 97-fold.[12] This finding suggests a similar link between the dysregulated gut innate immune system playing a significant role in the immunologic graft loss of the transplanted intestine. The recognition of potential intestinal transplant recipients with a NOD2 mutation, particularly those with Crohn's disease, is critically important to risk stratify these potential recipients appropriately.

Acute Volvulus

Unlike the typical case of volvulus, which usually occurs in infants with malrotation, adult cases of volvulus leading to a short gut and transplantation are not always related to the classic congenital mesenteric anatomic defects. Occasionally an adult who has suffered a volvulus as a child and has been maintained on parenteral nutrition until adult years, only to eventually suffer complications, is listed for an intestinal transplant. More commonly observed in the adult experience, however, is a surgically altered mesenteric anatomy that results in an acute volvulus event. An emerging observation of acute short gut has been reported in the Roux-en-Y gastric bypass population that has suffered an intestinal volvulus resulting in intestinal ischemia necessitating a life-saving total enterectomy. Rapid and massive weight loss after Roux-en-Y gastric bypass results in diminished mesenteric fat, which may increase the potential space between the jejunal limb and transverse mesocolon, allowing for a volvulus to occur (Petersen's hernia).[13] In addition, the standard use of the laparoscope in Roux-en-Y bypass has been implicated as a causative factor, because less adhesion formation may contribute to a larger open potential space.[14] In these particular cases, reestablishment of gastric continuity and removal of the jejunal limb, if it has survived the ischemic insult, is preferred before listing for intestinal transplantation.

Non–Short Gut Conditions Leading to Adult Intestinal Transplantation

Non–short gut conditions for the adult that lead to intestinal transplantation include intestinal motility disorders, tumors (chiefly desmoid tumors invading the base of the mesentery), and retransplantation.

Adult Motility Disorders

Motility disorders of the intestine are characterized by obstructive gastrointestinal symptoms without any evidence of mechanical occlusion of the gut lumen. Patients are typically symptomatic, with nausea, emesis, abdominal bloating, diffuse chronic abdominal pain, and weight loss. Stasis, bacterial overgrowth with malabsorption, and poor oral intake eventually lead to intestinal failure and the need for parenteral nutrition. Rehabilitative efforts are generally unsuccessful and do not provide any lasting enteral independence; these patients also undergo many futile surgeries, chiefly negative exploratory laparotomies for suspected bowel obstruction.[15] The evaluation includes first eliminating any possibility of a mechanical obstruction or possible causes of secondary forms of motility disorders, performing appropriate motility testing, and possibly a full-thickness biopsy or genetic testing. Typically, the symptoms evolve over many years presenting initially in the pediatric population and progressing into the adult years. It currently accounts for approximately 11% of all adult intestinal transplants.[2]

Intrabdominal Malignancy

Abdominal desmoid tumors account for the majority of intraabdominal tumors leading to intestinal transplantation in the adult. Desmoid tumors, although a benign fibromatous neoplasm, when it arises at the base of the mesentery, its infiltrative and locally invasive characteristics lead to a diffuse entrapment of the mesenteric vasculature, leading to intestinal complications such as obstruction and fistula formation. Conventional chemotherapy often proves unsatisfactory, and the treatment of choice is complete surgical resection that, owing to the location at the base of the mesentery, will uniformly result in ultrashort gut syndrome. In certain cases where the tumor has progressed and infiltrated cephalad to the root of the mesentery, complete exenteration of the foregut is mandatory, necessitating a modified multivisceral transplant. Recurrence of abdominal desmoids after intestinal transplantation have been reported, although usually are not associated with the transplanted graft and with no significant impact on survival after transplant.[16] Other intrabdominal malignancies have been considered for intestinal transplantation, although with much less frequency than the desmoid. Like with desmoid, the indication for intestinal replacement is usually due to the location of the tumor at the base of the mesentery, and those tumors with an indolent growth pattern, such as neuroendocrine tumors. In these cases, caution must be exercised when considering transplantation, because the biological behavior of many of these tumors, although low grade and indolent, is relatively unknown under long-term compulsory immunosuppression. Recent registry data report approximately 15% of all adult intestinal transplants were performed for malignancy.[2]

Adult Intestinal Retransplantation

Intestinal retransplantation in the adult population has increased over the past decade at a greater rate than adult primary transplants during the same time period. In an analysis of both adult retransplants from 2001 to 2009, adult retransplantation volume increased almost 5 times than the in preceding decade, whereas primary transplants only increased 3.2 times.[17] In addition, outcomes for retransplantations with an isolated intestine were significantly worse than primary transplants. Rejection, particularly humoral rejection, has been identified as a major barrier to successful retransplantation, primarily owing to the increased allosensitization that frequently accompanies the intestinal retransplant candidate. Adult intestinal retransplantation with a liver-inclusive graft, however, has not shown inferior results, possibly owing to the immunogenic protective effects of the liver allograft.[17] Current registry data report approximately 7% of all adult intestine transplants have been retransplants.[2]

INDICATIONS FOR ADULT INTESTINAL TRANSPLANTATION

Intestinal transplantation, despite the improvements in patient and graft survival over the past decade, has mostly been reserved for those suffering from the complications of parenteral nutrition or those with a physical inability to attain central venous access for the delivery of parenteral nutrition. Direct complications of parenteral nutrition include the development of overt liver disease, and indirect complications include frequent and/or life-threatening episodes of sepsis as well as loss of central venous access as described. Certain conditions have been recognized has having a high risk of death intrinsic to the disease state, such as abdominal desmoid tumors; congenital mucosal disorders, which are usually seen in pediatric population such as tufting enteropathy and microvillous inclusion disease; and those with a blind duodenum with retrograde biliopancreatic secretions drained from a gastrostomy tube or those adults with ultrashort bowel (<20 cm of jejunum). Other indications categorized as those with a high morbidity include those such as frequent hospitalizations, narcotic dependency, an inability to tolerate home parenteral nutrition, and those unwilling to accept long-term home parenteral nutrition (**Box 1**). These indications, published by the US Centers for Medicare and Medicaid Services in 2000 have largely been adopted worldwide as the standard for intestinal transplantation.[18] A more recent analysis performed by European intestinal transplant centers looking at the adult intestinal failure patient essentially parallels US guidelines specifically noting the increased risk of death in patients with parenteral nutrition associated liver disease (relative risk, 3.2) and invasive intrabdominal desmoids (relative risk, 7.1). This

---

Box 1
Centers for Medicare and Medicaid–approved indications for intestinal transplantation

Failure of parenteral nutrition

- Impending (total bilirubin 3–6 mg/dL, progressive thrombocytopenia, and progressive splenomegaly) or overt liver failure (portal hypertension, hepatosplenomegaly, hepatic fibrosis, or cirrhosis) because of parenteral nutrition liver injury

- Central venous catheter-related thrombosis of 2 central veins

- Frequent central line sepsis
  - Two episodes per year of systemic sepsis secondary to line infections requiring hospitalization
  - A single episode of line-related fungemia
  - Septic shock or acute respiratory distress syndrome

- Frequent episodes of severe dehydration despite intravenous fluid in addition to parenteral nutrition

High risk of death attributable to the underlying disease

- Desmoid tumors associated with familial adenomatous polyposis

- Congenital mucosal disorders

- Ultrashort bowel syndrome (residual bowel 20 cm in adults)

Intestinal failure with high morbidity or low acceptance of parenteral nutrition

- Frequent hospitalization

- Inability to function

- Patient unwillingness to accept long-term parenteral nutrition

Data from Department of Health and Human Services (DHHS) and Centers for Medicare and Medicaid Services (CMS). Intestinal and multi-visceral transplantation: program memorandum intermediaries/carriers. Pub #:60AB; CR #:1629. AB-02-040. 2002. Available at: https://www.cms.gov/Regulations-and-Guidance/Guidance/Transmittals/downloads/AB02040.pdf.

---

analysis, however, did not note an increased risk of death in adult patients with catheter-related complications or ultrashort bowel.[19]

SURGICAL PROCEDURE

The intestinal graft comes in many different forms and configurations depending on the needs of the recipient. Central to any type of intestinal graft is the jejunoileum component. Three major categories of intestinal transplant have been classically described: the isolated intestine, the liver–intestine, and the multivisceral transplant. In the adult intestinal recipient, the most common grafts used are the isolated intestine and the multivisceral grafts.

The major indication for isolated intestine transplant in both adult and pediatric patients are those patients with irreversible intestinal failure with preserved liver function who suffer from life-threatening complications of parenteral nutrition. The use of the nomenclature for the "liver–intestine" graft has differing meanings in the adult and pediatric populations. In pediatrics, the liver-intestine graft is generally understood to indicate a composite liver-pancreas-intestine graft and thus must be listed for a liver, pancreas, and intestine on the national United Network for Organ Sharing waiting list. In infants and small children, using the technique of foregut preservation and en bloc transplantation of the liver–pancreas–intestine, no reconstruction of the pediatric hepatic artery, portal vein, or common bile duct is necessary, greatly simplifying the transplant. In this case, because the native stomach, pancreatoduodenal complex, and spleen are preserved, a native portocaval shunt must be constructed before implantation of the organs.[20] This situation differs considerably from the adult recipient who requires a concomitant liver graft owing to parenteral nutrition associated liver disease. In these cases, the foregut anatomy is usually preserved and, with an intact and patent portal vein, and an isolated liver transplant can be performed in the standard fashion followed by an isolated intestine transplant. This graft is referred to as a "noncomposite" liver–intestine graft.[21]

Multivisceral graft transplantation entails total exenteration of the native stomach, pancreas, liver, spleen, and remaining intestine and replacement of all abdominal viscera with an en bloc graft. In many cases of adult multivisceral transplantation, the chief indication is the inability to safely delineate and preserve the foregut anatomy owing to multiple previous surgeries, which necessitate complete exenteration along with the diseased native liver. The most common indications for the adult multivisceral transplant is, as mentioned, portomesenteric thrombosis. Other indications in adults include abdominal desmoids infiltrating the foregut and motility disorders affecting the foregut. In those cases, where the liver is preserved and the foregut diseased, a "modified" multivisceral transplant is performed, transplanting only the stomach, duodenum, pancreas, and intestine. In the "modified" multivisceral transplant, the entire graft venous outflow is the inflow to the intact native liver.

All of these grafts, both pediatric and adult, can be with or without the inclusion of a colon component in continuity with the jejunoileum. Early poor outcomes in intestinal transplantation were thought to be attributed to the inclusion of the colon with the small intestine graft. Later colon inclusion experiences reported a 6% superior graft survival at 3 years ($P = .03$), a higher frequency of formed stool after stoma closure, improved quality of life, and a significantly greater likelihood of complete enteral independence after transplant.[22] The latest Intestinal Transplant Registry reports colon inclusion in intestinal allografts has increased from 10% in 2004 to almost 60% in 2015.[2]

Adult Isolated Intestine

The isolated intestine graft contains the jejunoileum with or without the colon (**Fig. 3**). Arterial inflow is established via the graft superior mesenteric artery, and venous

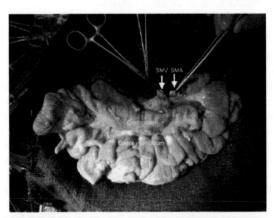

Fig. 3. En bloc adult intestine colon transplant graft with graft superior mesenteric artery (SMA) and superior mesenteric vein (SMV) labeled. (*From* Hawksworth J, Matsumoto S. Intestinal transplant techniques: from isolated intestine to intestine in continuity with other organs. In: Dunn SP, Horslen S, editors. Solid organ transplantation in infants and children, organ and tissue transplantation. Springer; 2017. p. 1–26; with permission.)

outflow via the graft superior mesenteric vein. Vascular conduits are universally used to facilitate the placement of the intestine graft without undue tension on the vessels as well as providing a more technically favorable condition for the vascular anastomoses, thus reducing the warm ischemic time. Arterial and venous conduits for adult intestinal recipients are obtained during the donor procedure from the donor external iliac artery and vein. In the common scenario of a simultaneous adult pancreas and liver procurement by separate teams, the external iliac artery is usually obtained from the liver donor vessels, and the external iliac vein obtained from the pancreas donor vessels.

There are 2 techniques for isolated intestine vascular reconstruction, either portal (orthotopic) or systemic (heterotopic) venous drainage (**Fig. 4**). In many cases of

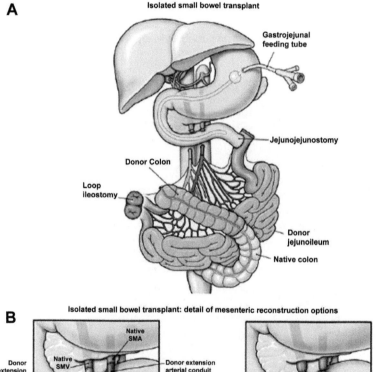

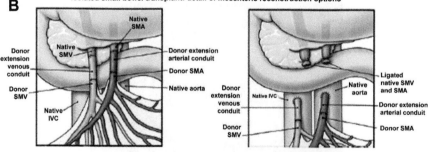

Fig. 4. (*A*) Isolated intestine transplant with the en bloc intestine colon graft implanted in a heterotopic position. (*B*) Isolated intestine transplant with details of the graft mesenteric reconstruction, either portal (orthotopic) or systemic (heterotopic). SMA, superior mesenteric artery; SMV, superior mesenteric vein. (*From* Hawksworth J, Matsumoto S. Intestinal transplant techniques: from isolated intestine to intestine in continuity with other organs. In: Dunn SP, Horslen S, editors. Solid organ transplantation in infants and children, organ and tissue transplantation. Springer; 2017. p. 1–26; with permission.)

recipients with short gut, the proximal native mesenteric pedicle is chronically occluded and atrophic, rendering the vessels unsuitable for the transplant graft. In those cases, systemic drainage is used by exposing the infrarenal aorta and vena cava. The donor iliac interposition grafts are anastomosed in an end-to-side fashion directed caudally (**Fig. 5**). Once the extension grafts are in place, the intestine graft is brought up into the field and the graft mesenteric vessels are anastomosed to the interposition grafts in and end-to-end fashion. It is critical that the interposition grafts are cut to an appropriate length to prevent undue tension on the vessels after reperfusion when the intestine graft size and weight increases significantly. After releasing the arterial clamp and before the release of the venous clamp, a blood flush is performed through the superior mesenteric vein anastomosis. After reperfusion and hemostasis, it critical to immediately affix the base of the graft mesentery to avoid graft volvulus of the mesenteric pedicle. In cases where the infrarenal vena cava is not patent owing to thrombosis from chronic indwelling femoral central venous lines, the suprarenal vena cava can be used for outflow. The extension graft is routed behind the mobilized duodenum to lie adjacent to the thrombosed infrarenal vena cava.

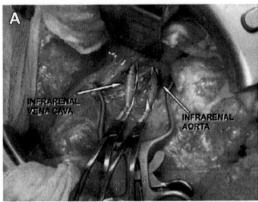

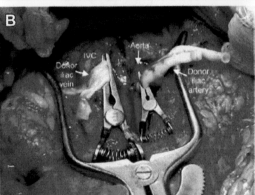

Fig. 5. (*A*) Exposure and clamping of the recipient infrarenal aorta and vena cava. (*B*) Donor interposition grafts anastomosed in a spatulated end-to-side manner. IVC, inferior vena cava. (*From* Hawksworth J, Matsumoto S. Intestinal transplant techniques: from isolated intestine to intestine in continuity with other organs. In: Dunn SP, Horslen S, editors. Solid organ transplantation in infants and children, organ and tissue transplantation. Springer; 2017. p. 1–26; with permission.)

In recipients with functional disorders such as pseudoobstruction, where the native intestine is typically preserved before transplantation, the mesenteric vascular pedicle can be suitable for use as inflow and outflow of the intestine graft. The undisturbed base of the small intestine mesentery allows for exposure of the proximal superior mesenteric artery and vein (**Fig. 6**). Extension grafts are used in a similar fashion and anastomosed to the native mesenteric vessels. Placement of the graft is performed with an end-to-end anastomosis to the graft mesenteric vessels and blood flush performed through the mesenteric vein anastomosis. Regardless of which anatomic venous drainage is used, however, no significant adverse outcomes have been reported with either technique.[23]

Graft Selection

Proper graft selection for the adult isolated intestinal recipient is paramount for a successful outcome. Many donor factors, all equally important, are evaluated on an individualized manner based on the recipient's condition at the time of the organ offer. In the current condition of adult intestine supply and demand, and in the absence of requiring a liver-inclusive graft, great latitude is afforded in selecting the most appropriate isolated intestinal graft for the stable adult recipient. General standard criteria such as donor normal gastrointestinal history and absence of any evidence of intestine trauma apply to all donors considered. Specific to the adult intestine donor, which need a high level of scrutiny before acceptance, are donor hemodynamic stability, graft size, and immunologic compatibility.

Hemodynamic stability must be established in the intestinal donor. The intestine is exquisitely sensitive to hemodynamic instability in the donor because splanchnic blood flow is reduced on a greater scale during periods of hypotension. In particular,

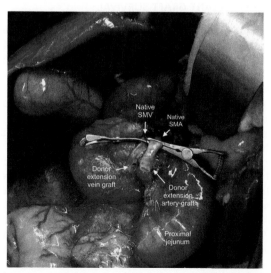

Fig. 6. Exposure of the native superior mesenteric artery (SMA) and superior mesenteric vein (SMV) with donor extension grafts for orthotopic placement of the isolated intestine graft. (*From* Hawksworth J, Matusumoto S. Intestinal transplant techniques: from isolated intestine to intestine in continuity with other organs. In: Dunn SP, Horslen S, editors. Solid organ transplantation in infants and children, organ and tissue transplantation. Springer; 2017. p. 1–26; with permission.)

donors who have suffered cardiopulmonary arrest and resuscitation pose a challenge to determine its suitability as a donor. Recent literature supports the successful use of intestinal grafts in carefully selected donors that who have undergone cardiopulmonary resuscitation.[24]

Size is a critical factor in the selection of the appropriate graft. In cases of short gut, significant loss of abdominal domain necessitates the placement of a smaller graft to achieve primary abdominal wall closure. In the adult recipient, this generally requires a donor size up to approximately one-half of the body weight of the recipient depending on the extent of the loss of domain. In a stable potential recipient, the benefits of primary closure with an appropriate-sized graft greatly outweigh the risks of a postoperative chronic open abdomen.

Intestinal transplants candidates, owing to a common history of multiple surgeries, infections, and blood transfusion often are sensitized to HLA antigens at the time of listing for transplantation. Evidence regarding the poor outcome with a positive cross-match in intestinal transplantation, as well as with other solid organ transplants, has been firmly established.[25] With a virtual cross-matching strategy, a negative cross-match can be accurately predicted, thus avoiding the adverse sequela of a preformed antibody at the time of transplantation. By using the virtual cross-match, an immunologically suitable intestine donor can be pursued with confidence over great distance without an actual cross-match. This serves to reduce or eliminate the logistical burden of traveling long distances with the uncertainty of obtaining a negative crossmatch in the highly sensitized recipient. Owing to the variable production of HLA antibody with each recipient, a successful negative virtual cross-match requires at least a monthly analysis of recipient serum for unacceptable antigens to accurately reflect the recipient's antibody profile at the time of transplantation.[26]

ADULT INTESTINAL TRANSPLANT GRAFT SURVIVAL

The evolution of immunosuppression, refinement of surgical techniques, earlier recognition of complications, and an increased overall experience in intestinal transplantation have improved patient and graft survival. Recent Organ Procurement and Transplantation Network/Scientific Registry of Transplant Recipients data have shown a decrease in graft failure rates for both adult and pediatric transplants that contain an intestinal transplant over the past 2 decades. Much of the decrease in graft failure rates, however, have occurred during the earlier period of the past 2 decades. Data from the past several years have observed a plateau in gains on graft survival for intestinal transplants with or without a liver component.[3] In the most recent Scientific Registry of Transplant Recipients report that covered the results from January 2014 through June 2016, in the 6 US centers that performed 10 or more adult intestinal transplants in 2016, the 1-year graft survival ranged from 60.5% to 83.0%. Including all centers that performed at least 1 adult intestinal transplant, the US 1-year graft survival average was 73.6%. The 3-year adult graft survival at these same centers ranged from 28.6% to 72.7% with a US average of 56.3%.[27] In an earlier reporting period from 2008 to 2010, the adult 1-year graft survival was 71.2%, illustrating the relatively modest gains achieved over this recent several year period[3] (**Fig. 7**).

SUMMARY

Adult intestinal transplantation is unique in many ways and differs significantly from pediatric intestinal transplantation. Indications for transplant have remained consistent since the introduction of the Centers for Medicare and Medicaid Services guidelines

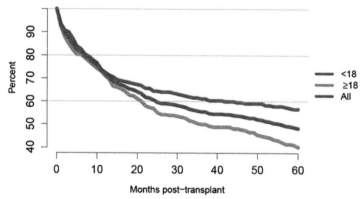

Fig. 7. Graft survival among intestine transplant recipients, 2008 to 2010, by transplant type. (*From* Smith J, Skeans M, Horslen S, et al. OPTN/SRTR 2015 annual data report: intestine. Am J Transplant 2017;17 Suppl 1:252–85; with permission.)

in 2000 particularly with regard to concomitant liver disease and intestinal failure; however, over the past 2 decades, with early improved results, indications for adults have expanded. Intestinal transplantation (multivisceral) for primary end-stage liver disease with portomesenteric thrombosis is a more frequent indication and intestinal transplantation for intraabdominal malignancies other than desmoids has been reported with good results. Graft type use in adult recipients depends on the distinct anatomic characteristics of the adult recipient, particularly in the cases liver-inclusive grafts and the recognition of the hazards of preformed and de novo antibody has led to the effective use of virtual cross-matching and improved pretransplant donor–recipient matching. Colon inclusion has increased over the past 2 decades with improved, sustainable results. Outcomes for adult recipients, as measured by graft survival, has seen a steady improvement since the 1990s; however, in the past several years, has slightly plateaued. Regardless, for adult intestinal transplant candidates, who have the highest pretransplant mortality, intestinal transplantation remains a mainstay therapy for those with complicated intestinal failure, as well as other life-threatening and debilitating conditions.

REFERENCES

1. Fishbein TM. Intestinal transplantation. N Engl J Med 2009;361(10):998.
2. Grant D, Abu-Elmagd K, Mazariegos G, et al. Intestinal transplant registry report: global activity and trends. Am J Transplant 2015;15:210.
3. Smith J, Skeans M, Horslen S, et al. OPTN/SRTR 2015 annual data report: intestine. Am J Transpl 2017;17(Suppl 1):252.
4. Vianna R, Mangus R, Kubal C, et al. Multivisceral transplantation for diffuse portomesenteric thrombosis. Ann Surg 2012;255(6):1144.
5. Organ Procurement and Transplantation Network(OPTN). OPTN national data: intestine. Website Available at: https://optn.transplant.org.gov. Accessed September 1, 2017.
6. Khan K, Desai C, Mete M, et al. Developing trends in the intestinal transplant waitlist. Am J Transpl 2014;14(12):2830.
7. Organ Procurement and Transplantation Network (OPTN). Policy 9.1.F liver and intestine candidates. Effective Date September 12, 2017. Available at: https://optn.transplant.hrsa.gov/media/1200/optn_policies.pdf. Accessed February 26, 2017.

8. Bala M, Kashuk J, Moore E, et al. Acute mesenteric ischemia: guidelines of the World Society of Emergency Surgery. World J Emerg Surg 2017;12:38.

9. Acosta S. Mesenteric ischemia. Curr Opin Crit Care 2015;21:171.

10. Singh S, Nguyen G. Management of Crohn's disease after surgical resection. Gastroenterol Clin North Am 2017;46:563.

11. Ogura Y, Bonen D, Inohara N, et al. A frameshift mutation in NOD2 associated with susceptibility to Crohn's disease. Nature 2001;411:603.

12. Fishbein T, Novitsky G, Mishra L, et al. NOD2 expressing bone marrow derived cells appear to regulate epithelial innate immunity of the transplanted human small intestine. Gut 2008;57:323.

13. Capella RF, Iannace VA, Capella JF. Bowel obstruction after open and laparo-scopic gastric bypass surgery for morbid obesity. J Am Coll Surg 2006;203:328.

14. Garza E Jr, Kuhn J, Arnold D, et al. Internal hernias after laparoscopic Roux-en-Y gastric bypass. Am J Surg 2004;188:796–800.

15. Masaki T, Sugihara K, Nakajima A, et al. Nationwide survey on adult type chronic intestinal pseudo-obstruction in surgical institutions in Japan. Surg Today 2012; 42(3):264.

16. Moon J, Selvaggi G, Nishida S, et al. Intestinal transplantation for the treatment of neoplastic disease. J Surg Oncol 2005;92(4):281.

17. Desai C, Khan K, Gruessner A, et al. Intestinal retransplantation: analysis of or-gan procurement and transplantation network database. Transplantation 2012; 93(1):120.

18. Department of Health and Human Services, Centers for Medicare and Medicaid Services. Program memorandum intermediaries/carriers. Intestinal and multi-visceral transplantation. AB-02–040. 2002. Available at: https://www.cms.gov/Regulations-and-Guidance/Guidance/Transmittals/Downloads/R58NCD.pdf. Accessed February 26, 2017.

19. Pironi L, Arends J, Bozzetti F, et al. ESPEN guidelines on chronic intestinal failure in adults. Clin Nutr 2016;35:247.

20. Sudan D, Iyer K, Deroover A, et al. A new technique for combined liver/small intestinal transplantation. Transplantation 2001;72(11):1846.

21. Fishbein T, Florman S, Gondolesi G, et al. Noncomposite simultaneous liver and intestinal transplantation. Transplantation 2003;75(4):564.

22. Matsumoto C, Kaufman S, Fishbein T. Inclusion of the colon in intestinal trans-plantation. Curr Opin Organ Transplant 2011;16(3):312.

23. Berney T, Kato T, Nishida S, et al. Portal versus systemic drainage of small bowel allografts: comparative assessment of survival, function, rejection, and bacterial translocation. J Am Coll Surg 2002;195(6):804.

24. Matsumoto C, Kaufman S, Girlanda R, et al. Utilization of donors who have suf-fered cardiopulmonary arrest and resuscitation in intestinal transplantation. Transplantation 2008;86(7):941.

25. Abu-Elmagd K, Wu G, Costa G, et al. Preformed and de novo donor specific an-tibodies in visceral transplantation: long-term outcome with special reference to the liver. Am J Transplant 2012;12(11):3047.

26. Hawksworth J, Rosen-Bronson S, Island E, et al. Successful isolated intestinal transplantation in sensitized recipients with the use of virtual crossmatching. Am J Transplant 2012;12(Supp4):S33.

27. Scientific Registry of Transplant Recipients (SRTR) Program Specific Reports. Available at: https://www.srtr.org/reports. Accessed September 1, 2017.

Pediatric Intestinal Transplantation

Neslihan Celik, MD[a], George V. Mazariegos, MD[a], Kyle Soltys, MD[a],
Jeffrey A. Rudolph, MD[b], Yanjun Shi, MD, MS[a], Geoffrey J. Bond, MD[a],
Rakesh Sindhi, MD[a], Armando Ganoza, MD[a],*

KEYWORDS

- Pediatric intestinal transplantation • Intestinal failure • Immunosuppression
- Short gut syndrome

KEY POINTS

- Intestinal transplantation is a successful procedure for children with life-threatening complications of irreversible intestinal failure.
- Intestinal transplantation has shown improvement in survival rates owing to advances of surgical techniques and immunosuppressive therapies.
- Infection and chronic rejection are the most common causes of graft loss after intestinal transplantation.
- Close monitoring, early recognition, and prompt treatment of viral infections have improved survival.
- Efforts are directed toward the prevention and management of immunosuppressant-related morbidities to achieve ideal outcomes in pediatric intestinal transplantation.

INTRODUCTION

Intestinal transplantation (ITx) has continued to be an important treatment modality for pediatric intestinal failure despite development of increasingly successful intestinal rehabilitation outcomes. Owing to challenges with long-term graft function due to chronic rejection, ITx has been generally reserved for children with irreversible intestinal failure suffering from complications of total parenteral nutrition.[1] Complications of total parenteral nutrition such as frequent sepsis, multiple central line infections, lack of intravenous access, and parenteral nutrition–associated liver disease are major factors for consideration of ITx in an patient with intestinal failure.

Disclosure Statement: The authors have nothing to disclose.
[a] Department of Surgery, Division of Pediatric Transplantation, Hillman Center for Pediatric Transplantation, Children's Hospital of Pittsburgh of UPMC, 4401 Penn Avenue, Pittsburgh, PA 15224, USA; [b] Department of Pediatrics, Division of Gastroenterology, Children's Hospital of Pittsburgh of UPMC, 4401 Penn Avenue, Pittsburgh, PA 15224, USA
* Corresponding author.
E-mail address: ganozaaj2@upmc.edu

Gastroenterol Clin N Am 47 (2018) 355–368
https://doi.org/10.1016/j.gtc.2018.01.007
0889-8553/18/© 2018 Elsevier Inc. All rights reserved.

gastro.theclinics.com

The initial trials for ITx developed by Lillehei in 1959 and Starzl in 1960 developed the experimental basis in dogs that established the technical cornerstones. In the cyclosporine era, experiences were mostly unsuccessful until the 1990s, when the long-term survival of patients with isolated small bowel transplantation occurred. The first human multivisceral transplant (MVT) was also performed by Starzl and colleagues[2–5] in 1983 and 1989 in 2 pediatric cases, but clinically reproducible results were not achieved until after the introduction of tacrolimus in 1989. The reasons for initial graft failure were mostly ascribed to unpredictable allograft rejection and recipient multiple organ disease severity as compared with isolated liver transplant recipients. The introduction of tacrolimus and then antibody conditioning with antithymocyte globulin or other antibodies significantly improved outcomes in pediatric ITx. However, chronic rejection and the prevention and management of immunosuppressant-related morbidities remain the most significant challenges to achieving ideal outcomes in this field.[6,7]

INDICATIONS

According to The Intestinal Transplant Registry (ITR) data, the main disease indications for ITx in the pediatric population are the presence of anatomic/surgical short gut and functional/motility disorders (**Box 1**). Between 1985 and February 2013, 1611 pediatric patients underwent ITx in 55 centers. Gastroschisis (22%), volvulus (16%), necrotizing enterocolitis (14%), and intestinal atresia (4%) were the main contributors of surgical short gut. Motility disorders (18%) were the major nonsurgical short gut indication with malabsorption (8%), with additional indications owing to tumors (1%) and re-ITx cases (8%).[8]

Box 1
Pediatric intestinal transplantation indications

Short gut syndrome

Volvulus

Gastroschisis

Necrotizing enterocolitis

Intestinal atresia

Ischemia

Trauma

Motility disorders

Primary pseudo-obstruction

Hollow visceral myopathy

Microvillus inclusion disease

Hirschsprung's disease

Other indications

Neuropathy with extensive involvement of gastrointestinal system with stomach

Gastrointestinal neoplastic disorders

Intestinal polyposis

Intestinal retransplantation

The traditional indications of loss of venous access, hepatic injury from total parenteral nutrition, and frequent sepsis remain the main indications for referral for transplantation, but revised indications may be necessary in the current era of hepatic-sparing parenteral nutrition and other advances in intestinal adaptation.[9]

ALLOGRAFT TYPES

Understanding the disease process and the extent of affected organs is crucial to decide on the appropriate transplantation technique with the proper graft. Radiologic, endoscopic, and histopathologic evaluation of the gastrointestinal system, motility studies, upper–lower extremity central venous system imaging, hematologic evaluation, liver function tests, and liver biopsy are the principal preoperative workup. It is also important to understand the terminology of intestine-containing transplantation allografts.[10] A summary of this allograft terminology is as follows and as shown in **Fig. 1**:

- Small intestine transplant: intestine graft without liver or stomach (**Fig. 1A**),
- Liver–small intestine transplant: intestine graft with liver but no stomach (**Fig. 1C**),
- Modified MVT: stomach and intestine graft without liver (**Fig. 1E**), and
- MVT: stomach, intestine and liver graft (**Fig. 1F**).

All of these graft types can include a segment of colon based on the disease indication. According to an ITR report, 36.2% of patients received isolated small bowel, 45.5% small bowel and liver, and 18.3% received modified multivisceral or multivisceral allografts.[8,11]

TECHNICAL ASPECTS
Donor Operation

The basic steps of donor operation with variations according to the organs that will be transplanted are as follows: (1) dissection of the liver, pancreas, spleen, stomach, duodenum, and intestine from diaphragm and retroperitoneum, (2) removal of the multivisceral graft proximally at the level of abdominal esophagus or proximal stomach and distally at the level of terminal ileum or descending colon, (3) transection of suprahepatic and infrahepatic vena cava, and (4) removal of the double central stem including celiac axis and superior mesenteric artery (SMA) with the extent of thoracic aorta (Carrel patch). The protection of kidneys for other recipients can be done in situ with careful dissection before the excision of the Carrel patch or by separation on the back table after total removal of multiviscera. The evaluation of the vascular anatomy is essential. The aorta is encircled proximally near the diaphragm and distally at or below the level of inferior mesenteric artery after careful dissection of the liver and its vascularity. The mobilization of colon, small bowel, and mesenteric root is followed by the cautious kocherization of the duodenum and mobilization of the spleen and stomach medially without compromising their vascular supply. The focus of the donor operation is appropriate in situ cooling of the subdiaphragmatic organs with preservation solution.[7] The cannulation is done through the abdominal aorta below the inferior mesenteric artery and the liver can be secondarily perfused by cannulation of the portal vein through the inferior mesenteric vein (see **Fig. 1**).

Isolated Intestinal Transplantation

Reserved for those patients with preserved liver function and isolated intestine failure, the isolated intestine graft is implanted either with systemic or portal drainage. Portal drainage is preferred when the SMV outflow and venous length is preserved, as is

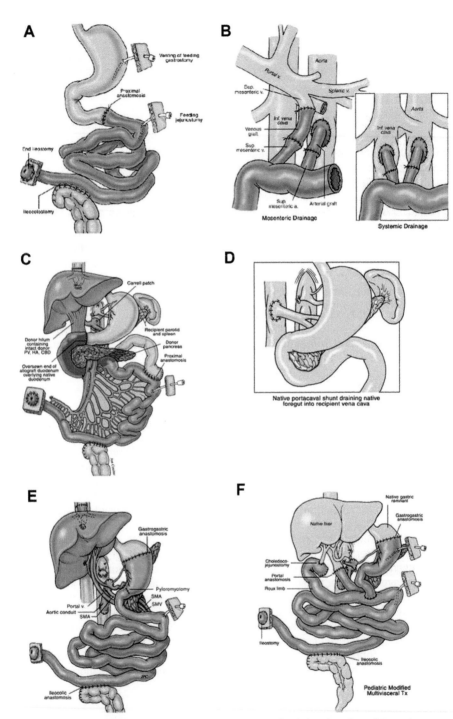

Fig. 1. Technical variations of intestinal containing grafts. (*A*) Isolated small intestine transplants. (*B*) Vascular reconstruction: the allograft superior mesenteric artery (SMA) and superior mesenteric vein (SMV) can be attached directly to the recipient SMA and SMV, but

often the case in pseudo-obstruction or motility disorders where native intestine length is often normal. Arterial inflow is either direct from the SMA or from an infrarenal aortic graft (see **Fig. 1**A, B), which is commonly placed to provide ease of arterial implantation in all the graft types.

Combined Liver–Intestine Transplantation

Liver and intestine allograft includes the C-loop of the duodenum and pancreas to preserve the biliopancreatic flow (see **Fig. 1**C). The arterial inflow is restored with an end-to-side anastomosis from the common aortic patch with the SMA and celiac trunk (Carrel patch) to the infrarenal aorta with the use of a segment of the donor thoracic aorta as an arterial conduit graft. Venous outflow of the complete graft is obtained by an anastomosis between the suprahepatic vena cava and the native hepatic veins confluence. During the anhepatic phase, the native foregut, including the stomach, pancreas, duodenum, and proximal jejunum, is preserved with its venous outflow directed systemically through an end-to-side portacaval shunt (see **Fig. 1**D). Intestinal reconstruction is accomplished proximally via a side-to-side anastomosis between the donor jejunum and recipient's upper gut and distally by an ileostomy or a colostomy accordingly. Depending on the needs of the patient, jejunostomy and gastrostomy tubes may be inserted. At the of this procedure, the recipient will have double duodenum and pancreas.

Complete Multivisceral Abdominal Transplantation

Irreversible intestinal failure or abdominal visceral neoplastic disorders including intestine with liver failure or portomesenteric thrombosis are the main causes for MVT. During donor organ procurement, en block removal of liver, stomach, duodenum, pancreas, and intestine is done with the vena cava and a Carrel patch or intact aorta. No portacaval shunt is necessary because the foregut is removed along with the other organs with the entire splanchnic circulation. On the recipient, the pancreas, spleen, the root of the intestinal mesentery, the stomach, and the liver are removed together, with preservation of the vena cava for piggyback allograft implantation (see **Fig. 1**E). The hepatic anastomosis with a piggyback technique is performed first and this enables venous outflow of the multiviscera. The arterial inflow is restored with an end-to-side anastomosis of the common aortic patch of the SMA and celiac trunk (Carrel patch) to infrarenal or supraceliac abdominal aorta with the use of the donor thoracic aorta as an arterial conduit graft (**Fig. 2**). The gastrointestinal tract continuity is established proximally by anastomosing the recipient 's distal esophagus or gastric stump to the graft stomach. The side-to-side or end-to-side anastomosis between terminal ileum or ascending/transverse/descending colon of the graft and remaining colon of the recipient allows distal connection or terminal ileostomy or colostomy can be

◄—————————————————————————————————————

mostly by interposition vascular conduits to the recipient vasculature, the arterial to the native aorta and the venous to the recipient SMV (portal drainage) or the inferior vena cava (systemic drainage). (*C*) Liver–small intestine and pancreas. The recipient stomach, native pancreas, and the remnant proximal gut (duodenum with or without a small amount of jejunum) is retained. (*D*) Native foregut venous outflow. Directed systemically via a permanent portacaval shunt. (*E*) Multivisceral transplantation. (*F*) Modified multivisceral transplantation. a., artery; CBD, common bile duct; HA, hepatic artery; inf., inferior; PV, pulmonary vein; Sup., superior; Tx, transplant; v., vein. (*From* Remaley L, Mc Ghee B, Reyes J, et al. Surgical procedures in pediatric abdominal transplantation. Appendix II. In: Remaley L, Mc Ghee B, Reyes J, editors. The pediatric transplant manual. 2nd edition. Hudson (OH): Lexi-Comp; 2009. p.255–59; with permission.)

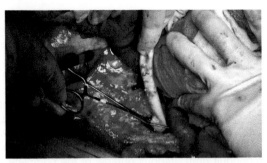

Fig. 2. Placement of infrarenal arterial graft by using donor thoracic aorta.

performed according to indication. A graft pyloroplasty is performed routinely to avoid gastric outlet obstruction owing to graft vagal denervation. Cholecystectomy, tube jejunostomy with or without gastrostomy, ileostomy, and colostomy complete the procedure.

Modified Multivisceral Abdominal Transplantation

Modified MVT was created for patients with diffuse gastrointestinal disorders but preserved hepatic function. Removal of native stomach, duodenum, pancreas, and spleen is performed. An infrarenal aortic graft is used for arterial inflow through a Carrel patch and venous outflow is maintained via an iliac vein graft between graft's SMV and native portal vein, SMV, or splenic vein. Early placement of arterial and venous grafts may allow for a shorter duration of warm ischemia. The near-total gastrectomy and removal of intestine are done with pancreaticoduodenal complex and splenic preservation technique.[12] The native pancreaticobiliary system remains patent in applicable cases because there are fewer biliary complication and less glucose intolerance, as well as immunologic benefits. The duodenum of the recipient and graft are anastomosed in a side-to-side fashion for native foregut continuity and the recipient remains with double duodenum and pancreas at the end of the procedure[13] (**Fig. 3**). The gastrointestinal tract continuity is maintained proximally by gastrogastric or esophagogastric anastomosis (see **Fig. 1**F). A pyloroplasty is performed to avoid gastric outlet obstruction, as described. The side-to-side or end-to-side anastomosis between terminal ileum or ascending/transverse/descending colon of the graft and remaining colon of the recipient restores the distal connection with a temporary ileostomy for the purpose of easy endoscopic follow-up. The gastrostomy and jejunostomy tube placement is done for postoperative decompression and early feeding concerns.

Living Donor Intestine Transplantation

The use of living donors in ITx remains controversial even though it is technically feasible and single-center experiences have shown acceptable outcomes.[14,15] Most of the intestinal transplants have been performed using grafts obtained from cadaver donors. Until 2013, only 63 small bowel transplants were performed from the 2887 intestinal transplants registered on the ITR.[11] Advantages related to intestinal transplants from living donors are the minimization of waiting time, the short cold ischemia time, and potentially better HLA matching. The technique describes the use of approximately 40% of the total bowel length in the donor. An important aspect is the preservation of the last 20 cm of the terminal ileum to avoid lipid or vitamin B_{12} malabsorption.[16,17] Combined live donor liver/intestine transplant seems to be a viable alternative, particularly for the small infant, in which appropriate size match is

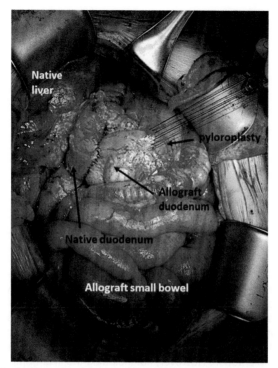

Fig. 3. Side-to-side duodenoduodenostomy in modified multivisceral transplantation.

challenging. Although living-related ITx represents an alternative for the treatment of intestinal failure in children,[18] further studies in a greater number of recipients is needed to validate single-center results.

Colon Inclusion

The colon plays an important role in the process of adaptation of the small intestine in the patient who has undergone extensive small intestinal resection. The most important functions of the colon include absorption of electrolytes and water, fermentation of complex carbohydrates, and residual proteins and storage of semisolid matter. Over the past 2 decades, the inclusion of the colon as part of an intestinal graft has changed significantly. In the early era of ITx, most centers avoided the use of a segment of colon after initial reports showed increased related medical and surgical complications.[8,19] Currently, there has been a significant increase in the colon inclusion rate to more than 40% (**Fig. 4**).

An ITR analysis showed that inclusion of the colon did not negatively affect survival; in fact, recipients with a colon segment showed a 5% higher rate of independence from supplemental parenteral nutrition.[8,11] Single-center experiences also demonstrated the benefit of including a segment of colon in a selective and cautious manner.[20–22]

RESULTS

According to ITR reports between 1985 and 2013, 2699 patients received 2887 visceral allografts in 82 centers worldwide. The overall patient survival rates in pediatric (n = 1611) and adult (n = 1088) population were 51% and 54.5%, respectively.

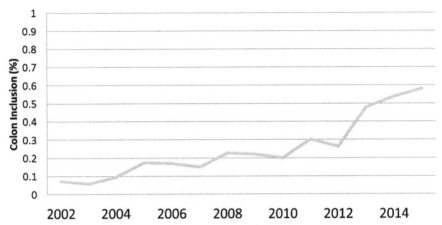

Fig. 4. Colon inclusion in pediatric intestinal transplant. (*From* Intestinal Rehabilitation and Transplant Association. Intestine transplant registry 2015 Bi-Annual Report; 2015; with permission.)

There was an improvement in the 1- and 5-year actuarial graft survivals according to the 2015 ITR report[11] (**Fig. 5**).

In recent years, there has been a significant trend toward intestinal transplant without a liver graft. This trend is most likely related to an improvement in early patient referrals for intestinal transplant evaluation, avoiding irreversible liver failure and the need for liver transplantation. However, not including the liver component may eventually affect negatively long-term graft survival, because the inclusion of the liver graft has shown significantly better graft survival.

Abu-Elmagd et al,[6] in a series of 500 intestinal transplants, reported a total of 47 retransplants (10%). In this series, rejection was the most common indication for retransplantation, with 37 patients (79%). The long-term cumulative survival was similar to the primary transplants with a 5-year survival rate of 47%. As in primary intestinal grafts, retransplantation with liver-containing intestinal allografts achieved better long-term survival with a 5-year survival of 61% compared with 16% of the liver-free intestinal grafts.[6] The 2015 ITR report showed a retransplantation rate of

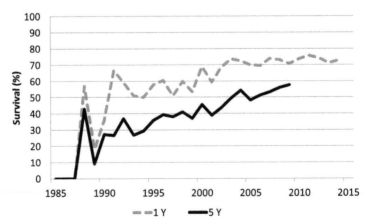

Fig. 5. Overall 1- and 5-year actuarial graft survivals. (*From* Intestinal Rehabilitation and Transplant Association. Intestine transplant registry 2015 Bi-Annual Report; 2015; with permission.)

8% with a second/third graft survival rate of 56% at 1 year and 35% at 5 years in pediatric and adult populations.[11]

POSTOPERATIVE MANAGEMENT AND COMPLICATIONS

Although improvements in graft outcomes have been achieved, long-term causes for mortality continue to be graft rejection, sepsis, and posttransplant lymphoproliferative disorder. Acute and chronic rejection, graft dysfunction, and primary nonfunction were the most frequent causes for graft loss. Arterial thrombosis (mostly at the Carrel patch; 2.4%), hepatic vein thrombosis (0.4%), aortic graft pseudoaneurysm (1.4%), and leakage from gastrointestinal–biliary anastomosis (2.2%) were early postoperative surgical complications in 500 visceral allografts reported at the University of Pittsburgh.[6]

The most common nonsurgical complications were stated as acute rejection, cytomegalovirus (CMV) infection, posttransplant lymphoproliferative disorder, and graft-versus-host disease. Hypertension, osteoporosis, diabetes, and chronic renal failure were the posttransplantation medication-related complications in 8.3-year median follow-up period. The original disease recurred in 6% of cases and 90% nutritional autonomy was achieved in surviving patients with a patent graft.[23]

Immunosuppression

Immunosuppressive therapy has evolved significantly over the past 20 years. Outcomes improved greatly after the introduction of tacrolimus in 1990.[24] Different protocols have been established among transplant centers, with the use of preconditioning with antithymocyte globulin or an interleukin-2 blocker in 72% of patients and tacrolimus monotherapy being used for maintenance in 92% of current survivors.[11] The use of a "secondary" agent like mycophenolate mofetil, steroids, azathioprine, or a mammalian target of rapamycin inhibitor is recommended after the presence of an episode of rejection.

Graft Monitoring and Rejection

Endoscopic mucosal biopsies remain the gold standard for the detection of immune-mediated rejection. A common protocol used is to take endoscopic ileal biopsies twice weekly for the first month, and then once a month or when symptoms of rejection develop for 3 to 6 months until stoma closure. The pathologic criteria of acute cellular rejection were formulated by consensus at the 8th International Small Bowel Transplantation Symposium in 2003[25] (**Table 1**). Over the past years, efforts have been made to develop a noninvasive test that can predict rejection. A cell-based assay using allospecific CD154$^+$ T-cytotoxic memory cells can predict acute cellular rejection after intestine transplantation with high sensitivity, specificity, and predictive values.[26,27] The clinical use of noninvasive assays to assist in the rapid diagnosis of acute rejection is still on early stages.

The etiology of graft loss and patient death has remained constant over time. Sepsis followed by rejection remain the leading causes of graft loss. Chronic rejection is a significant problem that jeopardizes long-term graft survival, particularly of the liver-free intestinal allografts and regardless of the currently used immunosuppressive protocols.[11,28] The diagnosis of chronic rejection is confirmed histopathologically by recognizing the obliterative arteriopathy changes in the submucosa, subserosa, and in the mesentery immediately adjacent to the bowel wall.[29] In recent years, there is more evidence that the formation of donor-specific antibodies (DSA) has an important role in the short- and long-term risks of rejection.[30,31] In 79 patients undergoing

Table 1
Pathologic criteria for acute cellular rejection

Grade	Criteria
Grade 0: no evidence of ACR	The tissue from the bowel allograft demonstrates unremarkable histological changes that are essentially similar to normal native bowel or pathologic changes are separate from ACR.
Indeterminate ACR	Minor amount of epithelial cell injury or destruction is present, principally manifested in the crypts. Increased crypt epithelial apoptosis but <6 apoptotic bodies/10 crypt cross-section.
Grade 1: mild ACR	Crypt injury. Increased mitotic activity, and/or crypt destruction with apoptosis (>6 apoptotic bodies/10 crypt cross-sections). Villus blunting and architectural distortion.
Grade 2: moderate ACR	Focal or diffuse crypt injury and destruction. >6 apoptotic bodies as described for 10 crypt cross-sections, with foci of confluent apoptosis. There can be focal superficial erosions of the surface mucosa.
Grade 3: severe ACR	A marked degree of crypt damage and destruction with crypt loss, there is diffuse mucosal erosion and/or ulceration with marked diffuse inflammatory infiltrate. If extended severe rejection exists, there is complete loss or the morphology of the bowel with granulation tissue and even fibropurulent exudate, with mucosal sloughing. The latter changes would be endoscopically defined as "exfoliative" rejection, which has a high risk for graft loss and increased mortality in children.[25]

Abbreviation: ACR, acute cellular rejection.
Data from Ruiz P, Bagni A, Brown R, et al. Histological criteria for the identification of acute cellular rejection in human small bowel allografts: results of the pathology workshop at the VIII International Small Bowel Transplant Symposium. Transplant Proc 2004;36(2)335–7.

intestinal/MVT, 28% of patients developed posttransplant DSA. These patients had increased risk of chronic rejection (14% vs 5%) and graft loss (18% vs 7%).[32] Cheng and colleagues[33] showed in a large series a direct association between DSA and accelerated intestinal allograft failure. Of their patients, 25% developed de novo DSA after ITx, and the probability of graft loss was close to 30% at 2 years after DSA detection.

Infections

Sepsis remains the most common cause of death after ITx. More than 90% of intestinal transplant recipients will develop a bacterial infection after transplantation.[34] Bacterial bloodstream infections remain the most common type of infection, with the central venous catheter and intraabdominal focus the most common sources of infection.[35]

Viral infections are very common and include CMV, Epstein-Barr virus (EBV), adenovirus, and rotavirus. CMV disease has been reported to be as high as 20%[36] with enteritis accounting for more than 80% of all episodes of symptomatic infections.[37] Treatment with ganciclovir and CMV-specific hyperimmunoglobulin remain the standard of care; however, in the event of resistance foscarnet is been used as a good alternative.[38]

EBV is a gamma herpesvirus that infects the B cells and causes infectious mononucleosis in immunocompetent people; it leads to EBV-driven systemic diseases in immunosuppressed individuals.[39] EBV viremia can progresses in immunosuppressed hosts to invasive EBV disease and can then transform to polyclonal and monoclonal lymphoproliferative diseases and lymphoma. EBV disease and posttransplant lymphoproliferative disorder was reported in up to 25% of recipients in the early era of ITx.[40] Patients with nonmalignant EBV disease and elevated EBV viral loads in the peripheral blood are amenable to preemptive treatment with intravenous ganciclovir, CMV intravenous immunoglobulin, and reduction in immunosuppression. The use of this combined approach along with evolution in immunosuppression algorithms for these patients has resulted in decreases in the incidence, morbidity, and mortality attributable to EBV disease and posttransplant lymphoproliferative disorder in this population.[41]

Graft-Versus-Host Disease

This complication is more frequent in ITx than other solid organs owing to the large lymphoid burden present in the allograft intestine. The overall incidence is 5% to 7%.[42] Risk factors include younger age, transplantation of multivisceral organs, immune deficiency disorders, and a history of splenectomy. The diagnosis is made by detecting in the peripheral blood donor cell chimerism or tissue-invading donor leukocytes in the recipient. The majority of cases of graft-versus-host disease can be treated with steroid administration and optimization of tacrolimus immunosuppression.

Quality of Life

Survival After ITX has improved significantly over the last decades with rates varying from 80% to 93% in recent studies.[6,23] In adults, intestinal transplant recipients have showed significant improvements in quality of life and functional status, as well as decreased anxiety and sleep difficulties compared with patients on parenteral nutrition.[43] In children, however, studies have demonstrated lower values in psychological health using the Pediatric Quality of Life Inventory despite being off parenteral nutrition and resuming normal daily activities.[44] ITx allows a more normal life for most patients, allowing them to join society and participate in age-appropriate activities.[45]

SUMMARY

Pediatric ITx has been improved over the past decades as a result of sophisticated multidisciplinary team work, and advances in immunosuppression and infectious disease monitoring. Improvement in immunomodulatory strategies have given the biggest change in outcomes and practice. The induction, preconditioning, and better maintenance therapies have enabled lesser graft loss and infection rates, and minimization of posttransplant immunosuppressive use for the benefit of posttransplant lymphoproliferative disorder. However, chronic rejection with allograft vasculopathy and the prevention and management of immunosuppressant-related morbidities remain the most significant challenges to achieve ideal outcomes in pediatric ITx. Newer regimens such as those proposed by Ceulemans and colleagues[46] or true tolerance-inducing regimens will be needed to lead to more dramatic improvements in ITx outcomes.

REFERENCES

1. Kaufman SS, Atkinson JB, Bianchi A, et al. Indications for pediatric intestinal transplantation: a position paper of the American Society of Transplantation. Pediatr Transplant 2001;5(2):80–7.

2. Mazariegos GV, Steffick DE, Horslen S, et al. Intestine transplantation in the United States, 1999-2008. Am J Transplant 2010;10(4 Pt 2):1020–34.
3. Starzl TE, Kaupp HA Jr. Mass homotransplantation of abdominal organs in dogs. Surg Forum 1960;11:28–30.
4. Starzl TE, Kaupp HA Jr, Brock DR, et al. Homotransplantation of multiple visceral organs. Am J Surg 1962;103:219–29.
5. Starzl TE, Todo S, Tzakis A, et al. Multivisceral and intestinal transplantation. Transplant Proc 1992;24(3):1217–23.
6. Abu-Elmagd KM, Costa G, Bond GJ, et al. Five hundred intestinal and multivisceral transplantations at a single center: major advances with new challenges. Ann Surg 2009;250(4):567–81.
7. Starzl TE, Todo S, Tzakis A, et al. The many faces of multivisceral transplantation. Surg Gynecol Obstet 1991;172(5):335–44.
8. Ganoza AJ, Farmer DG, Marquez MA, et al. Intestinal transplantation: international outcomes. Clin Transpl 2014;49–54.
9. Burghardt KM, Wales PW, de Silva N, et al. Pediatric intestinal transplant listing criteria - a call for a change in the new era of intestinal failure outcomes. Am J Transpl 2015;15(6):1674–81.
10. Todo S, Tzakis A, Abu-Elmagd K, et al. Abdominal multivisceral transplantation. Transplantation 1995;59(2):234–40.
11. Grant D, Abu-Elmagd K, Mazariegos G, et al. Intestinal Transplant Registry report: global activity and trends. Am J Transpl 2015;15(1):210–9.
12. Abu-Elmagd KM. Preservation of the native spleen, duodenum, and pancreas in patients with multivisceral transplantation: nomenclature, dispute of origin, and proof of premise. Transplantation 2007;84(9):1208–9 [author reply: 1209].
13. Cruz RJ Jr, Costa G, Bond G, et al. Modified "liver-sparing" multivisceral transplant with preserved native spleen, pancreas, and duodenum: technique and long-term outcome. J Gastrointest Surg 2010;14(11):1709–21.
14. Gruessner RW, Sharp HL. Living-related intestinal transplantation: first report of a standardized surgical technique. Transplantation 1997;64(11):1605–7.
15. Testa G, Panaro F, Schena S, et al. Living related small bowel transplantation: donor surgical technique. Ann Surg 2004;240(5):779–84.
16. Benedetti E, Holterman M, Asolati M, et al. Living related segmental bowel transplantation: from experimental to standardized procedure. Ann Surg 2006;244(5):694–9.
17. Garcia Aroz S, Tzvetanov I, Hetterman EA, et al. Long-term outcomes of living-related small intestinal transplantation in children: a single-center experience. Pediatr Transpl 2017;21(4):e12910.
18. Testa G, Holterman M, Abcarian H, et al. Simultaneous or sequential combined living donor-intestine transplantation in children. Transplantation 2008;85(5):713–7.
19. Todo S, Tzakis A, Reyes J, et al. Small intestinal transplantation in humans with or without the colon. Transplantation 1994;57(6):840–8.
20. Goulet O, Colomb-Jung V, Joly F. Role of the colon in short bowel syndrome and intestinal transplantation. J Pediatr Gastroenterol Nutr 2009;48(Suppl 2):S66–71.
21. Kato T, Selvaggi G, Gaynor JJ, et al. Inclusion of donor colon and ileocecal valve in intestinal transplantation. Transplantation 2008;86(2):293–7.
22. Matsumoto CS, Kaufman SS, Fishbein TM. Inclusion of the colon in intestinal transplantation. Curr Opin Organ Transplant 2011;16(3):312–5.

23. Abu-Elmagd KM, Kosmach-Park B, Costa G, et al. Long-term survival, nutritional autonomy, and quality of life after intestinal and multivisceral transplantation. Ann Surg 2012;256(3):494–508.
24. Starzl TE, Todo S, Fung J, et al. FK 506 for liver, kidney, and pancreas transplantation. Lancet 1989;2(8670):1000–4.
25. Ruiz P, Bagni A, Brown R, et al. Histological criteria for the identification of acute cellular rejection in human small bowel allografts: results of the pathology workshop at the VIII International Small Bowel Transplant Symposium. Transplant Proc 2004;36(2):335–7.
26. Ashokkumar C, Soltys K, Mazariegos G, et al. Predicting cellular rejection with a cell-based assay: preclinical evaluation in children. Transplantation 2017;101(1): 131–40.
27. Sindhi R, Ashokkumar C, Higgs BW, et al. Allospecific CD154 + T-cytotoxic memory cells as potential surrogate for rejection risk in pediatric intestine transplantation. Pediatr Transpl 2012;16(1):83–91.
28. Martinez Rivera A, Wales PW. Intestinal transplantation in children: current status. Pediatr Surg Int 2016;32(6):529–40.
29. Parizhskaya M, Redondo C, Demetris A, et al. Chronic rejection of small bowel grafts: pediatric and adult study of risk factors and morphologic progression. Pediatr Dev Pathol 2003;6(3):240–50.
30. Berger M, Zeevi A, Farmer DG, et al. Immunologic challenges in small bowel transplantation. Am J Transpl 2012;12(Suppl 4):S2–8.
31. Abu-Elmagd KM, Wu G, Costa G, et al. Preformed and de novo donor specific antibodies in visceral transplantation: long-term outcome with special reference to the liver. Am J Transpl 2012;12(11):3047–60.
32. Kubal C, Mangus R, Saxena R, et al. Prospective monitoring of donor-specific anti-HLA antibodies after intestine/multivisceral transplantation: significance of de novo antibodies. Transplantation 2015;99(8):e49–56.
33. Cheng EY, Everly MJ, Kaneku H, et al. Prevalence and clinical impact of donor-specific alloantibody among intestinal transplant recipients. Transplantation 2017;101(4):873–82.
34. Guaraldi G, Cocchi S, Codeluppi M, et al. Outcome, incidence, and timing of infectious complications in small bowel and multivisceral organ transplantation patients. Transplantation 2005;80(12):1742–8.
35. Kusne S, Furukawa H, Abu-Elmagd K, et al. Infectious complications after small bowel transplantation in adults: an update. Transpl Proc 1996;28(5):2761–2.
36. Manez R, Kusne S, Green M, et al. Incidence and risk factors associated with the development of cytomegalovirus disease after intestinal transplantation. Transplantation 1995;59(7):1010–4.
37. Florescu DF, Langnas AN, Grant W, et al. Incidence, risk factors, and outcomes associated with cytomegalovirus disease in small bowel transplant recipients. Pediatr Transpl 2012;16(3):294–301.
38. Kalil AC, Freifeld AG, Lyden ER, et al. Valganciclovir for cytomegalovirus prevention in solid organ transplant patients: an evidence-based reassessment of safety and efficacy. PLoS One 2009;4(5):e5512.
39. Green M, Michaels MG. Epstein-Barr virus infection and posttransplant lymphoproliferative disorder. Am J Transpl 2013;13(Suppl 3):41–54 [quiz: 54].
40. Abu-Elmagd KM, Mazariegos G, Costa G, et al. Lymphoproliferative disorders and de novo malignancies in intestinal and multivisceral recipients: improved outcomes with new outlooks. Transplantation 2009;88(7):926–34.

41. Green M, Reyes J, Webber S, et al. The role of antiviral and immunoglobulin therapy in the prevention of Epstein-Barr virus infection and post-transplant lymphoproliferative disease following solid organ transplantation. Transpl Infect Dis 2001;3(2):97–103.
42. Mazariegos GV, Abu-Elmagd K, Jaffe R, et al. Graft versus host disease in intestinal transplantation. Am J Transpl 2004;4(9):1459–65.
43. DiMartini A, Rovera GM, Graham TO, et al. Quality of life after small intestinal transplantation and among home parenteral nutrition patients. JPEN J Parenter Enteral Nutr 1998;22(6):357–62.
44. Ngo KD, Farmer DG, McDiarmid SV, et al. Pediatric health-related quality of life after intestinal transplantation. Pediatr Transpl 2011;15(8):849–54.
45. Andres AM, Alameda A, Mayoral O, et al. Health-related quality of life in pediatric intestinal transplantation. Pediatr Transpl 2014;18(7):746–56.
46. Ceulemans LJ, Braza F, Monbaliu D, et al. The Leuven immunomodulatory protocol promotes T-regulatory cells and substantially prolongs survival after first intestinal transplantation. Am J Transpl 2016;16(10):2973–85.

Living Donor Intestinal Transplantation

Ivo G. Tzvetanov, MD*, Kiara A. Tulla, MD, Giuseppe D'Amico, MD,
Enrico Benedetti, MD

KEYWORDS

- Intestinal failure • Pediatric recipients • Living donor small bowel transplantation
- Combined living donor intestinal/liver transplantation

KEY POINTS

- Living donor intestinal transplantation is compatible for appropriate candidates with deceased donor transplant graft and patient survival.
- Wait-time mortality has increased the viability of this procedure.
- Combining living donor intestinal/liver transplantation in pediatric recipients with organ failure allows for the reduction in waiting time, which is a large factor in the mortality rate of candidates on the deceased waiting list.
- Identical twins or human leukocyte antigen (HLA)-identical siblings have a significant immunologic advantage.
- ABO incompatibility and cross-match–positive transplants have been completed with success.

INTRODUCTION

Intestinal failure is defined as insufficient functional gut mass needed for adequate digestion and absorption of nutrient and fluid requirements for maintenance of adult nutrition in adults and growth in children.[1] Most cases of intestinal failure are due to loss of the small bowel as a result of surgical resection and approximately 10% are due to functional defects of absorption or motility.[2] In the United States, it has been estimated that approximately 225,000 patients require enteral or parenteral nutrition[3] as a result of short-term and long-term impaired intestinal absorption, the cost of which has been estimated to vary from $75,000 to $250,000 a year.[4] Thankfully advances in total parenteral nutrition (TPN) pharmacology and central line technology have allowed a decreased risk with use, but chronic use continues to pose a risk to end-organ damage, intestinal epithelial atrophy, and infectious risk.[5,6] Failure of

Disclosure: The authors have nothing to disclose.
Department of Surgery, University of Illinois at Chicago, 840 South Wood Street, Suite 402, Chicago, IL 60612, USA
* Corresponding author.
E-mail address: Itzveta@uic.edu

Gastroenterol Clin N Am 47 (2018) 369–380
https://doi.org/10.1016/j.gtc.2018.01.008
0889-8553/18/© 2018 Elsevier Inc. All rights reserved.

gastro.theclinics.com

medical intestinal rehabilitation with associated liver disease or concurrent failure is the primary indication for intestinal transplantation.[7]

The existing large gap between the number of potential recipients and available deceased donors (DDs) for liver and kidney transplantation has justified the significant expansion of living donor (LD) programs for those organs. This situation does not exist for adult recipients of intestinal transplantation, as the donor supply largely exceeds the current needs. However, there is a role for LD intestinal transplantation (LDIT) for pediatric patients with concomitant intestinal and liver failure.

According to United Network for Organ Sharing (UNOS) data, children (<10 kg) represent most (almost 70%) of the candidates on the intestinal transplantation waiting list in the United States. Most of them are listed for combined liver and bowel transplantation and 25% of pediatric patients worldwide die on the waiting list for an intestinal transplant.[8] The UNOS data and European Data sets show that this subset of patients still has the highest mortality rate on the waiting list compared with all the other categories of solid organ transplantation.[9,10] Small bowel transplantation (SBT) provides effective therapy for these patients and others with chronic, irreversible intestinal failure affected by subsequent life-threatening complications of TPN.

LDIT potentially can provide advantages, compared with DDs, including better tissue compatibility, shorter cold ischemia time, ability to implement desensitization protocols, and better donor bowel preparation. Probably the biggest advantage is that intestinal transplantation from a LD donor is a planned procedure, which is done at the optimal time for the recipient. The outcomes from LDIT in published literature are similar to those from DDs, which confirm the viability of the procedure.[11,12]

EARLY ATTEMPTS AT LIVING DONOR INTESTINAL TRANSPLANTATION

The first clinical intestinal transplant from an LD was reported in 1971. Alican and colleagues[13] described the case of an 8-year-old boy with the resection of the small bowel from the ligament of Treitz to the ileocecal valve secondary to strangulation. The transplant was performed with approximately 3 feet of ileum from his mother. However, the recipient's procedure was complicated by thrombosis of the vena cava, and the allograft had to be subsequently removed on the ninth posttransplant day. It was a new case and surgical attempt to save a child's life, whose case was incompatible with life without a transplant.

With the introduction of cyclosporine, the landscape of solid organ transplantation was revolutionized. However, the use of cyclosporine did not have as much of a benefit in intestinal transplantation as it did for other transplanted solid organs. Intestinal grafts are very susceptible to rejection because of high concentration of lymphoid tissue; therefore, a high level of immune suppression is required to prevent rejection, which can lead to serious and life-threatening sepsis. In the cyclosporine era, only 2 intestinal transplants from LDs were reported by Deltz and colleagues,[14,15] with both recipients receiving a 60-cm segment of jejunum. The first recipient was a boy, 4 years of age, with volvulus, who received the graft from his mother; unfortunately, the graft was removed due to an intractable rejection. The second recipient was a 42-year-old woman with a subtotal small bowel resection secondary to the thrombotic occlusion of mesenteric veins. She was on full enteral intake 2 weeks postoperatively and was weaned off parenteral nutrition until 1990, when chronic rejection caused the loss of the graft function. At that point in time, it was the first successful living intestinal transplant with a long-term function of more than 2 years.

The 1990s provided the introduction of tacrolimus as an immunosuppressive agent that allowed intestinal transplantation to become a clinically viable procedure with standardization of the methods.[15] Benedetti and colleagues[16] from the University of Minnesota studied the technical aspects of LDIT in a pig model. Subsequently, they performed the first LDIT, from which they concluded the following: (1) the ileum was the best option because of its greater absorptive capacity of bile acids, vitamins, fat, and water; (2) the terminal ileum (20–30 cm), the ileocecal valve, and the cecum should remain in the donor to minimize morbidity; (3) a vascular pedicle should be used consisting of only 1 artery and vein (either the ileo-colic artery and vein, or the terminal branches of the superior mesentery artery and superior mesentery vein); and (4) the bowel continuity should be restored with a proximal bowel anastomosis and a distal ileostomy (to allow access to graft for monitoring via biopsy). Before published guidelines, in 1995 Morris and colleagues[17] described an LDIT in an adult patient with a desmoid tumor, whose donor was his monozygotic twin. They transplanted the distal ileum, ileocecal valve, and portion of the cecum, unfortunately making the donor vitamin B12 deficient. Around the same time, the first two successful LDITs were completed at the University of Minnesota, excluding the terminal ileum and ileocecal valve, and the group published their respective guidelines in 1997,[18] as a standardized technique for intestinal transplants.

Following the US innovation in the procedure, Asia followed suit in living-related intestinal transplantation because of the difficulty with access to DDs. In 1998, Uemoto and colleagues[19] reported LDIT in Japan in a 2.5-year-old boy who had short bowel syndrome and recurrent line sepsis underwent LDIT using a segmental graft from his mother. They resected her distal ilium (100 cm) from her 460 cm of small intestine. The vessels were anastomosed to the recipient's infrarenal aorta and vena cava, respectively. The donor was discharged on postoperative day 15 without any surgical or medical complication. Ishii and colleagues,[20] reported in 2006 their experience with 2 cases of LDIT. The first patient was a 14-year-old boy with TPN-dependent short bowel syndrome associated with hypoganglionosis. The second patient was a 27-year-old woman who had undergone massive bowel resection due to volvulus. Up to one-third (150 cm in case 1, 210 cm in case 2) of the total small intestine was harvested from the ileum, preserving 30 cm of terminal ileum proximal to the ileocecal valve in the donors. The vessels were connected to the recipient infrarenal aorta and inferior vena cava. Both donors experienced no postoperative complications and were discharged at 10 days after the operation.

In 2004, Lee and colleagues[21] described the first experience at Catholic University of Korea, Seoul. The patient was a 57-year-old woman with short bowel syndrome. A 150-cm distal ileum graft from a 27-year-old living-related donor was successfully transplanted; the graft vessels were anastomosed to the recipient's inferior mesenteric vessels. The donor and recipient recovered without complications. Complications were described, after the first LDIT in India, by Kumaran and colleagues[22] in 2012. The patient required massive bowel resection for gangrene due to thrombosis of the superior mesenteric artery. LDIT was performed using 200 cm of small intestine from the patient's son. The graft was based on the continuation of the superior mesenteric vessels beyond the ileocolic branch. The artery was anastomosed directly to the aorta and the vein to the vena cava. The graft functioned well, and he was weaned off parenteral nutrition; however, he later developed complications (wound dehiscence and enterocutaneous fistula) and sepsis. He succumbed to sepsis with a functioning graft 6 weeks after the transplant. The donor recovered uneventfully and was discharged on the fourth postoperative day.

By the early 2000s, the successful completion of LDIT both on the national and international stage shifted the focus to optimize post-operative care for recipients and further develop donor selection. HLA and ABO compatibility were nearly a prerequisite in all these cases where success was claimed. In parallel, advances in immunosuppression would later prove indispensable for improvements in graft survival and prevent the early threats of acute cellular rejections faced by many of these candidates.

DONOR SELECTION

The field of solid organ transplantation has realized many technical milestones and functional advances with regards to the complex medical management of DDs and the techniques needed to safely perform living donation. During the mid-1980s, transplantation of whole or segmental grafts procured from live donors became a reality. Concurrent with the development and application of sophisticated open and minimally invasive techniques. Furthermore, few areas in medicine have seen surgical innovation and minimally invasive surgery directly influence long-term patient outcomes in the setting of end-stage organ functions as transplantation has with the steady expansion of DD intestinal transplantation (ITx) in the 1990s, occurred as LD liver and kidney transplantation were becoming more common across North America. Interestingly, ITx from living-related donors had only rarely been attempted[17,23–25] before the first report of a standardized surgical approach that was reported by Gruessner and Sharp[18] from the University of Minnesota in 1997. To minimize the incidence of complications and increase the rate of success, it is necessary to choose the donor carefully:

- Comprehensive analysis of medical and surgical history, review of systems, physical examination, current medications, history of malignancy, and previous intestinal surgery
- ABO compatibility, HLA type, lymphocytotoxic cross-match
- Comprehensive metabolic panel, levels of vitamins A, D, E, K, and B12
- Prothrombin time, partial thromboplastin time, alpha-fetoprotein, ammonia
- Chest radiograph, electrocardiogram
- Serology (cytomegalovirus [CMV], Epstein-Barr virus [EBV], varicella zoster virus [VZV], human immunodeficiency virus [HIV], hepatitis C virus [HCV], hepatitis B e antigen [HBeAg], hepatitis B surface antigen [HBsAg], antibody to HBsAg [HBsAb]), complete blood count, urine and stool cultures
- Anesthesia history, surgical procedures, and drug allergies
- Psychiatry evaluation, social work consultation
- An interview with a member of the institutional ethics committee to discuss with the potential donor about motivations and understanding of the risk involved
- Computed tomography (CT) scan of the abdomen or 3-dimensional [3D]-angio-CT-scan

The technical aspects of LDIT were standardized and the authors note the importance of obtaining angiographic images of the superior mesenteric artery to evaluate the caliber and distribution of the ileocolic artery that will be transected to become the vascular pedicle for the future graft.[18] Further technical validations with donor outcomes were verified and reviewed in later years in a larger sample size with efficacy; citing nor patient morbidity, changes in quality of life, or mortality.[26]

Mechanical preparation of the intestinal graft is completed 1 day before surgery with a bowel preparation and antibiotics. Two doses of 45 mL phosphosoda are given 4 hours apart on the afternoon before the surgery. Antibiotics are used in most protocols with 3 doses of neomycin 1 g, and metronidazole 500 mg given 18, 17, and 10 hours before the operation with perioperative antibiotics administered before the incision.[26]

DONOR: SURGICAL TECHNIQUE AND POSTOPERATIVE CARE

The surgical approach begins with entering the abdominal cavity through a relatively short (15 cm) midline incision and explored. The entire length of the small bowel from the ligament of Treitz to the ileocecal valve is measured. Subsequently, the cecum and the terminal ileum are identified and marked approximately 30 cm proximal from the ileocecal junction. The donor operation consists of harvesting 200 cm of distal ileum (160 cm for pediatric recipients), preserving at least 20 to 30 cm of terminal ileum and ileocecal valve to avoid macrocytic anemia and to shorten transit time. The vascular pedicle of the graft is formed by the ileocolic artery and vein. These vessels will be anastomosed to the infrarenal aorta and vena cava of the recipient, respectively.

If the procedure is a combined intestinal and liver transplantation, the donor operation becomes more complex. Combined LD intestinal and liver transplants have been successful for pediatric patients. The liver is transplanted first and if the patient is stable enough, the intestinal procurement (and consequently the transplant) can be performed; otherwise, a sequential approach can be followed in which the incision is closed, and the intestinal transplant is rescheduled, preferably within the first 2 weeks after the liver transplant.

Donor postoperative care includes close monitoring of patient recovery concurrent to graft viability and surveillance. After discharge, donors need to be evaluated on a monthly basis and then annually to review their nutritional and bowel habits, as well as signs of surgical complications. The donor also should undergo vitamin B12 assays at 1, 6, and 12 months after donation to ensure adequate vitamin B12 absorption.

Reviewing donor data at one institution, Ghafari and colleagues[27] reported a case of chronic diarrhea among their donors, controlled with medical therapy consisting of Imodium and cholestyramine. For 11 donors, of their total cohort of combined LD liver and LDIT, the investigators also reported a 36.4% reduction in low-density lipoprotein and a 22.3% decrease in total cholesterol levels when compared with their respective predonation lipid profiles, and they noted that the difference was statistically significant.[27] However, a further follow-up in a larger cohort should be completed to conclude the impact of this finding.

Although the number of LDITs is relatively small, there have been no reports of donor mortality or life-threatening complications, with many small case analyses completed.[28,29] Nevertheless, a more extensive follow-up is necessary to determine the presence of postsurgical complications, such as intestinal adhesions and obstructions.

PEDIATRIC INTESTINAL TRANSPLANTATION

Registry data suggest that the patient and graft survival rates are similar for both LD and DD intestinal transplants, making LDIT a viable option to reduce the mortality rate for those on the waiting list, which is especially high for candidates younger than 5 years of age.[9,30] This is due to the associated end-stage liver failure that approximately 15% of patients receiving TPN for more than 1 year acquire. In children, the incidence of liver disease is higher, especially in patients with less than 30 to 40 cm of remnant bowel.[31] Liver disease remains the leading indication for performing intestinal transplantation in children, but loss of central venous access to provide parenteral nutrition has also become an indication for intestinal transplantation.

The indications for intestinal transplantation in pediatric patients were updated in 2010 by Avitzur and Grant[32]:

- Loss of 50% of available central venous accesses due to thrombosis
- Recurrent septic episodes, resulting in multiorgan failure, shock, and metastatic infectious loci (more than 2 episodes per year)
- Imminent or overt end-stage liver disease
- Ultra-short bowel syndrome
- High risk of death attributable to the underlying disease
- Frequent hospitalization
- Severe dehydration episodes
- Lack of family support or unwillingness to accept long-term TPN

Due to the high mortality of children in need of combined intestinal/liver transplants, LD transplants present an opportunity to further serve this marginalized population. Benedetti and colleagues,[11] initially discussed in 2009 and later published follow up data in Garcia-Aroz,[33] in 2017, documented their experience with 6 combined intestinal/liver transplants at the University of Illinois Hospital. The transplants were performed between 2004 and 2007, with a total of 6 children (average age 13.5 months) having received the grafts from one of their parents (most from the mother). Three of these recipients had a simultaneous transplantation, whereas the other 3 recipients had a staged procedure, with an average interval of 6 days based on hemodynamic stability after the liver graft was implanted. None of the donors had any perioperative mortality or morbidity; all donors were discharged home on a regular diet. Five of the 6 children are still alive with adequate graft function, whereas 1 recipient died due to plasmoblastic lymphoma, albeit with functioning graft.

RECIPIENT EVALUATION

A multidisciplinary evaluation of the patient with intestinal failure is essential to assess adequate candidacy for transplantation and to ensure best outcomes. The evaluation process must elucidate the following: (1) the failure of TPN as compared with other surgical therapy strategies besides transplantation; (2) the need of intestine or combined liver/intestine transplantation; (3) the state of the remnant intestine and the patency of great vessels; and (4) the absence of absolute contraindications or associated disease that can put at risk the procedure and postoperative course. All the aspects of the recipient evaluation are summarized as follows:

- Comprehensive analysis of medical and surgical history, review of systems, physical examination, current medications, current nutrition requirements
- Blood group, HLAa type, panel of reactive antibody
- Upper and lower gastrointestinal barium study, esophagogastroduodenoscopy and colonoscopy, CT scan abdomen and pelvis, motility studies (if indicated)
- Height, weight, anthropometric measurements, nutritional support, comprehensive metabolic panel, zinc
- Prothrombin time, partial thromboplastin time, alpha-fetoprotein, ammonia
- Doppler ultrasound of liver and liver biopsy (if indicated)
- Electrocardiogram, chest radiograph, echocardiogram, stress test if more than 50 years of age or with cardiac history, and risk factors (hypertension, diabetes mellitus)
- Abdominal ultrasound with size of kidneys, triple renal scan, 24-hour creatinine clearance
- Doppler ultrasound of veins of upper and lower extremities

- History of infection episodes, immunization, serology (CMV, EBV, VZV, HIV, HCV, HBeAg, HBsAg, HBsAb, measles, rubella, and mumps titers), complete blood count
- Blood, urine, and stool culture
- Anesthesia history, surgical procedures, and drug allergies
- Child life and development
- Psychiatry evaluation, social work consultation
- Doppler ultrasound of great vessels and angiography or MRI or 3D-angio-CT-scan (if indicated)

Although the criteria used for listing DD and LD candidates are the same, we believe that certain patients may have a greater benefit from the LD option. Adults with an identical twin or HLA-identical sibling as a donor candidate should be transplanted without delay. In our experience, using donors with at least 1 haplotype match has been extremely favorable, with no acute rejection episodes during the first year post-transplant. In children affected by ultra-short bowel syndrome with slim possibilities of successful weaning of TPN, LDIT should be considered early to avoid progression to end-stage liver disease. For children who present TPN-related cirrhosis, the option of combined liver-bowel transplantation from an adult donor may minimize the probability of death on the waiting list, which is extremely high in this population.

RECIPIENT: SURGICAL TECHNIQUE AND POSTOPERATIVE CARE

Similar to the approach of the donor, the abdomen is entered through a midline incision with mobilization of the remaining small bowel to expose the infrarenal aorta and vena cava. They are identified and dissected from the renal vessels down to the iliac bifurcation. The arterial anastomosis is completed first, because it is more technically challenging due to the small diameter of donor's artery. The arteriotomy of the anterior wall of the aorta is made at the level between the origins of the inferior mesenteric artery and the renal arteries. Given the small size of the ileocolic artery of the graft, the end-to-side (ileocolic artery-to-infrarenal aorta) anastomosis is constructed in an interrupted fashion. Continuing with the venous anastomosis, an appropriate site on the vena cava is chosen for the venotomy, usually 2 to 3 cm proximal to the arterial anastomosis. The venous anastomosis is done with the quadrangulation technique, and the end-to-side (ileocolic vein to infrarenal cava) anastomosis is completed with a continuous technique. The proximal end of the intestinal graft is anastomosed to the remaining recipient duodenum/jejunum. All 3 forms of anastomosis are completed with no preference or advantage known (end-to-end, end-to-side, or side-to-side fashion). At the University of Illinois, the preference has been to complete a hand-sewn, two-layer side-to-side anastomosis to the remaining recipient duodenum/jejunum. The hand-sewn technique decreases the risk of intraluminal anastomotic bleeding, as compared with a stapled anastomosis. Except with identical twins, a loop ileostomy (or end ileostomy when applicable) is fashioned proximal to the distal anastamosis between the graft and recipient colon (if present). This allows for easy access for surveillance endoscopy and biopsy during the postoperative period.

The first 24 to 48 hours are critical for examination of the transplant, due to the interplay of inflammation caused by surgical trauma, the degree of ischemia affecting end-organ function, reperfusion injury, and the initiation of immunosuppression. Vital signs, color of the ostomy, and laboratory parameters are monitored every 4 hours. An important element to immediately monitor posttransplantation is systemic anticoagulation: due to the small diameter of the ileocolic vessels of the LD graft, they are more prone to vascular thrombosis. On posttransplant day 7, a small bowel follow-through contrast study is performed to confirm an anastomotic seal; and, on the next day, the first graft biopsy is performed. After an anastomotic leak is ruled out, recipients begin a clear liquid diet. For recipients of a combined LD liver and intestinal transplant, postoperative care is initially dictated by the liver graft function. Once liver function has stabilized, attention can be directed to the intestinal graft function. The immunosuppression and follow-up of the LDIT recipient does not differ significantly from DD recipients.

RECIPIENT OUTCOMES FOR ALL INTESTINAL TRANSPLANTS (LIVING DONOR AND DECEASED DONOR)

Graft survival has improved since the early 1990s, but has plateaued over the past decade. For intestine transplants with or without a liver in 2008 to 2010, 1-year and 5-year graft survival was 72.6% and 56.8%, respectively, for recipients aged younger than 18 years, and 71.2% and 40.3%, respectively, for recipients aged 18 years of age or older. One-year and 5-year graft survival was 71.5% and 45.2%, respectively, for recipients of intestines without a liver, and 70.2% and 50.0%, respectively, for intestine-liver recipients. The number of recipients alive with a functioning intestine graft has steadily increased since 2004, to 1099 in 2015; 43.3% were pediatric intestine-liver transplants. The incidence of first acute rejection in the first posttransplant year varied by era, age group, and transplant procedure. It is highest in the pediatric intestine recipients (55.2%) and lowest in the adult intestine-liver recipients (23.9%). Pediatric and adult patient survival was superior for intestine recipients compared with intestine-liver recipients. Patient survival continues to be the lowest for adult intestine-liver recipients (1-year and 5-year survival 68.6% and 35.7%, respectively) and highest for pediatric intestine recipients (1-year and 5-year survival 88.1% and 74.6%, respectively).[34]

As with many other transplanted organs, graft failure increases as the organ ages. The graft failure rate among intestine transplant recipients was 19.3% at 6 months, 24.5% at 1 year (2013–2014 transplants), 42.4% at 3 years (2011–2012 transplants), 54.8% at 5 years (2009–2010 transplants), and 66.2% at 10 years (2003–2004 transplants). Among intestine-liver transplant recipients, the graft failure rate was 17.6% at 6 months, 27.0% at 1 year, 33.8% at 3 years, 48.7% at 5 years, and 50.9% at 10 years. Between the first and third year after transplantation, graft failure doubles for patients with intestinal transplant alone. Reviewing the intestinal graft failure statistics during the 2000s, approximately 50% of all grafts fail between 3 to 5 years after transplantation. However, graft and patient survival data continues to improve over the past decade (**Table 1**).[34]

The application of immune induction agents in intestinal transplant/multivisceral organ recipients, like antithymocyte globulin,[35] anti-interleukin receptor globulin such as daclizumab (currently basiliximab is more commonly used),[36] and the latest therapy, anti-CD54 monoclonal antibody alemtuzumab (Campath),[37] has significantly reduced the incidence of early rejection and almost eliminated early graft loss.

Table 1 Graft failure data					
Graft Failure (SRTR 2015)	**6 mo**	**1 y**	**3 y**	**5 y**	**10 y**
Intestinal transplant, %	19.3	24.5	42.4	54.8	66.2
Combined intestine-liver, %	17.6	27.0	33.8	48.7	50.9

Data from Scientific Registry of Transplant Recipients (SRTR). 2015 Annual data report. Available at: http://srtr.transplant.hrsa.gov/annual_reports/Default.aspx. Accessed September 30, 2017.

In the pediatric population in 2013, Ueno and colleagues[30] reported a comparison in follow-up of intestinal transplants between 1996 and 2012 of DD (n=4) and LD (n=10) graft patients. The overall 1-year and 5-year patient survival rates were 77% and 57%, respectively. In transplants performed after 2006 (n = 6), the patient 1-year and 5-year survival and the graft 1-year and 5-year survival rates were all 83%. The living-related transplant survival rate was 80% at 1 year and 68% at 2 years, compared with 67% and 67% for cadaveric transplant recipients. There was no statistically significant difference in patient and graft survival rates.

CURRENT STATUS OF INTESTINE TRANSPLANTATION

According to UNOS data, the total number of registrations on the intestine waiting list in 2015 were 259, with 196 new patients added in 2015. More patients are waiting for an intestinal transplant than combined intestinal-liver transplant (63.3% vs 36.7%, respectively). The highest volume of patients listed for transplant persist to be children younger than 6 for both intestine alone and combined (66.5% vs 62.1%, respectively), although the past decade has seen an increase in the age distribution of candidates from primarily pediatric patients to increasing proportions of adults.

In 2015, 52.5% of candidates were on the waiting list for less than 1 year, and of candidates removed from the intestine-without-liver waiting list in 2015, most (78.6%) underwent DD transplant, and 2.4% underwent LD transplant (2 patients total) with 6.0% deaths. Similarly, in patients removed from the intestine-liver waiting list, most underwent DD transplant (64.4%), whereas 14.4% died and 3.8% were considered too sick to undergo transplantation, and 1.9% refused transplantation or 6.7% were delisted for clinical improvement. Among candidates listed in 2014 to 2015, median time to transplantation ranged from 3.8 to 6.7 months depending on age and transplant organ colisting. Pretransplant mortality was highest for adult candidates (19.6 per 100 waitlist years) and lowest for children younger than 6 years (3.5 per 100 waitlist years). However, the number of patients on the waiting list younger than 18 years remained higher as compared with those who were 18 years or older (194 vs 65, respectively, for candidates on the waiting list in 2015).[34] These data further indicate that pediatric patients have a higher risk of life-threating complications secondary to TPN, when compared with adults.

The implementation of surgical and medical protocols for transplantation have seen a greater than 2-fold increase in intestinal transplants. In 2009, there were a total of 180 intestinal transplants at its peak, with 141 performed in 2015. More than 70% of children listed for intestine transplant have concomitant liver failure. Recipients of a combined graft experience better graft survival outcomes compared with those who received an isolated intestinal transplant.[11,12]

According to UNOS, between 1990 and 2013, the rate of DD intestinal transplants had increased from 0.2% to 4.3%. However, the rate of LD intestinal transplants remains very low, with only 2 transplants performed in 2015 in comparison with the 133 DD intestinal transplants. Since 1995, the total number of LD intestinal transplants in the United States is 44, 26 of which were performed by the team at the University of Illinois at Chicago. Our longest LD intestinal graft survival is 15 years (Benedetti, unpublished data, 2017). However, the experience with LD intestinal transplants remains limited, with a very small number of procedures having been performed worldwide.

We recently analyzed most recent data by conducting a retrospective review. Between 1998 and March 2016, a total of 33 living-related donor bowel transplants were performed at the University of Illinois at Chicago (Benedetti, unpublished data, 2017 in concordance with[33]). The 1-year, 3-year, and 5-year patient and graft survival rates were 83%, 70%, and 50%, respectively. Among 10 pediatric recipients, 4 with isolated LD intestinal transplant and 6 with combined LD liver/intestine transplant, the 1-year, 5-year, and 10-year patient survival rates were 90%, 80%, and 70%, and graft survival rates were 80%, 60%, and 60%, respectively. Seven children are currently alive with perfectly functioning graft, oral diet without any requirement for TPN (6 with more than 10 years of follow-up and the other with 3 years of follow-up). Six children are currently enrolled in school and 1 child is homeschooled. All children report good quality of life. Their related donor and all their families report great satisfaction with their accomplishments.

NEW INNOVATIONS

LDIT is performed most commonly with well-matched HLA grafts. The significance of HLA matching in intestinal transplantation is still to be determined. In fact, experienced programs have obtained good outcomes and low rate of rejection with poorly matched deceased intestine transplants.[35,38] In 2015, an ABO-incompatible LDIT was completed by Fan and colleagues,[39] who were able to perform the transplant with aggressive immunotherapy and follow-up with 2 episodes of rejection that were treated well and at 2 years posttransplant, the patient is thriving. Similarly, the first reported cases of LDIT with cross-match–positive recipients was completed and published in 2016.[40] Garcia-Roca and colleagues[40] implemented desensitization protocols that were used to decrease the levels of alloantibodies and to convert an initial positive cross-match to prospective donors into a negative cross-match. No evidence of humoral rejection has occurred in either recipient. Both patients had successful ileostomy reversal at 6 and 9 months, respectively, and are tolerating oral intake. These successes provide a new avenue to further treat the many transplant candidates who are in need of an intestine transplant and who are deteriorating before a suitable organ is available for them.

SUMMARY

Intestinal transplantation continues to be in a state of flux, and with the improvement in medical management of short gut syndrome, many patients are able to survive without transplantation and wait for an allocated deceased organ. Unfortunately, waiting creates the unwanted complication of potential liver failure due to TPN administration and access issues, which brings to the forefront the application and need for continued use of LDIT as a treatment option for these patients. The marginal population can be allowed time to be medically optimized without the danger of decline during the unknown waiting period because it is a planned surgical procedure. It also serves as a way to transplant a patient with high levels of antibodies by applying desensitization protocols to allow for successful transplantation. The use of LDIT in the setting of pediatric transplantation has been legitimized with the combination of LD intestine-liver transplantation for combine end organ failure. For these potential recipients, the virtual elimination of waiting time can reduce the frequency of mortalities. Finally, in the specific case of available identical twins or HLA-identical siblings, LD intestinal transplantation has a significant immunologic advantage and should be offered.

REFERENCES

1. Goulet O, Ruemmele F. Causes and management of intestinal failure in children. Gastroenterology 2006;130(2 Suppl 1):S16–28.

2. Ueno T, Fukuzawa M. Current status of intestinal transplantation. Surg Today 2010;40(12):1112–22.
3. Howard L, Ament M, Fleming CR, et al. Current use and clinical outcome of home parenteral and enteral nutrition therapies in the United States. Gastroenterology 1995;109(2):355–65.
4. Sudan D. Cost and quality of life after intestinal transplantation. Gastroenterology 2006;130(2 Suppl 1):S158–62.
5. Vassallo M, Dunais B, Roger PM. Antimicrobial lock therapy in central-line associated bloodstream infections: a systematic review. Infection 2015;43(4):389–98.
6. Jeppesen PB. Pharmacologic options for intestinal rehabilitation in patients with short bowel syndrome. JPEN J Parenter Enteral Nutr 2014;38(1 Suppl):45S–52S.
7. Pironi L, Joly F, Forbes A, et al. Long-term follow-up of patients on home parenteral nutrition in Europe: implications for intestinal transplantation. Gut 2011;60(1):17–25.
8. Lauro A, Panaro F, Iyer KR. An overview of EU and USA intestinal transplant current activity. J Visc Surg 2017;154(2):105–14.
9. (OPTN/SRTR) OPaTNaSRoTR. OPTN/SRTR 2012 annual data report. 2013. https://srtr.transplant.hrsa.gov/annual_reports/2012/Default.aspx. Accessed September 30, 2017.
10. Giovanelli M, Gupte GL, McKiernan P, et al. Impact of change in the United Kingdom pediatric donor organ allocation policy for intestinal transplantation. Transplantation 2009;87(11):1695–9.
11. Gangemi A, Tzvetanov IG, Beatty E, et al. Lessons learned in pediatric small bowel and liver transplantation from living-related donors. Transplantation 2009;87(7):1027–30.
12. Testa G, Holterman M, Abcarian H, et al. Simultaneous or sequential combined living donor-intestine transplantation in children. Transplantation 2008;85(5):713–7.
13. Alican F, Hardy JD, Cayirli M, et al. Intestinal transplantation: laboratory experience and report of a clinical case. Am J Surg 1971;121(2):150–9.
14. Deltz E, Mengel W, Hamelmann H. Small bowel transplantation: report of a clinical case. Prog Pediatr Surg 1990;25:90–6.
15. Stratta P, Quaglia M, Cena T, et al. The interactions of age, sex, body mass index, genetics, and steroid weight-based doses on tacrolimus dosing requirement after adult kidney transplantation. Eur J Clin Pharmacol 2012;68(5):671–80.
16. Benedetti E, Pirenne J, Chul SM, et al. Simultaneous en bloc transplantation of liver, small bowel and large bowel in pigs–technical aspects. Transplant Proc 1995;27(1):341–3.
17. Morris JA, Johnson DL, Rimmer JA, et al. Identical-twin small-bowel transplant for desmoid tumour. Lancet 1995;345(8964):1577–8.
18. Gruessner RW, Sharp HL. Living-related intestinal transplantation: first report of a standardized surgical technique. Transplantation 1997;64(11):1605–7.
19. Uemoto S, Fujimoto Y, Inomata Y, et al. Living-related small bowel transplantation: the first case in Japan. Pediatr Transplant 1998;2(1):40–4.
20. Ishii T, Wada M, Nishi K, et al. Two cases of living-related intestinal transplantation. Transplant Proc 2006;38(6):1687–8.
21. Lee MD, Kim DG, Ahn ST, et al. Isolated small bowel transplantation from a living-related donor at the Catholic University of Kore-a case report of rejection -free course-. Yonsei Med J 2004;45(6):1198–202.

22. Kumaran V, Mehta NN, Varma V, et al. Living donor intestinal transplant using a standardized technique: first report from India. Indian J Gastroenterol 2012; 31(4):179–85.
23. Fortner JG, Sichuk G, Litwin SD, et al. Immunological responses to an intestinal allograft with HL-A-identical donor-recipient. Transplantation 1972;14(5):531–5.
24. Deltz E, Schroeder P, Gebhardt H, et al. First successful clinical small intestine transplantation. Tactics and surgical technic. Chirurg 1989;60(4):235–9 [in German].
25. Pollard SG, Lodge P, Selvakumar S, et al. Living related small bowel transplantation: the first United Kingdom case. Transplant Proc 1996;28(5):2733.
26. Benedetti E, Holterman M, Asolati M, et al. Living related segmental bowel transplantation: from experimental to standardized procedure. Ann Surg 2006;244(5): 694–9.
27. Ghafari J, Tzvetanov I, Spaggiari M, et al. The effect of small bowel living donation on donor lipid profile. Transpl Int 2012;25(1):e19–20.
28. Gruessner RWG, Benedetti E. Living donor organ transplantation. McGraw Hill professional. New York: McGraw-Hill Medical; 2008. Available at: http://ezproxy. library.arizona.edu/login?url=http://www.mhebooklibrary.com/reader/living-donor-organ-transplantation.
29. Ji G, Chu D, Wang W, et al. The safety of donor in living donor small bowel transplantation–an analysis of four cases. Clin Transplant 2009;23(5):761–4.
30. Ueno T, Wada M, Hoshino K, et al. Impact of pediatric intestinal transplantation on intestinal failure in Japan: findings based on the Japanese intestinal transplant registry. Pediatr Surg Int 2013;29(10):1065–70.
31. Kelly DA. Liver complications of pediatric parenteral nutrition–epidemiology. Nutrition 1998;14(1):153–7.
32. Halme L, Eklund B, Kyllonen L, et al. Is obesity still a risk factor in renal transplantation? Transpl Int 1997;10(4):284–8.
33. Garcia Aroz S, Tzvetanov I, Hetterman EA, et al. Long-term outcomes of living-related small intestinal transplantation in children: a single-center experience. Pediatr Transplant 2017;21:e12910.
34. Smith JM, Skeans MA, Horslen SP, et al. OPTN/SRTR 2015 Annual Data Report: Intestine. American journal of transplantation: official journal of the American Society of Transplantation and the American Society of Transplant Surgeons 2017;17(Suppl 1):252–85.
35. Reyes J, Mazariegos GV, Abu-Elmagd K, et al. Intestinal transplantation under tacrolimus monotherapy after perioperative lymphoid depletion with rabbit antithymocyte globulin (thymoglobulin). Am J Transplant 2005;5(6):1430–6.
36. Abu-Elmagd K, Fung J, McGhee W, et al. The efficacy of daclizumab for intestinal transplantation: preliminary report. Transplant Proc 2000;32(6):1195–6.
37. Tzakis AG, Kato T, Nishida S, et al. Campath-1H in intestinal and multivisceral transplantation: preliminary data. Transplant Proc 2002;34(3):937.
38. Langnas AN. Advances in small-intestine transplantation. Transplantation 2004; 77(9 Suppl):S75–8.
39. Fan DM, Zhao QC, Wang WZ, et al. Successful ABO-incompatible living-related intestinal transplantation: a 2-year follow-up. Am J Transplant 2015;15(5):1432–5.
40. Garcia-Roca R, Tzvetanov IG, Jeon H, et al. Successful living donor intestinal transplantation in cross-match positive recipients: initial experience. World J Gastrointest Surg 2016;8(1):101–5.

Endoscopic Follow-up of Intestinal Transplant Recipients

Robert E. Carroll, MD

KEYWORDS

- Intestine transplant • Magnification endoscopy • Acute rejection
- Post-transplant lymphoproliferative disorder • Twin transplants
- Intestinal transplant complications • Research directions in intestine transplants

KEY POINTS

- Magnification endoscopy is an asset in evaluating the integrity of post-transplant intestine but does not replace information obtained from biopsy.
- Ruling out acute rejection of the intestinal graft is a time-critical procedure; endoscopic evidence of rejection merits treatment while awaiting biopsy confirmation.
- Ischemia is a grave diagnosis with respect to graft survival.
- Chronic complications of intestinal transplants include motility disorders of the stomach and native duodenum. The cause may be multifactorial.
- Future directions should include better understanding the microbiome post-transplant; the role of newer Crohn therapies in modulating rejection; and use of growth factors, such as GLP-2, in enhancing surgical adaptation of the intestinal graft.

One never notices what has been done; one can only see what remains to be done.
—Marie Curie

INTRODUCTION

Intestinal transplantation has made significant strides in the last decade. Several centers, including our own at the University of Illinois Hospital, are reporting increased success in patient and graft survival because of technical improvements in surgery, better antirejection regimens, and improved mucosal surveillance protocols for early diagnosis of rejection.[1,2] Mucosal surveillance currently entails a series of fiberoptic ileoscopies with biopsy over 6 months at increasing spaced intervals as the transplant patient recovers from surgery. The seminal report on the endoscopic findings of rejection come from Kato and colleagues[3] at the University of Miami. Briefly, these authors

Disclosures: The author has nothing to disclose.
Department of Medicine, University of Illinois at Chicago, Chicago Veterans Administration Medical Center (West Side Division), 840 South Wood Street (M/C 787), Chicago, IL 60612, USA
E-mail address: rcarroll@uic.edu

Gastroenterol Clin N Am 47 (2018) 381–391
https://doi.org/10.1016/j.gtc.2018.01.012
0889-8553/18/© 2018 Elsevier Inc. All rights reserved.

in this and in an earlier report[4] described for the first time the use of zoom magnification endoscopy, endoscopic criteria for rejection, and a biopsy protocol to manage the transplant patient in the first 4 to 6 months post-transplant.[3] We have adopted almost all of their observations in the development of our own gastrointestinal (GI) support of an intestinal transplant program. This article expands on the observations of this benchmark investigation and discusses future directions for endoscopic research in the small but expanding group of patients who undergo intestinal transplantation.

MUCOSAL SURVEILLANCE FOR REJECTION

At the University of Illinois Hospital, our post-transplant rejection protocol is a bedside ileoscopy with conscious sedation in the Transplant ICU followed by endoscopy in the GI laboratory twice a week for Weeks 1 to 2 post-transplant, followed by once a week for Weeks 3 to 4. We then perform a biopsy every 2 weeks for the next 2 months, typically as an outpatient, and finally perform monthly biopsies until the stoma is closed, usually 6 months post-transplant.

We use a modification of the Miami endoscopic score for rejection and specifically record villous blunting, villous congestion, and villous background erythema in normal (**Fig. 1**A) and magnified mucosa (**Fig. 1**B).[3] We also record friability on biopsy or endoscopic trauma, as what is done at the University of Miami, but additionally look for the presence of spontaneous villous hemorrhage on immediate endoscope insertion and delayed or absent bleeding on biopsy (analogous to the assessment of capillary refill in nail beds). We expect blood to cover the biopsy site by the time we say, "intestinal transplantation," approximately 1.5 seconds in duration (**Fig. 1**C). These secondary findings we believe also are predictive of rejection. Similar to the Miami group report, with growing confidence in our endoscopic assessment of graft well-being, we have reduced our biopsy protocol from four single-pass biopsies in two endoscopic sites to one to two endoscopic biopsies per examination to confirm endoscopic findings with histology. We use a single-pass biopsy protocol with senior technicians trained

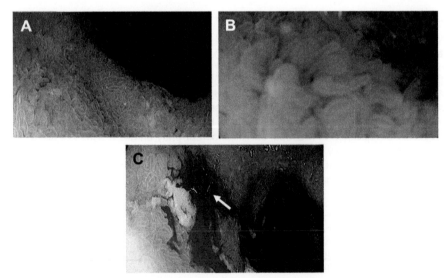

Fig. 1. Magnification endoscopic image of normal small intestine graft mucosa with standard magnification (*A*) and zoomed magnification (*B*). Bleeding postbiopsy is assessed independently at normal magnification (*C*). The arrow indicates biopsy location.

in the procedure to minimize forceps trauma to the graft mucosa. Endoscopic processing and reporting is obtained 6 to 8 hours postbiopsy with accelerated tissue processing protocols. In our facility, histologic grading of rejection is standardized using the VIII International Small Bowel Transplant Guidelines.[5]

Citrulline, an essential amino acid of the urea cycle, is not incorporated into protein and is synthesized in the small intestine. Plasma levels in postoperative patients are an accurate measure of enterocyte mass and predict subsequent independence from parenteral nutrition (PN).[6] Several reports have suggested citrulline levels might be useful as a marker of rejection.[7] We have not been able to obtain citrulline levels quickly enough (<6 hour) to use in evaluating acute rejection. In recovery, however, we do see a rising trend.

ENDOSCOPIC MANAGEMENT OF REJECTION

Suspicion of acute intestinal rejection is often based on mucosal changes in the exposed ileal stoma or the common clinical manifestations of fever, pain, abdominal tenderness, diarrhea, and/or elevated white blood cell count. This is treated at our institution as an endoscopic emergency with urgent endoscopy performed within 2 to 6 hours, depending on inpatient or outpatient status. Similar to the role of endoscopy in acute intestinal ischemia,[8] in which most urgent examinations are negative for the pathology sought, one should not be complacent regarding the timing of future or subsequent examinations. The reward for eternal vigilance is not liberty but the subsequent relief of patients and transplant physicians alike.

Biopsies should be obtained from suspicious areas of intestinal mucosa based on blunting, graft edema, and villous hemorrhage if no frank ulceration is identified. Inflamed ulcerated mucosa should be biopsied from intact mucosal areas adjacent to ulcers and from uninvolved areas, if any, for comparison (**Fig. 2**). We implement treatment of moderate to severe rejection at the time of endoscopic diagnosis, because tissue histology is delayed by processing protocols and initial biopsy findings may lag in severity to endoscopic findings. Once rejection is suspected and subsequently confirmed by histology, standard treatment protocols with high-dose intravenous (IV) steroids, infliximab, and/or thymoglobulin are initiated. Repeat biopsy is obtained about 72 hours after treatment to assess response of inflammation. Graft recovery or regeneration is documented with repeat examination one to two times per week until villous recovery is documented by endoscopy and confirmed by biopsy. Methylene blue staining to estimate mucosal regeneration and villous recovery is useful in this setting. We use a 0.05% methylene blue solution applied through a spray catheter (**Fig. 3**A) to

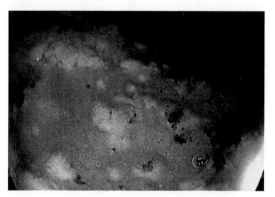

Fig. 2. Endoscopic image of a small intestinal graft with moderate acute rejection. Biopsies would be obtained from the nonulcerated areas to make a diagnosis of rejection.

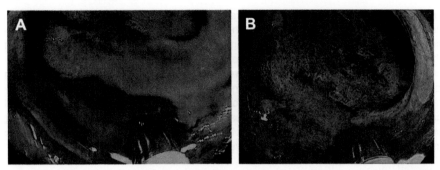

Fig. 3. Magnification endoscopic image of the small intestine graft mucosa during application of a 0.05% methylene blue solution (A). The dye does not adhere to denuded areas or exposed submucosa postwashing (B), allowing assessment of mucosal damage.

involved graft mucosa. Methylene blue is taken up by epithelial cells and does not adhere to exposed submucosa or denuded areas after washing (Fig 3B). This allows the endoscopist to assess extent of mucosal damage and recovery more accurately and confidently than assessment with zoom magnification alone.

INTESTINAL ISCHEMIA

We have seen early rejection associated with delayed bleeding postbiopsy. A more ominous finding is scant or undetectable bleeding on a background of pale edematous mucosa (**Fig. 4**). This may be painless and should prompt immediate Doppler examination of the stoma for adequate Doppler signal to assess perfusion. Urgent re-exploration for faint or reduced Doppler signal is indicated, but outcomes are poor in this situation. The biopsy shows thrombosed capillaries and submucosal hemorrhage, but typically the fate of the graft is established before the availability of the biopsy for review. In an isolated case, graft ischemia was identified 9 months post-transplant and found to be associated with stenosis of the arterial anastomosis. Chronic abdominal pain and weight loss caused by aversion to eating likely represented intestinal angina,[9] and in retrospect would have benefited from earlier evaluation of the vascular anastomosis.

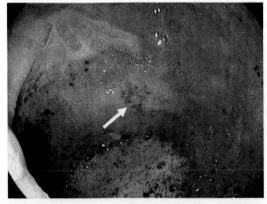

Fig. 4. Endoscopic image of absence of bleeding after forceps biopsy in an ischemic small intestinal graft. The arrow indicates biopsy location. Pale, edematous mucosa with absence of bleeding postbiopsy is a harbinger of vascular thrombosis or stenosis of the vascular anastomosis. This is in contrast to bleeding in the normal small intestine graft, as shown in **Fig. 1C**.

Urgent vascular stent placement for revascularization resulted in immediate graft reperfusion, but chronic graft ischemia with stricture, fistula, and perforation resulted in multiple resections and salvage surgery, ultimately requiring relisting for transplantation.

GASTROINTESTINAL BLEEDING AND FISTULA

Overt GI bleeding is not typically associated with acute rejection, although oozing and slow decline in hematocrit from graft ulceration in a severe rejection episode is not infrequent. Acute rejection is associated with hemodynamically significant GI bleeding if the graft is directly anastomosed to the stomach and responds to an IV pantoprazole drip and judicious application of bipolar cautery. The severe ulceration and bleeding is confined to the graft mucosa adjacent to the stomach, analogous to marginal ulceration in a Roux-en-Y gastrostomy.[10] Significant gastric and native duodenal ulceration have also occurred after small bowel graft removal for tacrolimus-induced Thrombotic Thrombocytopenic Purpura (TTP),[11] perhaps caused by the elevated gastrin levels and increased gastric acid secretion after massive intestinal resection, as reported by Straus and colleagues.[12] Finally, isolated small bowel bleeding with ulceration and visible vessels is seen remotely post-transplant in association with chronic fibrostenotic rejection and abdominal fistula formation. NOD-2 mutations, which in bone marrow transplantation (BMT) patients are associated with intestinal graft-versus-host disease (GVHD),[13] were not identified in all patients. These lesions were difficult to identify and not amenable to endoscopic treatment. Bleeding was ultimately controlled with endoscopic visualization in the operating room and surgical oversewing of the vessel.

Bleeding from fistula or stoma sites may also occur at the skin level and should be treated with silver nitrate stick application or oversewn if arterial in nature. If endoscopic examinations do not reveal an intestinal bleeding source, careful examination of the abdominal wall with all adhesive stomal material removed should be performed.

Obscure GI bleeding with hypotension and shock was also found in a single transplant pediatric patient. A small bowel source was suspected by repeated negative upper and lower GI endoscopy. Following an unrevealing angiography, GI bleeding was controlled with a 72-hour octreotide infusion followed by chronic depot octreotide with one recurrence of bleeding from transient interruption of therapy 1 year later. Long-acting or depot octreotide has been used chronically in bleeding from portal hypertension in pediatric patients[14] and is safe. Finally, a bleeding Dieulafoy lesion in the native duodenum adjacent to the graft in a pediatric liver/small bowel sequential transplantation, complicated by hepatocellular carcinoma formation and portal hypertension, occurred in a single patient. This required multiple transfusions (>20 units) and repeated endoscopy with ultimate control by endoscopic clip and cautery of the elusive vascular lesion. An OVESCO (OTSC Systems, Cary, NC) clip procedure was attempted but aborted, because the device was unable to pass through the narrow, intubated pharynx. The juvenile recipient subsequently expired in home hospice care fortunately with bleeding controlled.

FISTULA AND STRICTURE

We have used the OVESCO over-the-scope clip with success in closing a complex infected gastroileal cutaneous fistula that had developed immediately postoperatively after a second transplantation for chronic rejection about 13 years after successful living donor transplantation. The subsequent use of this device in an internal enteroenteral fistula after graft ischemia failed to provide long-term closure, presumably because of fibrosis of the graft and inability of the clip to adhere submucosally. We have used traditional coated stents (Wilson-Cook, Limerick, Ireland) fluoroscopically placed and through the scope (Daewoo, Seoul, Korea) to cover fistulous tracts with limited long-term success.

Endoscopic balloon dilation with through-the-scope TTS balloons (Wilson Cook) has been successful in dilation of proximal and distal transplant graft anastomotic strictures. We use a modified protocol with a reduced maximal balloon size and inflation time, compared with what is used in a standard stricture on nonimmunosuppressed patients, to prevent the occurrence of perforation. We have not had an endoscopic perforation in approximately 1000 endoscopic procedures performed at our institution, but it remains a constant concern.

POST-TRANSPLANT LYMPHOPROLIFERATIVE DISORDER

GVHD involving the integument of small bowel transplant recipients[15] has been seen in pediatric and adult transplants in our institution. However, post-transplant lymphoproliferative disorder has only occurred in our pediatric transplant population. Unlike previous GI reports describing ulcerated intestinal masses with late presentation,[16] we have made the diagnosis with earlier presentation on endoscopic biopsy precipitated by the presence of fevers and rising Epstein-Barr virus titers. Endoscopically, the mucosa is normal with only isolated mucosal edema around the site of enlarged Peyer patches. Initially, we removed the graft and patients were retransplanted after 6 months of chemotherapy (modified CHOP) and negative computed tomography scanning, but reduction in immunosuppression with rituximab therapy has allowed salvage of the graft and resolution of the lymphoproliferative state. Close collaboration with pediatric oncology and pediatric intensivists is critical to the successful treatment of these complicated patients. A recently published series discusses the current management of these cases in detail.[17]

IDENTICAL TWINS

We have performed transplant in identical twins with complete 10/10 HLA matching.[18] Although they require no immunologic surveillance for rejection, they still require postoperative endoscopic monitoring of the integrity of the anastomosis and adequacy of graft perfusion. Recently, we have foregone ileal stoma creation in these patients and instead perform a limited colonoscopy to reach and evaluate the graft at its distal anastomosis. This can successfully be performed at the bedside in the Transplant ICU, but positioning and sedation in the early postoperative period is more challenging than traditional ileoscopy and requires more time and endoscopic prudence at the newly created anastomosis. We typically perform biopsies across the anastomosis, with the colonoscope positioned entirely on the colonic side for the first 2 weeks, and only attempt to endoscopically traverse the surgical anastomosis after postoperative day 12 to 14.

GASTROPARESIS

Gastroparesis is a prevalent, almost ubiquitous complication following intestinal transplant. Response to metoclopramide is modest at best and erythromycin use to stimulate motilin receptors is complicated by drug interaction with tacrolimus, resulting in toxicity.[19] Causes for this complication in small bowel transplant have not been systematically investigated or reported but likely include developmental, surgical, and medical factors.

These patients have typically had multiple surgeries before this operation; often take opioid narcotics on a routine basis; and some have had intestinal developmental anomalies, particularly gastroschisis, which may be associated with abnormal foregut neural development and dysmotility.[20]

Whipple surgery, both traditional and pylorus sparing, are associated with gastropare-sis,[21] with the latter perhaps having better outcomes.[22] Catastrophic infarction of the small bowel caused by superior mesenteric artery (SMA) thrombosis post–Whipple sur-gery has led to intestinal transplant in two patients in our institution, both of whom had marked gastroparesis postoperatively. More recently, bariatric Roux-en-Y gastric bypass operations for weight loss have become increasingly associated with catastrophic intes-tinal loss and short bowel syndrome[23] This operation, although it often corrects gastro-paresis,[24] is often reversed as part of the technical repair post-transplant and may recur.

Additionally, because allogeneic BMT,[25] lung,[26] and heart-lung[27] transplantation are associated with gastroparesis, factors associated with immunosuppression are also likely relevant to this complication. Comparison of incidence and severity in the small bowel transplanted identical twin population would be potentially useful.

DUODENAL STASIS

The native duodenum post-transplant often becomes markedly dilated, and intestinal stasis with bacterial overgrowth can interfere with nutrient absorption, cause weight loss, and is a potential source of bacterial translocation and line infection. The motility disorder may respond to octreotide.[28] The bacterial overgrowth is typically responsive to short course of the nonabsorbable antibiotic rifaximin. Quantitative bacterial culture in a dedicated microbiology laboratory can often direct antibiotic coverage for opportu-nistic fungal infections, such as *Nocardia asteroids*, or unique and difficult bacterial path-ogens, such as *Ochrobactrum anthropi* and *Stentrophomonas maltophilia*. The gut has been accepted heuristically for some time as the engine of sepsis and infection from bacterial translocation. Recent studies suggest gut flora is specifically linked to distinct aspects of systemic inflammatory response syndrome entities, including line sepsis,[29] acute respiratory distress syndrome,[30] and pneumonia.[31] Mechanistic studies including the use of fecal microbiota transplant as potential therapy should be pursued.[32]

INTESTINAL INFLAMMATION AND INCLUSIONS

Melanosis of the proximal segment of the transplanted graft has been noted in two subjects with chronic anemia on iron supplementation. Prussian blue staining for hemo-siderin confirmed iron deposition (**Fig. 5**). The most recent patient was converted to IV iron-sucrose formulations with some improvement in the intestinal "melanosis." We believe this finding is similar to pseudomelanosis duodeni observed in chronic renal failure

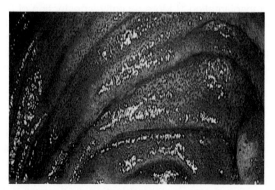

Fig. 5. Endoscopic image of "melanosis" of the proximal small intestine graft. Staining for he-mosiderin with Prussian blue confirmed iron deposition. Patient was switched to an intravenous iron-sucrose formulation.

patients.[33] The role of chronic inflammation and hepcidin inhibition of mucosal iron absorption, and the recently characterized factor erythroferrone,[34] is likely germane to intestinal transplant patients. The mucosal inflammation seen on biopsy does not resemble that seen in intestinal rejection because crypt apoptosis and villous blunting are not observed.

Following recovery from rejection episodes, we have seen isolated mucosal patches devoid of villi with evidence of gastric metaplasia on biopsy of the transplanted ileum from gastric and colonic sides of the anastomosis. This metaplastic transformation has been described in Crohn patients after treatment of severe inflammation and likely represents an altered intestinal stem cell response to severe inflammation.[35] It is an isolated anomaly and does not require treatment or surveillance.

FUTURE DIRECTIONS

In addition to endoscopic support, gastroenterologists typically manage PN and transition to oral diets. The transition off PN and cessation of electrolytes (mostly magnesium) and fluid supplementation with removal of central line access is driven by the speed and adequacy of intestinal adaptation. Intestinal adaptation post-transplant usually occurs 3 to 6 weeks postoperatively and is likely analogous to the physiologic adaptation of the bowel to resection with villous hypertrophy and increased crypt proliferation.[36] The hormonal factors underlying these processes are not well understood. We believe the GLP-2 agonist teduglutide, perhaps by upregulating insulin growth factor and keratinocyte growth factor,[37] in the perioperative transplant period may enhance and speed intestinal adaptation. Studies in animal transplant models would confirm this and perhaps justify a multicenter trial.

Low-dose infliximab infusion is now a standard part of our rejection treatment protocol.[38] There is an isolated report of a similar benefit with adalimumab.[39] The use of vedolizumab, a newer Crohn therapy,[40] prevents host lymphocyte tracking to the graft and may also be beneficial in complicated rejection in our limited experience. Mongersen, an oligonucleotide antisense molecule that inhibits transforming growth factor-β inflammation signaling through SMAD-7,[41] has early reports of benefit in Crohn patients.[42] Successful drugs in the treatment of Crohn patients, and possibly intestinal GVHD in BMT patients, should be considered for use in prevention and treatment of severe acute and chronic small intestinal rejection, because pathologically these lesions are similar.

Bacterial overgrowth has been described in the transplant graft even in the early days of intestinal transplantation.[43] More recently, constriction of the microbiome in Crohn disease has been associated with disease flare[44] and likely linked to defects in autophagy and innate immune signaling.[45] Further work on the microbiome of the small bowel transplant patient should be entertained with modern metagenomic analysis[46] to understand its potential role in reducing chronic rejection and promoting immune tolerance.[47]

SUMMARY

Short bowel syndrome is an orphan disease (Orphanet#104008) with unique presentation and complications. The even smaller population requiring intestinal transplant is unique and challenging for gastroenterologists to support and evaluate.[48] Individual transplant patients each require multiple (some >100) endoscopic procedures and interventions in the course of preoperative evaluation, postoperative care, and subsequent management of acute and chronic problems post-transplant. Evaluation of rejection and recovery requires a trained eye to detect subtle changes in the endoscopic mucosa, and a mental image or eidetic memory of the previous examination, to assess resolution of inflammation and adequacy of recovery. This is a slow, laborious process with experience gained from individual patients over time. It requires working intimately with transplant surgeons with rapid and frank dialogue regarding clinical thought processes and endoscopic assessment. It is the author's belief that the best care for these patients requires a single or small coterie of dedicated gastroenterologists with a thorough knowledge of the individual patient's current and past medical and surgical course. This work and these patients to be well-cared for cannot be left to rotating inpatient teams, on-call physicians, or local hospitals. It requires a commitment that extends beyond call schedules, weekdays, and daylight hours but is one that is immensely rewarding to those who care for these patients. However, as Madame Curie said, "much remains to be done."

ACKNOWLEDGMENTS

The author thanks Alvin T. George for his assistance in the composition of this article.

REFERENCES

1. Lauro A, Zanfi C, Ercolani G, et al. Twenty-five consecutive isolated intestinal transplants in adult patients: a five-yr clinical experience. Clin Transplant 2007; 21(2):177–85.
2. Dijkstra G, Rings EH, Bijleveld CM, et al. Intestinal transplantation in The Netherlands: first experience and future perspectives. Scand J Gastroenterol Suppl 2006;(243):39–45.
3. Kato T, Gaynor JJ, Nishida S, et al. Zoom endoscopic monitoring of small bowel allograft rejection. Surg Endosc 2006;20(5):773–82.
4. Kato T, O'Brien CB, Nishida S, et al. The first case report of the use of a zoom videoendoscope for the evaluation of small bowel graft mucosa in a human after intestinal transplantation. Gastrointest Endosc 1999;50(2):257–61.
5. Ruiz P, Bagni A, Brown R, et al. Histological criteria for the identification of acute cellular rejection in human small bowel allografts: results of the pathology workshop at the VIII International Small Bowel Transplant Symposium. Transplant Proc 2004;36(2):335–7.
6. Crenn P, Messing B, Cynober L. Citrulline as a biomarker of intestinal failure due to enterocyte mass reduction. Clin Nutr 2008;27(3):328–39.
7. Ruiz P, Tryphonopoulos P, Island E, et al. Citrulline evaluation in bowel transplantation. Transpl Proc 2010;42(1):54–6.
8. Brandt LJ, Feuerstadt P, Longstreth GF, et al, American College of Gastroenterology. ACG clinical guideline: epidemiology, risk factors, patterns of presentation, diagnosis, and management of colon ischemia (CI). Am J Gastroenterol 2015; 110(1):18–44 [quiz: 5].
9. Nuzzo A, Corcos O. Management of mesenteric ischemia in the era of intestinal stroke centers: the gut and lifesaving strategy. Rev Med Interne 2017;38(9): 592–602 [in French].
10. Rasmussen JJ, Fuller W, Ali MR. Marginal ulceration after laparoscopic gastric bypass: an analysis of predisposing factors in 260 patients. Surg Endosc 2007;21(7):1090–4.
11. Al-Nouri ZL, Reese JA, Terrell DR, et al. Drug-induced thrombotic microangiopathy: a systematic review of published reports. Blood 2015;125(4):616–8.
12. Straus E, Gerson CD, Yalow RS. Hypersecretion of gastrin associated with the short bowel syndrome. Gastroenterology 1974;66(2):175–80.

13. Rogler G, Holler E. Can NOD2/CARD15 mutations predict intestinal graft-versus-host disease and aid our understanding of Crohn's disease? Nat Clin Pract Gastroenterol Hepatol 2004;1(2):62–3.

14. O'Meara M, Cicalese MP, Bordugo A, et al. Successful use of long-acting octreotide for intractable chronic gastrointestinal bleeding in children. J Pediatr Gastroenterol Nutr 2015;60(1):48–53.

15. Cruysmans C, Ferneiny MG, Fraitag S, et al. Severe skin complications after small bowel transplantation: graft-versus-host disease, dress, virus, or drug toxicity? Transplantation 2016;100(10):2222–5.

16. O'Connor JA, Cogley C, Burton M, et al. Posttransplantation lymphoproliferative disorder: endoscopic findings. J Pediatr Gastroenterol Nutr 2000;31(4):458–61.

17. Lauro A, Arpinati M, Pinna AD. Managing the challenge of PTLD in liver and bowel transplant recipients. Br J Haematol 2015;169(2):157–72.

18. Schena S, Testa G, Setty S, et al. Successful identical-twin living donor small bowel transplant for necrotizing enterovasculitis secondary to Churg-Strauss syndrome. Transpl Int 2006;19(7):594–7.

19. Padhi ID, Long P, Basha M, et al. Interaction between tacrolimus and erythromycin. Ther Drug Monit 1997;19(1):120–2.

20. Phillips JD, Raval MV, Redden C, et al. Gastroschisis, atresia, dysmotility: surgical treatment strategies for a distinct clinical entity. J Pediatr Surg 2008;43(12): 2208–12.

21. Hanna MM, Gadde R, Tamariz L, et al. Delayed gastric emptying after pancreaticoduodenectomy: is subtotal stomach preserving better or pylorus preserving? J Gastrointest Surg 2015;19(8):1542–52.

22. Hanna MM, Tamariz L, Gadde R, et al. Delayed gastric emptying after pylorus preserving pancreaticoduodenectomy: does gastrointestinal reconstruction technique matter? Am J Surg 2016;211(4):810–9.

23. McBride CL, Petersen A, Sudan D, et al. Short bowel syndrome following bariatric surgical procedures. Am J Surg 2006;192(6):828–32.

24. Papasavas PK, Ng JS, Stone AM, et al. Gastric bypass surgery as treatment of recalcitrant gastroparesis. Surg Obes Relat Dis 2014;10(5):795–9.

25. Eagle DA, Gian V, Lauwers GY, et al. Gastroparesis following bone marrow transplantation. Bone Marrow Transpl 2001;28(1):59–62.

26. Hooft N, Smith M, Huang J, et al. Gastroparesis is common after lung transplantation and may be ameliorated by botulinum toxin-A injection of the pylorus. J Heart Lung Transplant 2014;33(12):1314–6.

27. Sodhi SS, Guo JP, Maurer AH, et al. Gastroparesis after combined heart and lung transplantation. J Clin Gastroenterol 2002;34(1):34–9.

28. Nakada K, Ikoma A, Suzuki T, et al. Amelioration of intestinal dysmotility and stasis by octreotide early after small-bowel autotransplantation in dogs. Am J Surg 1995;169(3):294–9.

29. Carl MA, Ndao IM, Springman AC, et al. Sepsis from the gut: the enteric habitat of bacteria that cause late-onset neonatal bloodstream infections. Clin Infect Dis 2014;58(9):1211–8.

30. Dickson RP, Singer BH, Newstead MW, et al. Enrichment of the lung microbiome with gut bacteria in sepsis and the acute respiratory distress syndrome. Nat Microbiol 2016;1(10):16113.

31. Schuijt TJ, Lankelma JM, Scicluna BP, et al. The gut microbiota plays a protective role in the host defense against pneumococcal pneumonia. Gut 2016;65(4): 575–83.

32. Gupta S, Allen-Vercoe E, Petrof EO. Fecal microbiota transplantation: in perspective. Therap Adv Gastroenterol 2016;9(2):229–39.
33. Siderits R, Hazra A, Mikhail N, et al. Endoscopically identified pseudomelanosis duodeni: striking yet harmless. Gastrointest Endosc 2014;80(3):508–10.
34. Vallet N, Club du Globule Rouge et du Fer. The role of erythroferrone in iron metabolism: from experimental results to pathogenesis. Rev Med Interne 2017 [pii:S0248-8663(17)30525-8]. [in French].
35. Kushima R, Borchard F, Hattori T. A new aspect of gastric metaplasia in Crohn's disease: bidirectional (foveolar and pyloric) differentiation in so-called "pyloric metaplasia" in the ileum. Pathol Int 1997;47(6):416–9.
36. Sukhotnik I, Siplovich L, Shiloni E, et al. Intestinal adaptation in short-bowel syndrome in infants and children: a collective review. Pediatr Surg Int 2002;18(4): 258–63.
37. Drucker DJ, Yusta B. Physiology and pharmacology of the enteroendocrine hormone glucagon-like peptide-2. Annu Rev Physiol 2014;76:561–83.
38. Pascher A, Klupp J, Langrehr JM, et al. Anti-TNF-alpha therapy for acute rejection in intestinal transplantation. Transpl Proc 2005;37(3):1635–6.
39. Rao B, Jafri SM, Kazimi M, et al. A case report of acute cellular rejection following intestinal transplantation managed with adalimumab. Transpl Proc 2016;48(2): 536–8.
40. Eriksson C, Marsal J, Bergemalm D, et al. Long-term effectiveness of vedolizumab in inflammatory bowel disease: a national study based on the Swedish National Quality Registry for Inflammatory Bowel Disease (SWIBREG). Scand J Gastroenterol 2017;52(6–7):722–9.
41. Yan X, Liu Z, Chen Y. Regulation of TGF-beta signaling by Smad7. Acta Biochim Biophys Sin (Shanghai) 2009;41(4):263–72.
42. Feagan BG, Sands BE, Rossiter G, et al. Effects of mongersen (GED-0301) on endoscopic and clinical outcomes in patients with active Crohn's disease. Gastroenterology 2018;154(1):61–4.e6.
43. Abu-Elmagd K, Todo S, Tzakis A, et al. Intestinal transplantation and bacterial overgrowth in humans. Transpl Proc 1994;26(3):1684–5.
44. Hofer U. Microbiome: bacterial imbalance in Crohn's disease. Nat Rev Microbiol 2014;12(5):312.
45. Henderson P, Stevens C. The role of autophagy in Crohn's disease. Cells 2012; 1(3):492–519.
46. Oulas A, Pavloudi C, Polymenakou P, et al. Metagenomics: tools and insights for analyzing next-generation sequencing data derived from biodiversity studies. Bioinform Biol Insights 2015;9:75–88.
47. Shreiner AB, Kao JY, Young VB. The gut microbiome in health and in disease. Curr Opin Gastroenterol 2015;31(1):69–75.
48. Carroll RE, Benedetti E, Schowalter JP, et al. Management and complications of short bowel syndrome: an updated review. Curr Gastroenterol Rep 2016;18(7):40.

Composite and Multivisceral Transplantation

Nomenclature, Surgical Techniques, Current Practice, and Long-term Outcome

Guilherme Costa, MD[a], Neha Parekh, MS, RD[a],
Mohammed Osman, MD[a], Sherif Armanyous, MD[c],
Masato Fujiki, MD, PhD[a], Kareem Abu-Elmagd, MD, PhD[a,b],*

KEYWORDS

- Liver-intestinal transplantation • Multivisceral transplantation
- Visceral transplantation • Intestinal failure • Portomesenteric venous thrombosis
- Surgical technique

KEY POINTS

- Composite and multivisceral transplantation is a life-saving procedure for patients with combined abdominal organ and gut failure.
- The observed continual improvement in survival outcome is the result of innovative surgical techniques, novel immunosuppressive protocols, and state-of-art postoperative care.
- Reestablishment of long-term nutritional autonomy with restored quality of life and socioeconomic milestones is achievable in most survivors.
- Further progress is anticipated with better in-depth understanding of innate immunity, adaptive gut alloimmunity, allograft tolerance, and the biology of gut microbiota.

INTRODUCTION

For nearly 4 decades, the abdominal viscera was considered a forbidden organ for clinical transplantation because of the associated massive lymphoid tissue, high antigenicity, and microbial colonization.[1,2] The late 1980s witnessed successful sporadic attempts under cyclosporine-based immunosuppression.[3] However, the practical application of the procedure was only feasible after the 1989 advent of tacrolimus.[4] Despite waves of enthusiasm and disappointment, the continual

Disclosure Statement: The authors have nothing to disclose.
[a] Center for Gut Rehabilitation and Transplantation, Cleveland Clinic, 9500 Euclid Avenue, Desk A100, Cleveland, OH 44195, USA; [b] Cleveland Clinic Lerner College of Medicine, Cleveland Clinic, 9500 Euclid Avenue, Desk A100, Cleveland, OH 44195, USA; [c] Department of Nephrology, Cleveland Clinic, 9500 Euclid Avenue, Desk A100, Cleveland, OH 44195, USA
* Corresponding author.
E-mail address: abuelmk@ccf.org

Gastroenterol Clin N Am 47 (2018) 393–415
https://doi.org/10.1016/j.gtc.2018.01.013
0889-8553/18/© 2018 Elsevier Inc. All rights reserved.

evolution of the procedure was achievable as a result of continuous interplay between new advances in surgical techniques, immunosuppressive strategies, and postoperative management.[2,5]

Establishment of the current distinctive nomenclature has largely stemmed from the anatomic and surgical principles described with the original multivisceral transplant operation.[6–8] Elucidation of the mechanisms of allograft acceptance, along with the availability of new immunosuppressive agents, has been behind the introduction of novel immunosuppressive, immunomodulatory, and preconditioning strategies.[9,10] The cumulative increase in clinical experience with advances in molecular diagnostic techniques and the availability of new antimicrobial agents enhanced postoperative care.[1]

In 2000, the Centers for Medicare and Medicaid Services qualified intestinal and multivisceral transplantation as the standard of care for patients with irreversible gut failure who no longer can be maintained on parenteral nutrition (PN).[11] With the subsequent increase in worldwide experience, practical guidelines, including expansion of the initial indications, have evolved in recent years.[12] Despite the continual improvement in outcome, the procedure is still limited to patients with nutritional failure who no longer can be maintained on PN. In addition, most health care providers also mandate failure of gut rehabilitative efforts as a prerequisite for transplantation. However, it is imperative to emphasize that early transplantation, at centers of excellence, has been associated with many therapeutic advantages, including better survival with successful restoration of nutritional autonomy and quality of life.[5] Furthermore, halting the PN-associated native liver damage with early transplantation optimizes the deceased donor liver utilization for patients with isolated hepatic failure.

HISTORICAL EVOLUTION

Traced back to the pioneer experimental work of the 1912 Nobel Prize winner Alexis Carrel,[13] the modern history of multivisceral transplantation was assigned by the innovative experimental work and initial clinical attempts of Thomas Starzl.[14,15] In 1983, 20 years after his first successful canine multivisceral transplant, Starzl performed the first 2 multivisceral transplantations in humans with en bloc inclusion of the stomach, duodenum, pancreas, intestine, colon, and liver.[16] Both cases were children with gut and liver failure associated with short bowel syndrome, which were transplanted under cyclosporine-based immunosuppression. Although the first case died perioperatively from multisystem organ failure, the second multivisceral recipient survived more than 6 months with a fully functioning graft only to die from progressive post-transplant lymphoproliferative disease (PTLD).

In 1990, Grant and colleagues[17] published the first successful case of a lesser composite visceral allograft in humans. The combined liver-intestinal allograft was transplanted under cyclosporine-based immunosuppression using the simultaneously transplanted donor liver as an immunoprotective shield to the transplanted intestine. The replaced native liver had normal structural and synthetic functions but with antithrombin III deficiency. Ironically, FK-506, currently known as tacrolimus, was introduced in the same year by the Pittsburgh team, allowing the successful clinical transplantation of the intestine-only allograft without the need for simultaneous hepatic replacement.[18] These successful initial efforts created a wave of enthusiasm that increased the clinical feasibility and practicality of the different types of visceral transplantation. In addition, new modifications were introduced to both the donor and recipient transplant procedures.[5,11,19,20]

Full details of the historical evolution of immunosuppression and postoperative care are beyond the scope of this article.[1,3] In brief, the clinical introduction of interleukin (IL)-2 receptor antibodies and the different antilymphocyte preparations have contributed significantly to the evolution of the immunosuppressive regimen. Meanwhile, new insights into the mechanism of allograft acceptance and transplant tolerance have guided the effective utilization of these agents for induction therapy and recipient or donor pretreatment.[1] Advances in postoperative care were the result of cumulative experience, introduction of new diagnostic and biologic tools, and availability of effective antimicrobial agents.[5]

NOMENCLATURE

In 1991, the many faces of multivisceral and composite visceral transplantation were eloquently described and illustrated by Starzl and colleagues.[7] In essence, the intestine is the central core of any visceral allograft and the nomenclature is based on the type and number of the organs that are transplanted en bloc with the intestine (**Fig. 1**).[8,21] Accordingly, the cluster operation that entails en bloc replacement of the liver, pancreas, duodenum, and small portion of jejunum, with or without the stomach (**Fig. 2**) is commonly misnamed as a multivisceral transplantation. It is also imperative to differentiate between the terms multiorgan transplantation and multivisceral transplantation. The term multiorgan transplantation is defined as simultaneous or sequential individual organ transplantation without inclusion of the intestine. The term multivisceral transplantation is defined as en bloc implantation of the abdominal visceral organs, including the stomach and intestine.[22]

Composite visceral transplantation is a broader term encompassing multivisceral transplantation and any other combination of the visceral allograft with en bloc inclusion of the liver and/or pancreas (see **Fig. 1**). The multivisceral transplantation can be full or modified, including the stomach, duodenum, pancreas, and intestine, with or

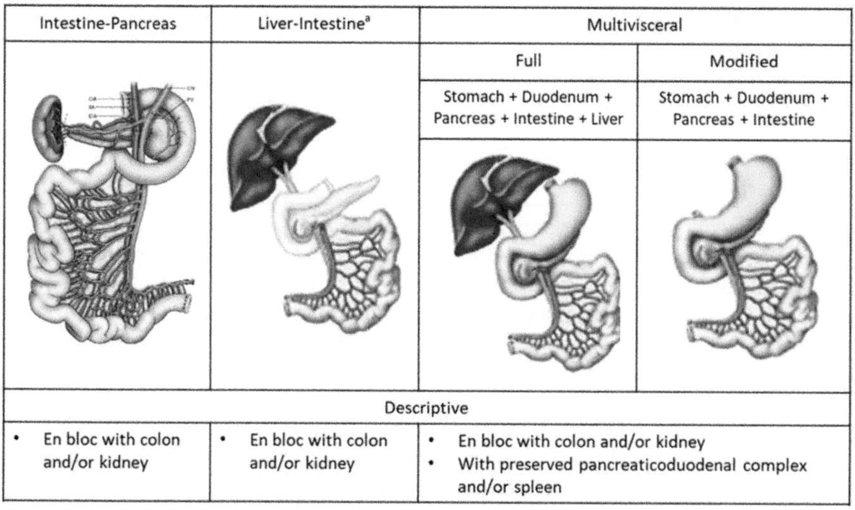

Intestine-Pancreas	Liver-Intestine[a]	Multivisceral	
		Full	Modified
		Stomach + Duodenum + Pancreas + Intestine + Liver	Stomach + Duodenum + Pancreas + Intestine
Descriptive			
• En bloc with colon and/or kidney	• En bloc with colon and/or kidney	• En bloc with colon and/or kidney • With preserved pancreaticoduodenal complex and/or spleen	

Fig. 1. Types of composite visceral allografts. [a] Inclusion of the pancreaticoduodenal complex is optional and commonly used for technical reasons. (*Adapted from* Fujiki M, Hashimoto H, Khanna A, et al. Technical innovation and visceral transplantation. In: Subramaniam K, Sakai T, editors. Anesthesia and perioperative care for organ transplantation. New York: Springer; 2017. p. 498; with permission.)

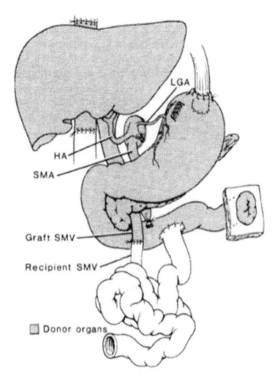

Fig. 2. Cluster graft, including stomach. HA, hepatic artery; LGA, left gastric artery; SMA, superior mesenteric artery; and SMV, superior mesenteric vein. (*From* Starlz TE, Todo S, Tzakis A. The many faces of multivisceral transplantation. Surg Gynecol Obstet 1991;172(5):340; with permission.)

without the liver, respectively (see **Fig. 1**). The other composite visceral allografts include the intestine and pancreas, with or without the liver (see **Fig. 1**). The donor colon, spleen, and/or kidney can always be retained as secondary organs with any of these allograft types without the need for any further substratification.[21]

TECHNIQUES
Donor Operation

The early challenges experienced with both donor and recipient surgery combined with organ shortage in the milieu of complex abdominal pathologic conditions stimulated relentless efforts toward various technical modifications. The quality of the visceral allograft is the Achilles heel of successful transplantation.[23] In brief, procurement of the composite visceral and multivisceral allografts from deceased donors is usually part of the standard multiorgan retrieval procedure.[11] The retrieval technique is based on the embryology and vascular blood supply of the gut organs (**Fig. 3**).[24] In recent years, Benedetti and colleagues introduced the living donor composite visceral transplantation with separate segmental liver and intestine.[25] It is fundamental for both deceased and live donor allografts to obtain good quality arterial and venous-free vascular grafts for the back table and in situ vascular reconstruction.

Recipient Surgery

The recipient operation with implantation of the different composite visceral allografts is often complex and technically challenging (**Fig. 4**).[26] The extent of abdominal

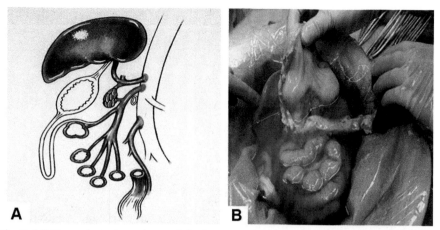

Fig. 3. (*A*) The embryonic anatomy of the foregut, midgut, and hindgut. (*B*) A multivisceral graft, including the stomach, duodenum, pancreas, liver, and intestine, in the ice cold organ preservation solution. Note that the spleen was used to handle the organs and was removed as part of the back table procedure. (*Courtesy of* Kareem Abu-Elmagd, MD, Cleveland, OH.)

dissection in patients who require a multivisceral transplantation is illustrated in **Fig. 5**. In selected patients with infected abdomen or extensive mesenteric desmoid tumor, an initial exploratory laparotomy is required as a first-stage operation to rescue candidacy for transplantation.[27,28] In the presence of limited central venous access, perioperative establishment of a reliable wide-bore venous access is required for prompt intraoperative resuscitation. Patients with multiple prior abdominal surgeries and organ failure often undergo careful major abdominal dissection with creation of a new abdominal domain. In addition, the extent of the abdominal evisceration procedure is modified according to the indications for transplantation, particularly in patients

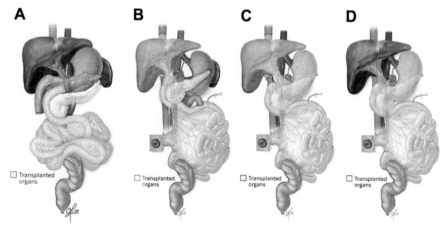

Fig. 4. Recipient operation; the different composite visceral allografts. (*A*) Intestine-pancreas. (*B*) Combined liver-intestine with en bloc pancreaticoduodenal complex. (*C*) Full multivisceral. (*D*) Modified multivisceral. (*Reprinted with permission*, Cleveland Clinic Center for Medical Art & Photography © 2018. All Rights Reserved.)

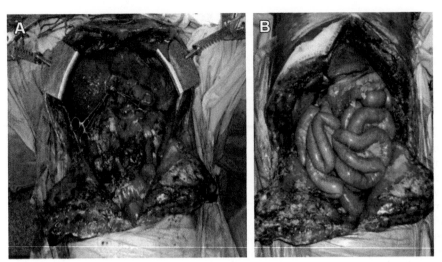

Fig. 5. Multivisceral transplantation. (*A*) Removal of diseased organs. (*B*) Reperfusion of new organs.

with gut dysmotility and Gardner syndrome.[20] When technically feasible, the native pancreaticoduodenal complex or the splenic compartment is preserved in those who are in need of full and modified multivisceral transplantation with merit to reduce risk of infection, PTLD, and diabetes (**Fig. 6**).[19,20,29]

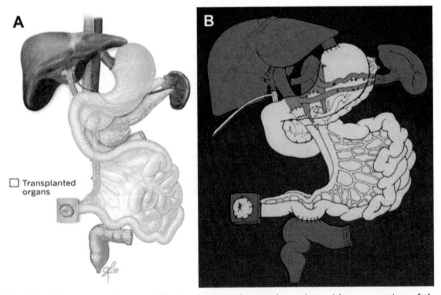

Fig. 6. Recipient operation; modified multivisceral transplantation with preservation of the native spleen. (*A*) With preservation of the native pancreas. (*B*) With inclusion of pancreas in the donor allograft. ((*A*) *Reprinted with permission*, Cleveland Clinic Center for Medical Art & Photography © 2018. All Rights Reserved; and (*B*) *From* Abu-Elmagd K, Khanna A, Fujiki M, et al. Surgery for gut failure: Auto-reconstruction and allo-transplantation. In: Fazio V, Church JM, Delaney CP, Kiran RP, eds. Current Therapy in Colon and Rectal Surgery. Philadelphia, PA: Elsevier, Inc.; 2017. p. 379; with permission.)

The vascular reconstruction is technically demanding using back table and in situ techniques. The back table arterial reconstruction is required to establish a single or bifurcated arterial conduit for the allograft celiac and superior mesenteric arteries. A segment of the donor descending aorta is used for the single conduit, applying the Carrel-patch technique (**Fig. 7**). The donor common iliac artery with its external and internal arterial branches can be used for the bifurcated arterial conduit, particularly for the combined intestinal and pancreas composite visceral allograft (see **Fig. 1**).

In preparation for visceral allograft implantation, a free arterial graft using another segment of the donor descending thoracic aorta is placed on the infrarenal and, less frequently, the supraceliac native aorta (**Fig. 8**). Such a technique was introduced by the senior author to ensure an easy and safe vascular reconstruction before bringing the voluminous allograft into the operative field.[30] An interposition vein graft with proper orientation is also often needed to restore the venous drainage of the modified multivisceral and combined intestine-pancreas composite graft (see **Fig. 8**). The free common iliac donor vein graft is commonly placed on 1 of the recipient's major portal tributaries or the infrarenal vena cava. In patients who are in need of simultaneous liver replacement (liver-intestine or full multivisceral) with preservation of the native left upper quadrant organs, a permanent native portocaval shunt is created before or immediately after completion of the native hepatectomy (**Fig. 9**).

Visceral allograft implantation is initiated by the in vivo vascular reconstruction of both the arterial inflow and venous outflow of the en bloc contained organs (see **Fig. 4**). With liver-free composite allografts, including the intestine-duodenum-pancreas (combined intestine-pancreas) and stomach-duodenum-pancreas-intestine (modified multivisceral), the bifurcated or Carrel-patch arterial conduit is

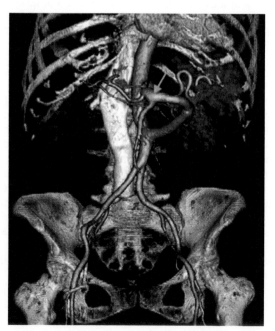

Fig. 7. A 3-dimensional reconstruction of computed tomography angiogram in a multivisceral recipient. Note the Carrel-patch reconstruction (*arrow*) that was performed on the back table containing both the celiac and superior mesenteric origin.

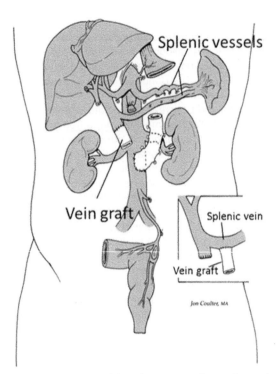

Fig. 8. Placement of interposition arterial and venous grafts on the native infrarenal aorta and the remnant stump of the native superior mesenteric vein or splenic vein, respectively. (*From* Cruz RJ, Costa G, Bond G, et al. Modified "liver-sparing" multivisceral transplant with preserved native spleen, pancreas, and duodenum: technique and long-term outcome. J Gastrointest Surg 2010;14:1714; with permission.)

anastomosed to the placed infrarenal aortic or common iliac free arterial vascular graft. The venous reconstruction is guided by the allograft type. With simultaneous hepatic replacement, the venous drainage is established by anastomosing the donor suprahepatic cava to the main confluence of the native hepatic veins because most of these patients undergo hepatectomy using the piggyback technique (see **Fig. 4**B, C). With liver-free visceral transplantation, the bifurcated vein graft (intestine-pancreas) or the retained main portal vein stump (modified multivisceral) is anastomosed to the interposition vein graft that is commonly placed on the recipient portal vein or 1 of its main tributaries (see **Fig. 8**). In a few of these liver-free allograft recipients, the venous drainage is established into the native infrarenal inferior vena cava, particularly in those with hepatic parenchymal changes and mild elevation of the portal venous pressure.[31]

The gastrointestinal reconstruction is commonly dictated by the surgical anatomy of the retained native gut organs and type of visceral allograft. Foregut reconstruction is part of the full or modified multivisceral transplantation. The residual native stomach or abdominal esophagus is anastomosed to the anterior wall of the allograft stomach with pyloroplasty or pyloromyotomy performed as a drainage procedure (see **Fig. 4**C, D). In recipients of liver-intestinal allografts and those with preserved pancreaticoduodenal complex, midgut reconstruction is required to restore continuity between the native and transplanted gut. With liver-intestinal transplant, the very

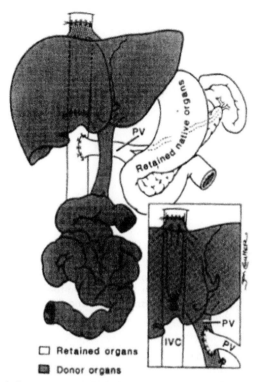

Fig. 9. Drainage of the venous outflow of the retained native viscera in liver-intestinal recipients into their inferior vena cava (IVC) by portocaval shunt. PV, portal vein. (*From* Starzl TE, Todo S, Tzakis A. The many faces of multivisceral transplantation. Surg Gynecol Obstet 1991;172(5):336; with permission.)

proximal allograft jejunum is anastomosed to the retained short segment of the native jejunum in end-to-end, end-to-side, or side-to-side fashion (**Fig. 10**). With retained native duodenum, a piggyback duodenoduodenal reconstruction is performed (see **Figs. 4**A and **6**A).

Hindgut reconstruction is commonly performed in recipients with residual colon or rectum, with creation of a diverting chimney (**Fig. 11**A) or simple loop ileostomy (**Fig. 11**B) to facilitate surveillance biopsies. In patients with pseudoobstruction, a hindgut reconstruction is still performed with total abdominal colectomy and creation of an ileosigmoid anastomosis. Patients with previous proctocolectomy who are not candidates for a pull-through operation receive a permanent allograft end ileostomy (**Fig. 11**C). Surgical closure of the temporary vents is generally performed within 6 months of transplantation, guided by the postoperative course and functional recovery of the visceral graft.

In recent years, colonic conduits were used for foregut and hindgut reconstruction. An interposition segment of the native colon is used for foregut reconstruction to reduce the number of required allograft organs (**Fig. 12**A). The donor colon was also used en bloc with the visceral allograft to restore hindgut reconstruction and eliminate the need for lifelong end ileostomy (**Fig. 12**B).With technical details described elsewhere, inclusion of the donor colon in the visceral graft improves functional outcome and quality of life when it is clinically indicated.[32]

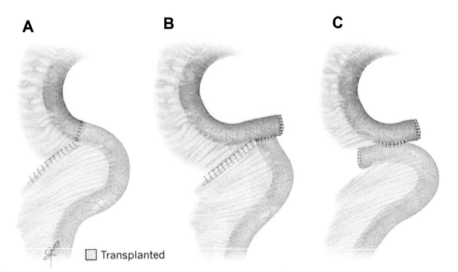

Fig. 10. Gastrointestinal reconstruction. Proximal allograft jejunum is anastomosed to the retained short segment of native jejunum in an (A) end-to-end, (B) end-to-side, or (C) side-to-side fashion. (*Reprinted with permission*, Cleveland Clinic Center for Medical Art & Photography © 2018. All Rights Reserved.)

Loss of the abdominal domain has been among the major surgical challenges in patients with short gut syndrome and complex abdominal pathologic conditions. With the morbidity and mortality commonly associated with exposed organs, several innovative surgical tactics have been introduced, including implantation of tissue expanders before transplant, use of small-for-size allografts, visceral allograft reduction, component separation techniques, myocutaneous flaps, acellular dermal allograft, synthetic mesh, and simultaneous vascularized abdominal wall or nonvascularized rectus fascia transplant.[33–37] Nonetheless, it has been the authors' experience that small-for-size allografts and judicious intraoperative fluid resuscitation allows successful primary skin closure in most recipients, without the need for immediate major abdominal wall reconstructive procedures.[28]

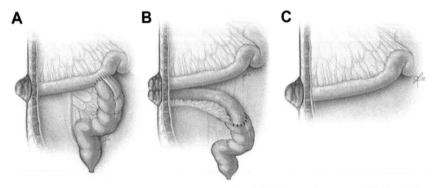

Fig. 11. Hindgut reconstruction with creation of a (A) chimney ileostomy, (B) simple loop ileostomy, or (C) end ileostomy. (*Reprinted with permission*, Cleveland Clinic Center for Medical Art & Photography © 2018. All Rights Reserved.)

A

B

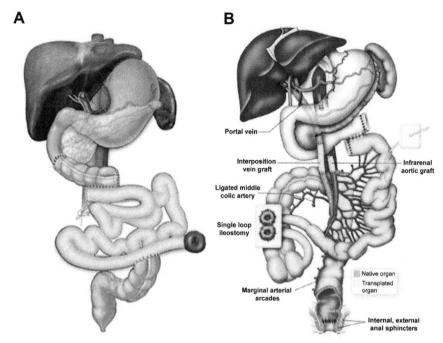

Portal vein

Interposition vein graft

Ligated middle colic artery

Single loop ileostomy

Marginal arterial arcades

Infrarenal aortic graft

Native organ
Transplanted organ

Internal, external anal sphincters

Fig. 12. (*A*) Foregut reconstruction with interposition segment of the native colon. (*B*) Hindgut pull-through reconstruction with en bloc colon and intestinal transplantation. ([*A*] *Reprinted with permission*, Cleveland Clinic Center for Medical Art & Photography © 2018. All Rights Reserved; and [*B*] *From* Hashimoto K, Costa G, Khanna A, Fujiki M, Quintini C, Abu-Elmagd K. Recent advances in intestinal and multivisceral transplantation. Adv Surg 2015;45:31–63.)

CURRENT CLINICAL PRACTICE
Indications

Visceral transplantation with different organ combinations has been successfully used for patients with gut failure due to a wide spectrum of structural and functional gastro-intestinal disorders.[11,38] It is also indicated for patients with complex abdominal pathologic conditions. According to the international Intestinal Transplant Registry and extensive single-center experience, the leading indication for visceral transplantation is short gut syndrome due to mesenteric ischemia, end-stage Crohn's disease in adults, and congenital disorders in the pediatric population.[5,38] Other common indications include global gut dysmotility, neoplastic disorders, and primary or secondary enterocyte dysfunction. Diffuse portomesenteric venous thrombosis and bariatric surgery-associated gut failure have recently emerged as infrequent indications for gut transplantation.[26]

Diffuse gastrointestinal disorders commonly dictate the need for multivisceral replacement with inclusion of the liver in those with concomitant liver failure and extensive portomesenteric venous thrombosis. Simultaneous replacement of the native liver without advanced cirrhosis or overt hepatic failure should not be entertained solely because of the biological privilege of the simultaneously transplanted liver.[5] However, replacement of a fully functioning native liver could be justified in selected patients with recurrent chronic rejection of an isolated intestinal allograft. As previously described, the recipient's native liver is given to another candidate requiring isolated liver transplantation using the well-described domino transplant procedure.[5] Different modalities of multivisceral transplantation are also used for patients who are in need of retransplantation, particularly those with a hostile abdomen. The combined en bloc intestine-pancreas transplant is required for patients with irreversible intestinal and beta cell failure. In patients with end-stage renal disease, the donor kidney is transplanted en bloc with the liver-intestine or multivisceral, and separately with the combined intestine-pancreas transplant.

In contrast to isolated intestinal transplantation, the need for or failure of PN therapy is not an essential prerequisite for some of the liver-free composite visceral allografts. In most of these patients, the indications for transplantation are commonly life-saving because of premalignant and diffuse gut disorders in the milieu of complex abdominal pathologic conditions. This is compounded by the lack of effective gut rehabilitation modalities for these complex patients.[27]

Contraindications

Significant cardiopulmonary insufficiency, incurable malignancy, persistent life-threatening intraabdominal or systemic infections, and severe immune deficiency syndromes with inability for pretransplant successful stem cell transplantation are absolute contraindications to visceral transplantation.[11,26] Lack of adequate social support has recently emerged as a relative contraindication owing to associated poor long-term survival. Accordingly, all efforts should be made to reestablish functional social support before considering transplantation.[39] The presence of long-standing, controlled neuropsychiatric disorders should not preclude transplantation as successful rehabilitation because visceral transplantation has recently been documented in both children and adults.[39] Similarly, history of gut malignancy, loss of central venous access, and older age should not be solely considered as a contraindication for transplantation.

Evaluation

All patients undergo a thorough evaluation process to assess extent of gut failure, candidacy for transplantation, type of required allograft, and presence of contraindications for transplantation. The assessment includes clinical, biochemical, radiologic, endoscopic, and histologic studies. Equally important is the thorough socioeconomic and psychiatric evaluation with the establishment of management tactics to address the underlying pathologic conditions and rescue candidacy for transplantation. Special attention should be paid to the absolute and relative transplant contraindications as previously discussed.

The cause of gut failure commonly dictates the need for special laboratory, endoscopic, and imaging studies. The innate and adaptive immune status should be evaluated in patients with hereditary or congenital disorders to assess the potential risk of graft-versus-host disease after transplantation. Pan endoscopy is performed in patients with hereditary neoplastic disorders to assess the extent of the dysplastic syndrome and coexistent malignancy. Central venous angiography of both upper and lower extremities is mandatory in patients with a history of central venous thrombosis to establish a reliable venous access plan at the time of transplant. Computerized tomography and/or standard abdominal visceral angiography is indicated for patients with history of portomesenteric venous thrombosis to assess candidacy for liver transplant alone, liver plus intestine with the technical feasibility of creating a native portocaval shunt, or multivisceral transplant with complete evisceration of the left upper quadrant abdominal organs with totally occluded splenic venous system. The surgical anatomy of the residual gastrointestinal tract, particularly of the hindgut, is radiologically and manometrically studied to assess potential candidacy for hindgut reconstruction or a pull-through operation.

Waiting List Management

The establishment of clinical guidelines for proper management of the composite and multivisceral candidates on the United Network of Organ Sharing (UNOS) waitlist has been comprehensively addressed elsewhere.[40] The complexity and dynamic nature of the clinical management of these challenging patients is emanating from the expected continual risk of PN-associated complications, including life-threatening infection, vanishing of central venous access, and progression of liver damage. Despite the periodic changes in the UNOS regulations and organ allocation, the log relative risk of mortality for liver-intestine continues to be 3-fold that of the liver-only candidates (**Fig. 13**).[40] Further development of central and portomesenteric venous thrombosis can potentially preclude or upgrade the type of required allograft, respectively. In contrast, recent advances in PN management have the potential to ameliorate cholestatic liver dysfunction and downgrade the type of required composite visceral graft with preservation of native liver.

Postoperative Care

Management of immunosuppression, monitoring of allograft function, and diagnosis with prompt treatment of recipient microbial infection are the 3 essential components of postoperative care. With the high immunogenicity of the gut allograft, concerted efforts have been made toward innovative immunosuppressive strategies.[27] One of the most important contributions has been the introduction of induction therapy and recipient preconditioning to the tacrolimus-based immunosuppression regimen.[1] The commonly used pharmacologic and biologic agents are cyclophosphamide,

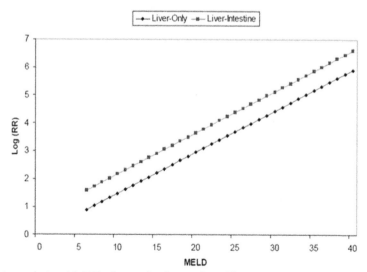

Fig. 13. Log relative risk (RR) of mortality for combined liver-intestine candidates compared with liver-only candidates on the Organ Procurement and Transplantation Network waiting list. (*From* Abu-Elmagd K. Intestinal and multivisceral transplant waiting list: clinical management according to allograft type and current organ allocation system. In: Kirk A, Knechtle S, Larsen C, editors. Textbook of organ transplantation. 1st edition. Oxford (United Kingdom): Wiley-Blackwell; 2014. p. 492; with permission.)

anti-IL-2 receptor humanized antibodies, rabbit antithymocyte globulin (rATG), and alemtuzumab. In addition, azathioprine, mycophenolate mofetil, and mammalian target of rapamycin (mTOR) inhibitors have been used as an adjunct maintenance therapy. Immunomodulatory strategies, including donor pretreatment, bone marrow augmentation, and allograft irradiation, have also been used to improve the outcome with multivisceral transplantation.[1,31,38] Interestingly, there have been no efforts among all major centers to tailor the immunosuppressive regimen according to the type of the visceral allograft, with or without inclusion of the liver. It is the authors' recommendation that future prospective studies are required to address the efficacy of different immunosuppressive protocols designed based on the type of the visceral allograft, with special reference to the liver.

Monitoring of the recipient alloimmune response and allograft functions has been the central core of postoperative care. Monitoring of graft rejection is achieved by protocol ileoscopies with multiple random intestinal biopsies and serial measurement of circulating donor-specific antibodies (DSA).[31,41] The diagnosis of acute cellular, humoral, and chronic rejection is established according to previously defined histopathologic criteria.[42,43] The diagnosis of liver rejection is suspected in patients with transaminitis and confirmed by the histopathologic examination of a Tru-Cut liver biopsy. Rejection of the pancreatic allograft is suspected in patients with significant elevation of serum amylase and lipase, without evident causes of nonimmunologic pancreatitis.

The dynamic process of graft-versus-host reaction with establishment of macrochimerism and microchimerism has been recently monitored by the serial detection of circulating donor cells in the recipient peripheral blood.[5] The diagnosis of graft-versus-host disease is confirmed by histopathologic and immunocytochemical studies that allow identification of donor leukocytes in the peripheral blood and targeted organs. The methodology includes polymerase chain reaction (PCR) techniques, in situ hybridization using Y-chromosome–specific probe, and the immunohistologic staining of donor-specific HLA antigens. In addition, the short tandem repeat technique has been more frequently used in recent years.[44]

The achievement of full nutritional autonomy has required flexible and complex management strategies. Enteric feeding is commonly initiated during the early postoperative period. In parallel, a stepwise reduction in intravenous nutrition is adopted with complete discontinuation of PN therapy within the first few weeks after transplantation. Temporary and intermittent reinstitution of PN support is often required in patients with severe allograft rejection and suboptimal nutritional status.

With cumulative clinical experience, advanced molecular diagnostic techniques, and new antimicrobial drugs, the outcome after multivisceral transplantation has substantially improved.[5] The availability of the PCR assay prompted early detection and serial monitoring of peripheral blood viremia with Epstein-Barr virus and cytomegalovirus. The introduction of new antimicrobial agents has also improved the efficacy of infection prophylaxis, preemptive therapy, and active treatment. Along with stepwise judicious reduction in maintenance immunosuppression, these developments have considerably reduced the risks of PTLD, cytomegalovirus, and fungal infections that were observed with the initial multivisceral transplant clinical experience.[5]

LONG-TERM OUTCOME

The growing global experience with visceral transplantation is a testimony of the continual improvement in the procedure's short-term and long-term efficacy over the last 3 decades. Such an achievement is a result of innovative surgical techniques, novel immunosuppressive protocols, and better postoperative management. The current results justify the recent elevation of the procedure level to that of other abdominal organs, with the privilege to permanently reside in a respected place in the surgical armamentarium.

Survival

The worldwide and largest single-center cumulative experience has repeatedly demonstrated steady improvement in 1-year and 5-year actuarial patient and allograft survival, with current rates comparable to pancreas and lung allografts (**Fig. 14**).[5,27,38] Beyond the 5-year milestone, the longest and largest single-center series documented a 10-year patient survival of 75% and 60% at 15 years with a respective graft survival of 59% and 50%.[39] Loss of graft function and complications of immunosuppression continue to be the major threat to long-term survival, with rejection, infection, and renal failure being the leading causes of death. Interestingly, the cumulative risk of infection has been significantly higher among the multivisceral recipients compared with other visceral allograft patients (**Fig. 15A**).[5] Meanwhile, the liver-free visceral allografts experienced a significantly higher risk of cumulative graft loss due to rejection (**Fig. 15B**).[5]

Several predictors of survival outcome for both patient and allograft have been recently published.[39] The lack of social support and absence of the liver as part of the composite and multivisceral grafts have emerged as highly significant risk factors for patient and graft survival, respectively (**Table 1**).[39] The immunoprotective effect of the liver can be potentially explained in the context of ameliorating the detrimental effect of DSA on the visceral allograft survival (**Fig. 16**).[41] Other important risk factors include early rejection, recipient sex and age, splenectomy, retransplantation, HLA mismatch, and type of immunosuppression, with variable weight of statistical significance.[5,39]

Graft Function

The ability to restore nutritional autonomy is the second most important indicator of successful visceral transplantation. A high rate of freedom from intravenous nutrition with

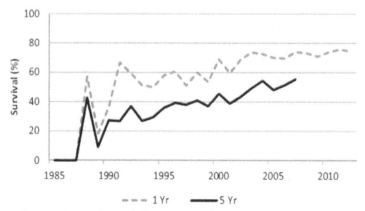

Fig. 14. A times series analysis of the 1-year and 5-year actuarial graft survival shows significant improvement over time (*P*<.001). (*From* Grant D, Abu-Elmagd K, Mazariegos G, et al. Intestinal transplant registry report: global activity and trends. Am J Transplant 2015;15:214; with permission.)

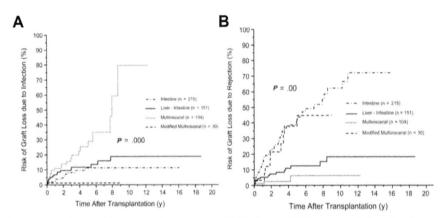

Fig. 15. Cumulative risk of graft loss due to (A) infection and (B) acute and chronic rejection according to type of visceral allograft. (*From* Abu-Elmagd KM, Costa G, Bond G, et al. Five hundred intestinal and multivisceral transplantations at a single center: major advances with new challenges. Ann Surg 2009;250:576; with permission.)

maintained nutritional status and significant improvement in body mass index has been documented in the literature (**Fig. 17**).[38,39] The adult recipients maintain normal serum albumin and trace elements with improved skeletal health (**Fig. 18**).[39] Most children experience fairly normal linear growth, with a few requiring hormonal replacement.

The failure to achieve full nutritional autonomy in a few of the composite and multi-visceral recipients is mainly due to persistent allograft dysmotility and steatorrhea resulting from allograft denervation and lymphatic disruption inherent to the transplant procedure. With the clinical availability of normothermic ex vivo perfusion technology, the unwanted effect of ischemia reperfusion could be ameliorated.[45] It is also

Table 1			
Long-term survival risk factors for visceral transplant			
Risk Factor	**P Value**	**Hazard Ratio**	**95% CI**
Patient			
Lack of social support	.000	6.132	3.370–11.160
Rejection <90 d	.016	2.363	1.172–4.765
Female recipient	.025	1.992	1.089–3.646
Recipient age >20 y	.025	2.014	1.093–3.711
Retransplantation	.026	2.053	1.089–3.873
No preconditioning	.046	2.013	1.013–4.997
Graft			
Liver-free allograft	.000	3.224	2.026–5.132
Splenectomy	.001	2.212	1.396–3.506
HLA mismatch	.040	1.258	1.011–1.565
Rejection <90 d	.046	1.601	1.008–2.541
PTLD	.085	1.638	0.934–2.872

From Abu-Elmagd K. The concept of gut rehabilitation and the future of visceral transplantation. Nat Rev Gastroenterol Hepatol 2015;12:114; with permission.

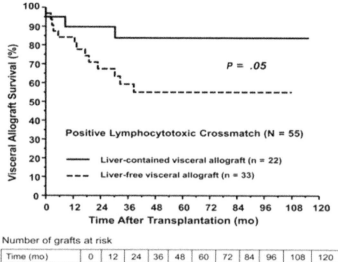

Fig. 16. The immunoprotective effect of the liver has been recently explained by ameliorating the detrimental effect of DSA on the visceral allograft survival. (*From* Abu-Elmagd KM, Wu G, Costa G, et al. Preformed and de novo donor specific antibodies in visceral transplantation: long-term outcome with special reference to the liver. Am J Transplant 2012;12:3054; with permission.)

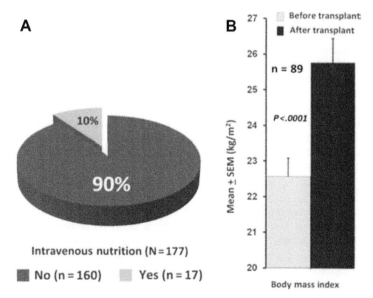

Fig. 17. Nutritional autonomy after visceral transplantation. (*A*) Achievement of enteric autonomy defined by freedom from intravenous nutrition and fluid supplement. (*B*) Body mass index before and after transplantation. (*From* Abu-Elmagd KM, Kosmach-Park B, Costa G, et al. Long-term survival, nutritional autonomy, and quality of life after intestinal and multivisceral transplantation. Ann Surg 2012;256:499; with permission.)

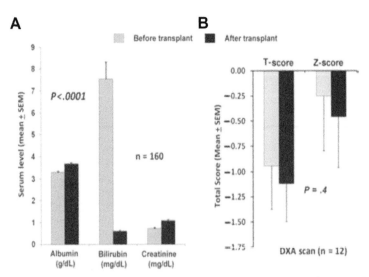

Fig. 18. (A) Physiologic biochemical measures and (B) skeletal health in a large single-center series before and after visceral transplantation. Skeletal health was measured by dual-energy x-ray absorptiometry (DXA). (*From* Abu-Elmagd KM, Kosmach-Park B, Costa G, et al. Long-term survival, nutritional autonomy, and quality of life after intestinal and multivisceral transplantation. Ann Surg 2012;256:500; with permission.)

reasonable to think that the altered allograft microbiota may play a significant role in allograft dysfunction and recipient wellbeing.

Morbidities

With long-term follow-up, multivisceral allograft recipients are at a relatively high risk of lymphoproliferative disorders and de novo malignancies.[39] Such formidable threats are most probably due to prolonged exposure to different environmental and nonenvironmental oncogenes with a foreseeable acquired state of impaired immune surveillance.[46] Impaired kidney function, glucose homeostasis, skeletal health, and cardiovascular integrity are also observed in some patients with suboptimal allograft function and chronic need for heavy maintenance immunosuppression. Regular tumor surveillance and other pertinent screening protocols have been effective in the early diagnosis and prompt management of these unique recipients, with sustained improvement in outcome and quality of life.[39]

Quality of Life

With improved survival outcome, quality of life has become among the primary therapeutic endpoints. A few scattered reports have been recently published among both children and adults.[47–58] Studies among children demonstrated physical and psychosocial functions similar to healthy normal children.[47,48] However, the parental proxy assessments were different with lower responses in certain categories than that given by children. In addition, lower values in the school functioning subcategories and psychological health summary score were reported compared with healthy children.[48] In adults, most published studies on health-related quality of life have demonstrated improvement in many of the domains, with better rehabilitative indices than PN.[39] Except for depression, successful transplantation offsets the deprived effect of both PN and disease gravity in most domains (**Fig. 19**).[39]

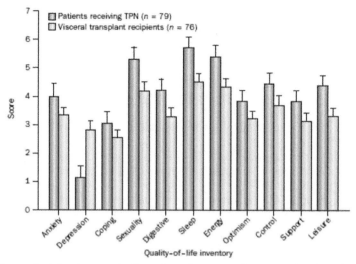

Fig. 19. Reversal of the depressed effect of total parenteral nutrition (TPN) on most quality of life domains, except depression, after visceral transplantation. (*From* Abu-Elmagd K. The concept of gut rehabilitation and the future of visceral transplantation. Nat Rev Gastroenterol Hepatol 2015;12:115; with permission.)

The socioeconomic milestones have also been used to assess the rehabilitative efficacy of visceral transplantation in all age groups.[39] A high education score was reported with sustained cognitive, psychosocial, and physical functions. In addition, the ability to create a nuclear family, along with high Lansky and Karnofsky performance scores, are demonstrated and comprehensively reported.[39] The data have also been in favor of early consideration for visceral transplantation to further improve quality of life by reducing the risk of organic brain-dysfunction–related morbidities associated with brain atrophy, cerebral vascular insufficiency, micronutrient deficiencies, trace element toxicities, and liver-failure.[59–62] Accordingly, early consideration of transplantation is strongly recommended for patients with irreversible gut failure who are not suitable candidates for autologous gut rehabilitation.

SUMMARY

Composite visceral and multivisceral transplantation continues to evolve as a life-saving therapy for patients with irreversible metabolic, parenchymal, and functional gut failure. The procedure has also been used to rescue patients with complex abdominal pathologic conditions that are not amenable to current conventional medical and surgical modalities. Despite all efforts, the field continues to face the challenges of immunologic monitoring and longevity of the liver-free visceral allografts. With new insights into the biology of gut immunity and mechanisms of transplant acceptance, the establishment of less complex postoperative care and the achievement of a drug-free allograft acceptance are within reach.

REFERENCES

1. Abu-Elmagd KM, Costa G, Bond GJ, et al. Evolution of the immunosuppressive strategies for the intestinal and multivisceral recipients with special reference to

allograft immunity and achievement of partial tolerance. Transpl Int 2009;22: 96–109.

2. Grant D, Abu-Elmagd K, Reyes J, et al. 2003 report of the intestine transplant registry: a new era has dawned. Ann Surg 2005;241:607–13.

3. Nassar A, Fujiki M, Khanna A, et al. The historic evolution of intestinal and multivisceral transplantation. In: Subramaniam K, Sakai T, editors. Anesthesia and perioperative care for organ transplantation. New York: Springer Science+Business Media LLC; 2017. p. 487–96.

4. Starzl TE. FK 506 for human liver, kidney, and pancreas transplantation. Lancet 1989;2:1000–4.

5. Abu-Elmagd KM, Costa G, Bond G, et al. Five hundred intestinal and multivisceral transplantations at a single center: major advances with new challenges. Ann Surg 2009;250:567–81.

6. Starzl TE, Kaupp HA Jr. Mass homotransplantations of abdominal organs in dogs. Surg Forum 1960;11:28–30.

7. Starzl TE, Todo S, Tzakis A, et al. The many faces of multivisceral transplantation. Surg Gynecol Obstet 1991;172:335–44.

8. Abu-Elmagd KM. Preservation of the native spleen, duodenum, and pancreas in patients with multivisceral transplantation: nomenclature, dispute of origin, and proof of premise. Transplantation 2007;84:1208–9.

9. Starzl TE, Demetris AJ, Trucco M, et al. Cell migration and chimerism after whole-organ transplantation: the basic graft acceptance. Hepatology 1993;17:1127–52.

10. Starzl TE, Zinkernagel RM. Transplantation tolerance from a historical perspective. Nat Rev Immunol 2001;1:233–9.

11. Abu-Elmagd K, Bond G, Reyes J, et al. Intestinal transplantation: a coming of age. Adv Surg 2002;36:65–101.

12. Abu-Elmagd K. Intestinal transplantation: indications and patient selection. In: Langnas AN, Goulet O, Quigley EM, et al, editors. Intestinal failure: diagnosis, management and transplantation. Malden, Massachusetts: Blackwell Publishing; 2008. p. 245–53.

13. Carrel A. La technique operatoire des anastmoses vaculaires et la transplantation des visceres. Lyon MEO 1902;98:859–64.

14. Starzl TE, Kaupp HA Jr, Brock DR, et al. Homotransplantation of multiple visceral organs. Am J Surg 1962;103:219–29.

15. Starzl TE, Miller C, Bronznik B, et al. An improved technique for multiple organ harvesting. Surg Gynecol Obstet 1987;165:343–8.

16. Starzl TE, Rowe MI, Todo S, et al. Transplantation of multiple abdominal viscera. JAMA 1989;261:1449–57.

17. Grant D, Wall W, Mimeault R, et al. Successful small-bowel/liver transplantation. Lancet 1990;335:181–4.

18. Todo S, Tzakis AG, Abu-Elmagd K, et al. Intestinal transplantation in composite visceral grafts or alone. Ann Surg 1992;216:223–34.

19. Cruz RJ, Costa G, Bond G, et al. Modified "liver-sparing" multivisceral transplant with preserved native spleen, pancreas, and duodenum: technique and long-term outcome. J Gastrointest Surg 2010;14:1709–21.

20. Cruz RJ, Costa G, Bond GJ, et al. Modified multivisceral transplantation with spleen-preserving pancreaticoduodenectomy for patients with familial adenomatous polyposis "Gardner's syndrome". Transplantation 2011;91:1417–23.

21. Fujiki M, Hashimoto H, Khanna A, et al. Technical innovation and visceral transplantation. In: Subramaniam K, Sakai T, editors. Anesthesia and perioperative care for organ transplantation. New York: Springer; 2017. p. 497–511.

22. Abu-Elmagd KM. The small bowel contained allografts: existing and proposed nomenclature. Am J Transplant 2011;11:184–5.
23. Nickkholgh A, Contin P, Abu-Elmagd K, et al. Intestinal transplantation: review of operative techniques. Clin Transpl 2013;27:56–65.
24. Abu-Elmagd K, Reyes J, Fung JJ. Clinical intestinal transplantation: recent advances and future consideration. In: Norman DJ, Turka LA, editors. Primer on transplantation. 2nd edition. Mt Laurel (NJ): American Society of Transplantation; 2001. p. 610–25.
25. Garcia-Roca R, Tzvetanov IG, Jeon H, et al. Successful living donor intestinal transplantation in cross-match positive recipients: initial experience. World J Gastrointest Surg 2016;8:101–5.
26. Abu-Elmagd K, Khanna A, Fujiki M, et al. Surgery for gut failure: autoreconstruction and allo-transplantation. In: Fazio V, Church JM, Delaney CP, et al, editors. Current therapy in colon and rectal surgery. Philadelphia: Elsevier, Inc; 2017. p. 372–84.
27. Abu-Elmagd K. The concept of gut rehabilitation and the future of visceral transplantation. Nat Rev Gastroenterol Hepatol 2015;12:108–20.
28. Hashimoto K, Costa G, Khanna A, et al. Recent advances in intestinal and multivisceral transplantation. Adv Surg 2015;49:31–63.
29. Abu-Elmagd K, Reyes J, Todo S, et al. Clinical intestinal transplantation: new perspectives and immunologic considerations. J Am Coll Surg 1998;186:512–27.
30. Abu-Elmagd K, Fung J, Bueno J, et al. Logistics and technique for procurement of intestinal, pancreatic and hepatic grafts from the same donor. Ann Surg 2000; 232:680–7.
31. Abu-Elmagd K, Reyes J, Bond G, et al. Clinical intestinal transplantation: a decade of experience at a single center. Ann Surg 2001;234:404–16.
32. Eid KR, Costa G, Bond GJ, et al. An innovative sphincter preserving pull-through technique with en bloc colon and small bowel transplantation. Am J Transplant 2010;10:1940–6.
33. Carlsen BT, Farmer DG, Busuttil RW, et al. Incidence and management of abdominal wall defects after intestinal and multivisceral transplantation. Plast Reconstr Surg 2007;119:1247–55.
34. Mangus RS, Kubal CA, Tector AJ, et al. Closure of the abdominal wall with acellular dermal allograft in intestinal transplantation. Am J Transplant 2012;12:S55–9.
35. Watson MJ, Kundu N, Coppa C, et al. Role of tissue expanders in patients with loss of abdominal domain awaiting intestinal transplantation. Transpl Int 2013; 26:1184–90.
36. Gondolesi G, Selvaggi G, Tzakis A, et al. Use of the abdominal rectus fascia as a nonvascularized allograft for abdominal wall closure after liver, intestinal, and multivisceral transplantation. Transplantation 2009;87:1884–8.
37. Levi DM, Tzakis AG, Kato T, et al. Transplantation of the abdominal wall. Lancet 2003;361:2173–6.
38. Grant D, Abu-Elmagd K, Masariegos G, et al. Intestinal transplant registry report: global activity and trends. Am J Transplant 2015;15:210–9.
39. Abu-Elmagd KM, Kosmach-Park B, Costa G, et al. Long-term survival, nutritional autonomy, and quality of life after intestinal and multivisceral transplantation. Ann Surg 2012;256:494–508.
40. Abu-Elmagd K. Intestinal and multivisceral transplant waiting list: clinical management according to allograft type and current organ allocation system. In: Kirk A, Knechtle S, Larsen C, editors. Textbook of organ transplantation. 1st edition. Oxford (United Kingdom): Wiley-Blackwell; 2014. p. 489–94.

41. Abu-Elmagd KM, Wu G, Costa G, et al. Preformed and de novo donor specific antibodies in visceral transplantation: long-term outcome with special reference to the liver. Am J Transplant 2012;12:3047–360.
42. Lee RG, Nakamura K, Tsamandas AC, et al. Pathology of human intestinal transplantation. Gastroenterology 1996;110:2009–12.
43. Wu T, Abu-Elmagd K, Bond G, et al. A clinicopathologic study of isolated intestinal allografts with preformed IgG lymphocytotoxic antibodies. Hum Pathol 2004; 35:1332–9.
44. Thiede C, Bornhauser M, Oelschlagel U, et al. Sequential monitoring of chimerism and detection of minimal residual disease after allogeneic blood stem cell transplantation (BSCT) using multiplex PCR amplification of short tandem repeat markers. Leukemia 2001;15:293–302.
45. Boehnert MU, Yeung JC, Bazerbachi F, et al. Normothermic acelluar ex vivo perfusion reduces liver and bile duct injury of pig livers retrieved after cardiac death. Am J Transplant 2013;13:1441–9.
46. Abu-Elmagd KM, Mazariegos G, Costa G, et al. Lymphoproliferative disorders and de novo malignancies in intestinal and multivisceral recipients: improved outcomes with new outlooks. Transplantation 2009;88:926–34.
47. Sudan D, Iyer K, Horslen S, et al. Assessment of quality of life after pediatric intestinal transplantation by parents and pediatric recipients using the child health questionnaire. Transplant Proc 2002;34:963–4.
48. Ngo KD, Farmer DG, McDiarmid SV, et al. Pediatric health-related quality of life after intestinal transplantation. Pediatr Transplant 2011;15:849–54.
49. DiMartini A, Rovera GM, Graham TO, et al. Quality of life after small intestinal transplantation and among home parenteral nutrition patients. JPEN J Parenter Enteral Nutr 1998;22:357–62.
50. Rovera GM, DiMartini A, Schoen RE, et al. Quality of life of patients after intestinal transplantation. Transplantation 1998;66:1141–5.
51. Rovera GM, DiMartini A, Graham TO, et al. Quality of life after intestinal transplantation and on total parenteral nutrition. Transplant Proc 1998;30:2513–4.
52. Stenn PG, Lammens P, Houle L, et al. Psychiatric psychosocial and ethical aspects of small bowel transplantation. Transplant Proc 1992;24:1251–2.
53. Cameron EA, Binnie JA, Jamieson NV, et al. Quality of life in adults following small bowel transplantation. Transplant Proc 2002;34:965–6.
54. Pironi L, Paganelli F, Lauro A, et al. Quality of life on home parenteral nutrition or after intestinal transplantation. Transplant Proc 2006;38:1673–5.
55. Sudan DL, Iverson A, Weseman RA, et al. Assessment of function, growth and development, and long-term quality of life after small bowel transplantation. Transplant Proc 2000;32:1211–2.
56. Golfieri L, Lauro A, Tossani E, et al. Psychological adaptation and quality of life of adult intestinal transplant recipients: University of Bologna experience. Transplant Proc 2010;42:42–4.
57. O'Keefe SJ, Emerling M, Koritsky D, et al. Nutrition and quality of life following small intestinal transplantation. Am J Gastroenterol 2007;102:1093–100.
58. Pironi L, Baxter JP, Lauro A, et al. Assessment of quality of life on home parenteral nutrition and after intestinal transplantation using treatment-specific questionnaires. Am J Transplant 2012;12:S60–6.
59. Idoate MA, Martinez AJ, Bueno J, et al. The neuropathology of intestinal failure and small bowel transplantation. Acta Neuropathol 1999;97:502–8.
60. Dekaban AS. Changes in brain weights during the span of human life: relation of brain weights to body heights and body weights. Ann Neurol 1978;4:345–56.

61. El-Tatawy S, Badrawi N, El Bishlawy A. Cerebral atrophy in infants with protein energy malnutrition. AJNR Am J Neuroradiol 1983;4:434–6.
62. Kawakubo K, Iida M, Matsumoto T, et al. Progressive encephalopathy in a Crohn's disease patient on long-term total parenteral nutrition: possible relationship to selenium deficiency. Postgrad Med J 1994;70:215–9.

Pancreas Transplantation for Patients with Type 1 and Type 2 Diabetes Mellitus in the United States: A Registry Report

Angelika C. Gruessner, MS, PhD[a],*, Rainer W.G. Gruessner, MD[b]

KEYWORDS

- Pancreas transplantation • Patient survival • Graft function • Technical failure
- Immunologic graft loss • Type 1 diabetes • Type 2 diabetes

KEY POINTS

- The registry shows improvement in patient survival and graft function.
- Trends show an increase in older recipients.
- Trends show an increase of younger donors.

Diabetes is a pandemic disease of the modern era. In the United States, 30.3 million people have diabetes, which represents 9.4% of the population. Type 1 diabetes makes up between 5% and 10% of those cases.[1] Diabetes is the seventh leading cause of death in the United States and it is among the main reasons for cardiovascular disease, stroke, amputation, and endstage renal disease. Despite the prevalence, morbidities, and the associated financial burden, treatment options have not changed very much since the introduction of injectable insulin. For patients who are not successfully treated with conservative insulin therapy and who developed brittle diabetes, a treatment option is pancreas transplantation.

From December16, 1966 to December 31, 2016, more than 50,000 worldwide and more than 30,000 pancreas transplants in the United States were reported to the International Pancreas Transplant Registry. Since the first transplant, tremendous progress was made in patient and graft survival. Pancreas transplantation is still the only method to achieve long-term insulin-independence and euglycemia. However, although the numbers increased steadily until 2004, the number of pancreas transplants then declined significantly (**Fig. 1**). This article analyses developments in pancreas transplantation in the United States between 2001 and 2016. This time

[a] Department of Nephrology, SUNY Downstate Medical Center, 450 Clarkson Avenue, MSC 40, Brooklyn, NY 11203, USA; [b] Department of Surgery, SUNY Downstate Medical Center, 450 Clarkson Avenue, MSC 40, Brooklyn, NY 11203, USA
* Corresponding author.
E-mail address: Angelika.Gruessner@Downstate.edu

Gastroenterol Clin N Am 47 (2018) 417–441
https://doi.org/10.1016/j.gtc.2018.01.009
0889-8553/18/Published by Elsevier Inc.

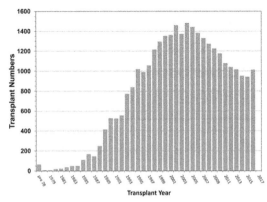

Fig. 1. Annual number of US pancreas transplants reported to IPTR/UNOS from 1966 to 2016.

period encompasses the peak of pancreas transplantation (2001–2005), the period of decline (2006–2010), and the period of slight recuperation (2011–2016). An overview of changes in patient and donor characteristics and outcome is given.

METHODS

All 16,419 patients with type 1 and type 2 diabetes mellitus who received a primary pancreas and/or pancreas and kidney transplant are included in this study. During this time, a total of 13 living donor pancreas transplants were performed (9 simultaneous pancreas and kidney [SPK], 1 pancreas after kidney [PAK], and 3 pancreas transplant alone [PTA]), which are were excluded from this study. All patients had a follow-up time of at least 6-months posttransplant.

Pancreas graft function was defined as complete insulin-independence. Partial function or dying with a functioning graft was counted as failure when not mentioned otherwise. Kidney graft failure was defined as being back on dialysis or dying with a functioning graft.

To measure the impact of risk factors on immunologic failure, only technically successful transplants were analyzed. Technical failures were primarily defined as early graft thrombosis or graft removal due to bleeding, anastomotic leaks, pancreatitis, or infections.

The impact on center volume was measured by defining low-volume, medium-volume, and high-volume centers. This was achieved by counting the number of transplants per center from 2001 to 2005 and defining the tertiles of these counts. A low-volume center performed a maximum of 14 and a high-volume center performed at least 40 transplants during a 5-year period.

A wide range of different antibody induction regimens were noted. For analyses, induction therapy was defined as the use of depleting (eg, rabbit antithymocyte globulin, alemtuzumab, anti-thymocyte globulin [equine]) and/or nondepleting (daclizumab, basiliximab) antibodies.

For maintenance therapy, a multitude of different drugs and combinations were recorded. The analyses focused on the most commonly used combinations of tacrolimus (Tac) in combination with mycophenolate mofetil (MMF) with or without steroids. Another category was protocols, which were based on sirolimus (Srl) in combination with other drugs. All the other possible combinations of monotherapy, duotherapy, or Cyclosporin A-based therapy (CsA), which represented only a very small percentage, were combined in a category called Other.

Patient survival and graft function were computed using the Kaplan-Meier method. Different time periods or groups were compared with the log-rank test using equal follow-up times (3 years). *P*-values for pairwise comparisons were corrected according to the Šidák correction.

Cox proportional and nonproportional hazard models were applied to compute adjusted survival and graft function rates, and to investigate the independent influence of risk factors. Time-dependent covariates were added for specific estimation of patient and graft survival. All statistics were obtained using the statistical analysis system, SAS 9.4 (SAS Institute, CARY, NC, USA).

RESULTS

The number of primary pancreas transplants from deceased donors declined from 6046 from 2001 to 2005, to 5214 from 2006 to 2010, and to 5159 from 2011 to 2016. The average number of transplants declined, therefore, from approximately 1200 down to 860 primary transplants per year.

Table 1 shows the development of recipient characteristics over the analyzed time. Relatively more SPK than solitary transplants were performed over time. From 2011 to 2016, 84% of all pancreas transplants in the diabetic population were SPK. Although the number of PTA remained relatively stable, a drop of 70% in PAK was noted.

Most recipients had type 1 diabetics but the number of recipients with type 2 diabetes increased significantly in SPK but declined in PTA over time. The age distribution changed in all 3 categories over time. There was a trend to accept older recipients, especially for solitary transplants. From 2011 to 2016, a significant age difference between solitary and SPK recipients was found; SPK recipients on average were younger. The 2 oldest patients at the time of transplant were each 71 years of age; 1 received an SPK and the other a PAK.

The rate of male recipients remained significantly higher in uremic SPK and posturemic PAK compared with PTA in which most were female recipients.

Most recipients were of white race but a shift over time was noted. An increasing number of black and Hispanic patients received an SPK or a PAK. In PTA, most patients were white. The change to more black patients in SPK was also due to the increase of type 2 diabetic recipients. The rate of black patients with type 2 diabetes getting a pancreas transplant was significantly higher compared with black patients getting the transplant for type 1.

Over time, the body weight of the recipients followed the national trend: the number of overweight or obese recipients increased significantly. From 2011 to 2016, 50% or more of the recipients were overweight or obese at the time of transplant.

The rate of sensitized recipients increased in all 3 categories over time. From 2011 to 2016 this accounted for 15% to 22% of all recipients.

The distribution of the different blood groups remained stable in solitary transplants. However, in SPK a slight shift to an increased number of transplants in patients with blood type O from 45% to 48% was noted.

The wait time between listing and transplant remained stable for PTA, with a median of 144 days from 2011 to 2016. The time on the waitlist decreased for SPK from a median of 536 days from 2001 to 2005, to 495 days from 2006 to 2010. No further decline was noted from the years 2006 to 2010 to the years 2011 to 2016 for SPK. In contrast, the wait time in PAK increased significantly from 183 days from 2001 to 2005, to up to 366 days from 2011 to 2016.

Over the analyzed time, the donor factors changed significantly (**Table 2**). A significant trend to younger donors was detected in all 3 categories. From 2011 to 2016, the

Table 1
Transplant recipient characteristics for primary deceased donor pancreas transplants performed from 2001 to 2005, 2006 to 2010, and 2011 to 2016

	SPK				PAK				PTA			
	2001–2005	2006–2009	2011–2016	P	2001–2005	2006–2009	2011–2016	P	2001–2005	2006–2009	2011–2016	P
# Primary Tx (%)	4192 (69)	4009 (77)	4342 (84)	—	1321 (22)	770 (15)	399 (8)	—	533 (9)	435 (8)	418 (8)	—
Diabetes												
Type1	3870 (92)	3699 (92)	3838 (88)	<.0001	1255 (95)	740 (96)	371 (93)	.07	508 (95)	426 (98)	412 (99)	.006
Type2	322 (8)	310 (8)	504 (12)		66 (5)	30 (4)	28 (7)		25 (5)	9 (2)	6 (1)	
Recipient Age (y)												
<18	2 (0)	0 (0)	1 (0)	<.0001	1 (0)	0 (0)	0 (0)	.0002	2 (0)	2 (0)	0 (0)	.011
18–29	332 (8)	302 (8)	264 (6)		72 (5)	42 (5)	24 (6)		64 (12)	61 (14)	45 (11)	
30–44	2490 (59)	2166 (54)	2453 (57)		779 (59)	384 (50)	203 (51)		276 (52)	203 (47)	171 (41)	
45–59	1325 (32)	1484 (37)	1560 (36)		458 (35)	324 (42)	160 (40)		175 (33)	153 (35)	180 (43)	
>60	43 (1)	57 (1)	64 (1)		11 (1)	20 (3)	12 (3)		16 (3)	16 (4)	22 (5)	
Gender												
Male	2588 (62)	2517 (63)	2719 (63)	.57	782 (59)	452 (59)	245 (61)	.66	206 (39)	178 (41)	158 (38)	.62
Race												
White	3165 (76)	2841 (71)	2582 (59)	<.0001	1111 (84)	647 (84)	288 (72)	<.0001	509 (96)	409 (94)	381 (92)	.07
Black	601 (14)	673 (17)	995 (23)		108 (8)	57 (7)	47 (12)		8 (2)	17 (4)	17 (4)	
Hispanic	343 (8)	392 (10)	594 (14)		83 (6)	59 (8)	52 (13)		12 (2)	8 (2)	18 (4)	
Asian	45 (1)	52 (1)	102 (2)		8 (1)	5 (1)	3 (1)		1 (0)	0 (0)	1 (0)	
Multiracial or Other	38 (1)	51 (1)	69 (2)		11 (1)	2 (0)	9 (2)		3 (0)	1 (0)	1 (0)	

Body Mass Index												
<18.5 (underweight)	100 (2)	75 (2)	75 (2)	<.0001	37 (3)	11 (1)	12 (3)	.02	13 (2)	8 (2)	5 (1)	.03
18.5–24.9 (normal)	2,233 (54)	1,989 (500)	2,098 (480)		654 (50)	349 (46)	173 (43)		251 (48)	203 (48)	162 (39)	
25–29.9 (overweight)	1349 (33)	1427 (36)	1663 (38)		446 (34)	300 (39)	148 (37)		199 (38)	157 (37)	179 (43)	
>30 (obese)	456 (11)	510 (13)	506 (12)		166 (13)	104 (14)	66 (17)		63 (12)	57 (13)	72 (17)	
Missing	54	8	0		18	6	0		7	10	0	
Recent PRA%												
0–19	3544 (94)	3567 (91)	3687 (85)	<.0001	1149 (96)	672 (90)	322 (81)	<.0001	437 (91)	328 (78)	328 (78)	<.0001
>20	208 (6)	364 (9)	469 (15)		52 (4)	74 (10)	77 (19)		52 (12)	90 (22)	90 (22)	
Missing	440	78	0		120	24	0		7	0	0	
Blood Group												
A	1628 (39)	1451 (36)	1541 (35)	.06	525 (40)	310 (40)	168 (42)	.42	220 (41)	200 (46)	171 (41)	.31
B	486 (12)	497 (12)	536 (12)		171 (13)	78 (10)	47 (12)		54 (10)	36 (10)	47 (11)	
AB	171 (4)	179 (4)	186 (4)		61 (4)	29 (4)	15 (4)		19 (4)	21 (5)	12 (3)	
O	1907 (45)	1882 (47)	2079 (48)		564 (43)	353 (46)	169 (42)		240 (45)	178 (41)	188 (45)	
Time to Tx (d)												
0<30	350 (8)	373 (9)	424 (10)	<.0001	166 (13)	62 (8)	30 (7)	<.0001	94 (18)	76 (18)	71 (17)	.32
30<180	1139 (27)	1279 (32)	1413 (33)		482 (36)	219 (28)	82 (21)		241 (45)	191 (44)	165 (40)	
180<360	957 (23)	920 (23)	919 (21)		293 (22)	181 (24)	83 (21)		93 (17)	93 (22)	93 (22)	
≥360	1746 (42)	1437 (36)	1586 (36)		380 (29)	308 (40)	204 (51)		105 (20)	89 (21)	89 (21)	

Abbreviatios: #, number; PRA, Panel reactivity assay; Tx, Transplant.

Table 2
Donor characteristics for primary deceased donor pancreas transplants performed from 2001 to 2005, 2006 to 2010, and 2011 to 2016

	SPK				PAK				PTA			
	2001–2005	2006–2009	2011–2016	P	2001–2005	2006–2009	2011–2016	P	2001–2005	2006–2009	2011–2016	P
# Primary Tx (%)	4,192 (69)	4009 (77)	4342 (84)	—	1321 (22)	770 (15)	399 (8)	—	533 (9)	435 (8)	418 (8)	—
Donor Age (y)												
<15	425 (10)	377 (9)	452 (10)	<.0001	167 (19)	70 (9)	62 (9)	<.0001	64 (12)	45 (10)	64 (15)	.0007
16–30	2407 (57)	2544 (63)	2961 (68)		793 (60)	533 (69)	270 (68)		313 (59)	287 (66)	282 (68)	
31–45	1078 (26)	918 (23)	837 (19)		300 (23)	142 (18)	63 (16)		124 (23)	82 (19)	62 (15)	
>45	282 (8)	170 (4)	92 (2)		61 (5)	25 (3)	4 (1)		32 (6)	21 (5)	10 (2)	
Donor Gender												
Male	2864 (68)	2747 (69)	3040 (70)	.18	915 (69)	534 (69)	294 (74)	.21	345 (65)	293 (67)	274 (66)	.68
Donor Race												
White	2958 (71)	2540 (63)	2671 (62)	<.0001	969 (73)	495 (64)	239 (60)	<.0001	394 (74)	300 (69)	275 (66)	.01
Black	573 (14)	750 (19)	852 (20)		145 (11)	124 (16)	74 (18)		54 (10)	64 (15)	75 (18)	
Hispanic	559 (13)	596 (15)	609 (14)		171 (13)	130 (17)	66 (12)		66 (12)	62 (14)	56 (13)	
Asian	62 (1)	75 (2)	94 (2)		19 (1)	15 (2)	11 (3)		6 (1)	4 (1)	8 (2)	
Multiracial or Other	40 (1)	48 (1)	116 (3)		17 (1)	6 (1)	9 (2)		13 (2)	5 (1)	4 (0)	
Donor Cause of Death												
Trauma	3139 (76)	3078 (78)	3410 (80)	<.0001	1001 (77)	589 (78)	304 (78)	.64	392 (75)	319 (75)	308 (76)	.25
CCV	976 (24)	845 (21)	856 (20)		295 (23)	166 (22)	86 (22)		126 (24)	106 (25)	89 (22)	
CNS Tumor	27 (0)	22 (1)	9 (0)		7 (1)	1 (0)	1 (0)		7 (1)	1 (0)	7 (2)	
Missing	2	4	4		18	8	8		8	9	16	
DCD Donor	55 (1)	129 (3)	113 (3)	<.0001	7 (1)	8 (1)	1 (0)	.21	10 (2)	12 (3)	13 (3)	.45

				p				p				p
Donor Body Mass Index												
<18.5 (underweight)	264 (6)	233 (6)	281 (6)	.07	81 (6)	34 (4)	27 (7)	.0007	37 (7)	26 (6)	39 (9)	.002
18.5–24.9 (normal)	2411 (58)	2301 (57)	2492 (58)		752 (57)	430 (56)	243 (61)		243 (61)	254 (59)	255 (61)	
25–29.9 (overweight)	1168 (28)	1169 (29)	1277 (29)		382 (29)	261 (34)	113 (28)		113 (28)	129 (30)	111 (27)	
>30 (obese)	347 (8)	302 (8)	288 (7)		106 (8)	45 (6)	16 (4)		16 (4)	25 (6)	12 (3)	
Missing	14	15	260		0	0	0		0	1	1	
HLA A, B, DR MM												
0	77 (2)	27 (1)	16 (0)	<.0001	19 (1)	4 (1)	1 (0)	<.0001	8 (2)	4 (1)	4 (1)	<.0001
1	55 (1)	13 (0)	23 (1)		33 (3)	14 (2)	5 (1)		26 (5)	9 (2)	6 (1)	
2	133 (3)	134 (3)	128 (3)		102 (8)	22 (3)	20 (5)		56 (11)	22 (5)	30 (7)	
3	556 (13)	481 (13)	520 (12)		235 (18)	121 (16)	54 (14)		125 (23)	70 (16)	72 (17)	
4	1071 (26)	1001 (25)	1170 (27)		361 (27)	198 (26)	105 (26)		112 (21)	113 (26)	104 (25)	
5	1457 (35)	1443 (36)	1527 (35)		360 (27)	267 (35)	147 (37)		131 (25)	136 (31)	120 (29)	
6	841 (20)	910 (23)	958 (22)		209 (16)	144 (19)	67 (17)		75 (14)	81 (19)	82 (19)	
Rec/Dnr CMV Status												
−/−	886 (23)	778 (21)	833 (20)	<.0001	257 (21)	137 (19)	66 (15)	.27	119 (24)	114 (28)	94 (23)	.04
−/+	1176 (30)	1,99 (32)	1168 (27)		309 (26)	211 (29)	101 (26)		153 (30)	109 (26)	148 (36)	
+/−	738 (19)	666 (18)	864 (20)		259 (22)	144 (20)	92 (24)		106 (21)	87 (21)	63 (15)	
+/+	1115 (28)	1148 (30)	1393 (33)		377 (31)	233 (32)	199 (33)		127 (25)	101 (25)	105 (26)	
Missing	227	218	84		119	45	11		28	8	8	

median donor age for solitary transplants was 21 years, for SPK it was 23 years. Only 25% of donors were older than 29 years of age during this time but older donors were still used. The oldest SPK donor was 72 years of age, the oldest solitary pancreas donor was 58 year old.

Most pancreas donors were white but over time the number of black and Hispanic donors increased significantly in all 3 categories. For most pancreas donors the cause of death was related to traumatic accidents. The rate remained stable in solitary transplants but increased significantly in SPK over time. More than three-quarters of donors had trauma reported as cause of death. Donation after circulatory death (DCD) donors are only very rarely used in pancreas transplantation and make up less than 3% of all transplants. The number of DCD donors is higher for SPK but very low in solitary transplants. Male donors were used significantly more frequently than female donors. This was because the rate of accidental death was significantly higher in male donors.

The importance of HLA antigen matching decreased over time. From 2011 to 2016, 57% of all SPK had a 5 or 6 antigen mismatch and the same trend was seen in PAK. Historically, in PTA, more emphasis was put on matching but the trend was also to less emphasis on matching. From 2011 to 2016, 48% of all PTA were performed with a 5 or 6 antigen mismatch.

The cytomegalovirus (CMV) status between donor and recipient changed significantly over time. In SPK and PAK more CMV-positive recipients received a pancreas transplant. In PTA, the rate of CMV-positive recipients went slightly down. The rate of CMV-positive donors accepted for transplantation did not change over time.

With the overall decline in the number of transplants, the distribution of transplants performed by low-volume, medium-volume, or high-volume centers changed in all 3 categories (**Table 3**). Fewer transplants were performed at high-volume centers over time. This was because the centers that were high-volume in the beginning became medium-volume centers. PTA was the transplant type that was mostly performed at high-volume centers and only very few PTA were reported from low-volume centers.

With the drop in transplant numbers, the preservation time in all 3 categories decreased significantly. From 2011 to 2016, the reported preservation time in greater than 50% of transplants was less than 12 hours. This trend to shorter preservation times was transplants highly significant, especially in SPK.

The use of bladder drainage for the management of the pancreatic duct decreased significantly in all 3 categories and was used in less than 10% of all transplants from 2011 to 2016. In most transplants, enteric drainage was used and duct injection was only occasionally chosen. In enteric-drained transplants, systemic venous drainage was the most common, whereas drainage into the portal vein declined, especially in solitary transplants.

Over time, more and more induction therapy was used in all 3 categories. The trend for using depleting antibody therapy increased significantly and made up greater than 80% of all cases from 2011 to 2016. Fewer and fewer nondepleting antibodies were used, and the combination of depleting and nondepleting antibodies became less common over time.

Most maintenance immunosuppressive protocols were based on tacrolimus in combination with MMF. From 2011 to 2016, greater than 90% of this combination was used in SPK and PAK; only in PTA was the rate lower. The promise of sirolimus-based protocol has not been kept and the rate declined in all 3 categories over time. The overall use of steroid free maintenance protocols increased in all 3 categories from 20% to 32% over time. The steroid-free protocol was most frequently used in combination with tacrolimus and MMF. All other drug combinations with

Table 3
Transplant characteristics for primary deceased donor pancreas transplants performed from 2001 to 2005, 2006 to 2010, and 2011 to 2016

Transplant Year	SPK 2001-2005	SPK 2006-2009	SPK 2011-2016	SPK P	PAK 2001-2005	PAK 2006-2009	PAK 2011-2016	PAK P	PTA 2001-2005	PTA 2006-2009	PTA 2011-2016	PTA P
# Primary Tx (%)	4192 (69)	4009 (77)	4342 (84)	—	1321 (22)	770 (15)	399 (8)	—	533 (9)	435 (8)	418 (8)	—
Tx Center Volume												
Low	239 (6)	215 (5)	274 (6)	<.0001	63 (5)	84 (11)	49 (12)	<.0001	10 (2)	7 (2)	22 (5)	<.0001
Medium	858 (20)	985 (25)	1030 (24)		329 (25)	193 (25)	114 (29)		49 (9)	84 (19)	58 (14)	
Large	3095 (74)	2809 (70)	2073 (70)		929 (70)	493 (64)	236 (59)		474 (89)	344 (79)	338 (81)	
Preservation Time (h)												
0-12	1491 (46)	2009 (65)	2705 (65)	<.0001	382 (37)	376 (54)	227 (59)	<.0001	117 (28)	205 (53)	218 (54)	<.0001
12-23	1636 (50)	1479 (41)	1374 (33)		610 (58)	306 (44)	150 (40)		283 (67)	175 (45)	184 (45)	
>24	132 (4)	102 (3)	76 (2)		51 (5)	12 (2)	2 (1)		25 (6)	7 (2)	4 (1)	
Missing	993	419	187		278	76	20		108	48	12	
Duct Management												
Enteric Drainage	3464 (85)	3548 (91)	3938 (92)	<.0001	967 (74)	639 (85)	357 (91)	<.0001	346 (66)	337 (79)	376 (91)	<.0001
Bladder Drainage	611 (15)	318 (8)	322 (8)		339 (26)	98 (13)	28 (7)		172 (33)	89 (21)	35 (9)	
Duct Injection	24 (0)	40 (1)	10 (0)		4 (0)	18 (2)	9 (2)		5 (1)	1 (0)	0 (0)	
Missing	93	103	72		11	15	5		10	8	7	

(continued on next page)

Table 3
(continued)

Transplant Year	SPK				PAK				PTA			
	2001–2005	2006–2009	2011–2016	P	2001–2005	2006–2009	2011–2016	P	2001–2005	2006–2009	2011–2016	P
Venous Management (ED Txs)												
Systemic Drainage	2731 (79)	2837 (80)	3140 (80)	.03	780 (81)	535 (84)	328 (92)	<.0001	257 (74)	298 (88)	336 (89)	<.0001
Portal Drainage	733 (21)	711 (20)	798 (20)		187 (19)	105 (16)	29 (8)		89 (26)	41 (12)	40 (11)	
Induction Therapy				<.0001				<.0001				<.0001
None	953 (23)	625 (16)	423 (10)		285 (22)	152 (20)	38 (10)		93 (18)	52 (12)	27 (7)	
Nondepleting AB	1019 (25)	414 (10)	308 (7)		177 (14)	68 (9)	16 (4)		33 (6)	26 (6)	21 (5)	
Depleting AB	1999 (48)	2770 (71)	3405 (80)		718 (55)	515 (69)	331 (85)		306 (59)	335 (80)	346 (86)	
Both	175 (4)	108 (3)	133 (3)		120 (9)	7 (1)	4 (1)		85 (16)	6 (1)	9 (2)	
Missing	46	92	73		21	28	10		16	16	15	
Maintenance Protocol				<.0001				<.0001				<.0001
Tac&MMF	230 (6)	880 (23)	1041 (25)		74 (7)	228 (31)	111 (29)		42 (8)	316 (34)	123 (31)	
Tac&MMF&Steroids	2598 (63)	2421 (62)	2854 (67)		735 (57)	362 (49)	238 (61)		281 (55)	156 (39)	203 (52)	
Srl-Based	372 (9)	277 (7)	150 (4)		69 (5)	55 (7)	18 (5)		56 (11)	74 (18)	51 (13)	
Srl-Based& Steroids	374 (9)	94 (2)	19 (0)		159 (12)	35 (7)	0 (0)		35 (7)	11 (3)	2 (0)	
Other	554 (13)	219 (6)	190 (4)		236 (18)	94 (19)	21 (5)		94 (19)	28 (7)	17 (4)	
Missing	74	118	78		28	25	11		25	30	22	

CsA and AZA were used less and less over time, and make up only a very small percentage of protocols.

OUTCOME
Patient Survival

The outcomes of pancreas transplantation improved significantly over time. Patient survival improved significantly at 1-year (3-year) posttransplant for SPK from 95.2% (91.0%) in 2001 to 2005 (91.0%), to 97.6% (94.6%) in 2011 to 2016 (**Fig. 2**A). Ten-year patient survival reached 71.6% for transplants performed from 2001 to 2005. The improvement was significant from time period to time period ($P<.008$).

For PAK, the improvement in patient survival occurred between the periods of 2001 to 2005 and 2006 to 2010 (**Fig. 2**B) and only there a significant improvement in patient survival was detected ($P = .05$). PAK patient survival at 10 years was 64.8% for transplants between 2001 and 2005.

PTA patient survival was the highest in the 3 categories (**Fig. 2**C). The improvement in patient survival was noted for transplants between the periods of 2001 to 2010 and 2011 to 2016. The increase in PTA patient survival between the time periods did not reach significance ($P = .11$). PTA patient survival at 10 years reached 72.3% for transplants from 2001 to 2005.

The distribution of the causes of death changed during the posttransplant time in all 3 categories. For the first 3 months, posttransplant cardiocerebrovascular events and infections were the main reason for patient death. Overall, in 11% of deaths the reason was unknown and those were most likely also cardiocerebrovascular accidents. During the next 9 months infections and unknown causes remained the main reason for

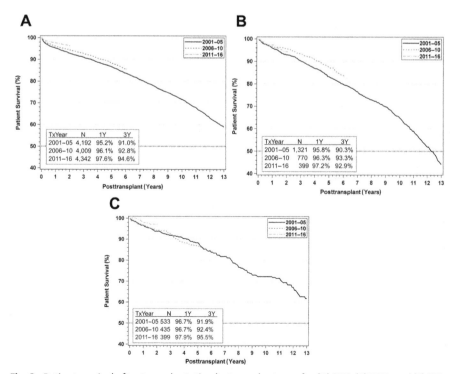

Fig. 2. Patient survival after transplantation by transplant year for (A) SPK, (B) PAK, and (C) PTA.

death. For the next 5 years, cardiocerebrovascular events (CCV) were the main reason, followed by infections. In one-third of all deaths, the reasons were unknown and these may also have been cardiocerebrovascular events. Malignancies made up for 7% of deaths during this time. The distribution of death causes did not change significantly over the analyzed time periods.

The multivariate risk factor analysis for patient survival after transplantation (**Table 4**) showed that losing a pancreas and/or a kidney graft represented the highest

Table 4
Risk factor analysis for patient death after pancreas transplantation performed from 2001 to 2005, 2006 to 2010, and 2011 to 2016

	SPK		PAK		PTA	
	RR (95% CI)	P	RR (95% CI)	P	RR (95% CI)	P
Transplant Year						
2001–2005	1.00	.0002	1.00	.31	1.00	.26
2006–2010	0.83 (0.71–0.97)		0.77 (0.54–1.08)		0.96 (0.59–1.58)	
2011–2016	0.68 (0.56–0.81)		0.86 (9.30–1.13)		0.58 (0.30–1.13)	
Recipient Age						
18–30	1.01 (0.79–1.28)	<.0001	0.91 (0.49–1.68)	.03	2.05 (1.08–3.91)	.005
31–45	1.00		1.00		1.00	
>45	1.65 (1.42–1.92)		1.46 (1.08–1.98)		2.29 (1.37–3.81)	
Recipient Gender						
Female	1.00	.57	1.00	.80	1.00	.67
Male	1.04 (0.90–1.20)		1.04 (0.77–1.40)		1.10 (0.70—1.74)	
Recipient Race						
White	1.00	.52	1.00	.13	1.00	.86
Black	0.96 (0.79–1.16)		1.37 (0.87–2.15)		0.61 (0.18–4.40)	
Hispanic	0.83 (0.64–1.07)		0.50 (0.23–1.08)		0.54 (0.17–3.94)	
Other	1.05 (0.71–1.55)		—		—	
Diabetes						
Type 1DM	0.99 (0.78–1.28)	.98	1.29 (0.63–2.66)	.51	0.44 (0.19–1.03)	.08
Type 2DM	1.00		1.00		1.00	
PreTx Dialysis						
No	1.0	.0001	—		—	—
Yes	1.38 (1.17–1.63)		—		—	
Pancreas Status						
Function	1.00	<.0001	1.00	<.0001	1.00	<.0001
Failed	2.56 (2.15–3.04)		2.15 (1.51–3.04)		3.65 (2.18–6.11)1.00	
Kidney Status						
Function	1.00	<.0001	1.00	<.0001	—	—
Failed	10.38 (8.63–12.49)		13.48 (8.69–20.90)		—	
Kidney Donor Type						
Living	—	—	1.00	.03	—	—
Deceased	—		1.46 (1.04–1.90)		—	
Center Volume						
Low	1.00	.12	1.00	.79	1.00	.59
Medium	0.75 (0.57–0.99)		0.82 (0.44–1.50)		1.63 (0.54–4.90)	
High	0.80 (0.62–1.03)		0.88 (0.50–1.54)		1.71 (0.61–4.77)	

relative risk to die. Losing a kidney was more life-threatening than losing the pancreas in SPK and in PAK.

Older recipient age at transplant was a risk factor. The relative risk to die increased with growing age in SPK and PAK. In PTA, the relative risk to die was also increased in pancreas transplant recipients younger than the age of 30 years. This is the group of patients with very brittle diabetes who have a high cardiocerebrovascular risk to die. In SPK, being on dialysis pretransplant increased the relative risk to die by 40%. In a separate analysis it could be shown that the relative risk to die increased by 9% for every year on dialysis.

Having received a previous living donor versus a deceased donor kidney in PAK decreased the relative risk to die. Having a deceased donor kidney raised the relative risk by 46%.

Diabetes type, recipient gender and race, and center volume did not significantly affect patient survival. The significant improvement of patient survival over time could only be verified by the multivariate analyses for SPK but not for the solitary transplants.

Graft Function

SPK pancreas graft function improved over the analyzed time significantly 1-year (3-year) to 89.9% (83.4%) from 2011 to 2016 (**Fig. 3**A). The improvement in pancreas graft function between the periods of 2001 to 2005 and 2005 to 2010 did not reach statistical significance ($P = .16$) but the progress between the periods of 2006 to 2010 and 2011 to 2016 was significant ($P = .001$). Ten-year SPK pancreas graft function reached 56.6% for 2001 to 2005 transplants. SPK kidney graft function improved accordingly (**Fig. 3**B). As in SPK transplantation, the significant changes happened between the periods of 2006 to 2010 and 2011 to 2016 ($P = .003$).

As shown in the figures, the most critical time for graft loss is the first year posttransplant. When only the SPK transplants were analyzed that reached the first year mark with a functioning graft, 3-year pancreas graft function reached greater than 92% and no difference could be found between the different time periods ($P = .17$). For SPK kidney graft function with greater than 1-year graft function in all 3 time periods, the outcome at 3 years was 93.5% and no differences between the time periods were noted ($P = .55$).

Overall, PAK pancreas graft function improved from period to period ($P<.0001$) (**Fig. 3**C) but only the progress between the periods of 2001 to 2005 and 2006 to 2010 reached statistical significance ($P = .01$) for the pairwise comparison. If only PAK were analyzed with pancreas graft function at 1 year, no statistical difference for the time periods could be found but the long-term outcome increased.

PTA pancreas function increased over time ($P = .004$) (**Fig 3**D). The significant improvement for the pairwise comparisons was between the periods of 2001 to 2005 and 2011 to 2016. The improvement remained significant when only PTA transplants with at least 1 year of graft function were analyzed. From 2011 to 2016, 3-year graft function reached 85.1% for those cases.

In all 3 categories, technical failures were the main reason for pancreas graft loss during the first 3 months, with greater than 70% of all losses followed by patient death. During the next 9 months the main reason for graft failure was patient death, especially in PAK and SPK, followed by immunologic losses and infections. In solitary transplants, immunologic pancreas graft losses were significantly higher compared with SPK. After the first year, immunologic graft loss remained the main reason for failure of SPK and PAK, followed by patient death. In PTA, the main reason remained immunologic graft loss.

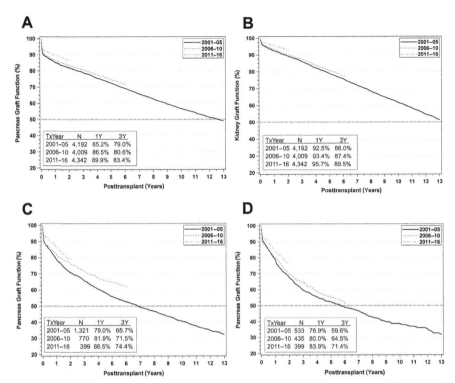

Fig. 3. Graft function by transplant year for (A) SPK pancreas, (B) SPK kidney, (C) PAK, and (D) PTA.

The results of the multivariate risk analyses for graft failure are shown in **Table 5**. In SPK, the main risk factors for graft failure were young age, black race, a body mass index of greater than 30 kg/m², older donor age, and longer preservation time. The use of induction therapy and a maintenance protocol based on Tac in combination with MMF decreased the relative risk of graft loss. Higher volume centers had a lower graft loss rate. For SPK, the relative risk for kidney graft loss was significantly lower when the pancreas was enteric-drained and not bladder-drained. The progress could be verified by the model with decreasing risk over time.

For PAK, younger recipient and older donor ages were the main risk factors for graft loss. Induction therapy and standard maintenance immunosuppression significantly lowered the relative risk. High-volume centers had better outcomes and the progress over time was confirmed.

For PTA, younger recipient age was the most influential factor, with an increased relative risk of greater than 2.0%. A maintenance protocol that was not based on tacrolimus in combination with MMF, or on sirolimus (SRL), also increased the relative risk of graft failure significantly. No significant improvement over time and no impact of center volume could be detected.

Technical Failures

Technical failure of the pancreas graft was a major problem in all 3 categories over the analyzed time (**Table 6**). It dropped in all 3 categories between the periods of 2001 to 2005 and 2011 to 2016, but this improvement was only significant in SPK and PAK. In

Table 5
Risk analysis for pancreas and kidney graft failure for transplants performed from 2001 to 2005, 2006 to 2010, and 2011 to 2016

	SPK				PAK		PTA	
	Pancreas		Kidney					
	RR (95% CI)	P	RR (95% CI)	P	RR (95% CI)	P	RR (95% CI)	P
Era								
2001–2005	1.00	.008	1.00	.01	1.00	.007	1.00	.34
2006–10	0.92 (0.82–1.02)		0.97 (0.89–1.08)		0.76 (0.64–0.91)		1.13 (0.89–1.44)	
2011–2016	0.83 (0.74–0.93)		0.82 (0.71–0.94)		0.76 (0.59–0.98)		0.94 (0.70–1.249)	
Recipient Age (y)								
18–29	1.26 (1.10–1.44)	.002	1.64 (1.45–1.86)	<.0001	1.58 (1.22–2.08)	.0002	2.04 (1.58–2.62)	<.0001
30–44	1.00		1.00		1.00		1.00	
>45	0.98 (0.89–1.08)		1.09 (0.92–1.27)		0.89 (0.76–1.05)		0.83 (0.69–1.05)	
Recipient Gender								
Female	1.00	.19	1.00	.004	1.00	.60	1.00	.13
Male	0.94 (0.87–1.03)		0.90 (0.83–0.97)		0.96 (0.83–1.11)		0.85 (0.62–0.97)	
Recipient Race								
White	1.00	.003	1.00	<.0001	1.00	.19	1.00	.65
Black	1.15 (1.03–1.28)		1.37 (1.24–1.50)		1.12 (0.87–1.43)		1.18 (0.70–2.00)	
Hispanic	0.86 (0.73–1.01)		0.84 (0.73–0.97)		1.02 (0.77–1.36)		—	
Other	1.15 (0.90–1.49)		1.18 (0.94–1.48)		0.46 (0.17–1.05)		—	
Recipient Bod Mass Index								
<30	1.00	<.0001	1.00	.0004	1.00	.74	1.00	.44
≥30	1.48 (1.31–1.67)		1.21 (1.09–1.35)		1.09 (0.90–1.36)		1.13 (0.83–1.51)	
Diabetes								
Type 1	0.96 (0.82–1.11)	.55	1.04 (0.91–1.18)	.61	1.42 (0.96–2.12)	.08	1.35 (0.76–2.41)	.16
Type 2	1.00		1.00		1.00		1.00	
PRA								
<20%	1.00	.28	1.00	.65	1.00	.40	1.00	.55
≥20%	1.08 (0.94–1.25)		1.05 (0.88–1.27)		1.12 (0.86–1.47)		1.10 (0.81–1.49)	

(continued on next page)

Table 5
(continued)

	SPK				PAK		PTA	
	Pancreas		Kidney					
	RR (95% CI)	P	RR (95% CI)	P	RR (95% CI)	P	RR (95% CI)	P
Donor Age (y)								
<15	0.94 (0.81–1.10)	<.0001	1.10 (0.97–1.25)	<.0001	1.09 (0.87–1.38)	.003	0.89 (0.66–1.21)	.48
16–30	1.00		1.00		1.00		1.00	
≥31	1.44 (1.32–1.58)		1.32 (1.09–1.59)		1.34 (1.13–1.58)		1.17 (0.93–1.47)	
Preservation Time (h)								
0–<12	1.00	.001	1.00	.17	1.00	.64	1.00	.30
12–<24	1.11 (0.99–1.24)		1.03 (0.96–1.11)		1.06 (0.87–1.28)		0.81 (0.61–1.06)	
24+	1.50 (1.18–1.90)		1.22 (0.99–1.50)		0.98 (0.80–1.20)		0.86 (0.66–1.13)	
Duct Management								
Bladder Drainage	1.00	.30	1.00	.001	1.00	.31	1.00	.04
Enteric Drainage	1.08 (0.94–1.24)		0.84 (0.75–0.93)		1.11 (0.91–1.34)		0.77 (0.61–0.99)	
Induction								
None	1.0	.10	1.0	.007	1.00	.009	1.00	.40
Nondepleting AB	0.90 (0.77–1.05)		0.81 (0.72–0.91)		0.91 (0.75–1.18)		1.25 (0.75–2.04)	
Depleting AB	0.88 (0.79–0.99)		0.89 (0.81–0.99)		0.75 (0.63–0.90)		1.16 (0.84–1.58)	
Both	1.06 (0.84–1.34)		0.95 (0.78–1.15)		0.66 (0.45–0.96)		1.47 (0.93–2.32)	
Maintenance Protocol								
Tac&MMF	0.98 (0.87–1.11)	<.0001	1.00 (0.89–1.12)	<.0001	1.00 (0.81–1.25)	.004	0.91 (0.65–1.20)	<.0001
Tac&MMF&Steroids	1.00		1.00		1.00		1.00	
Srl-Based	1.03 (0.96–1.27)		1.30 (1.13–1.49)		0.87 (0.68–1.10)		0.98 (0.73–1.31)	
Other	1.46 (1.28–1.68)		1.29 (1.14–1.45)		1.37 (1.12–1.67)		2.80 (2.14–3.66)	
Center Volume								
Low	1.00	<.0001	1.00	.02	1.00	.02	1.00	.29
Medium	0.79 (0.68–0.95)		0.89 (0.71–0.99)		0.74 (0.56–0.98)		0.65 (0.36–1.18)	
High	0.70 (0.59–0.82)		0.87 (0.79–0.96)		0.77 (0.52–0.89)		0.63 (0.36–1.08)	

Table 6
Technical failures in pancreas transplantation performed from 2001 to 2005, 2006 to 2010, and 2011 to 2016

	SPK				PAK				PTA			
	2001–2005	2006–2009	2011–2016	P	2001–2005	2006–2009	2011–2016	P	2001–2005	2006–2009	2011–2016	P
Technical Failure Rate (%)	6.7	7.0	5.6	.03	8.4	9.8	5.7	.03	7.5	9.2	6.1	.24
Graft Thrombosis (%)	4.6	4.7	4.2	—	5.9	7.7	4.4	—	5.2	7.3	4.9	—
Infection (%)	0.7	0.4	0.3		1.3	0.3	0.3		0.4	0.2	0.2	
Pancreatitis (%)	0.5	0.4	0.2		0.2	0.7	0.2		0.8	0.5	0.2	
Anastomotic Leak (%)	0.3	0.4	0.4		0.1	0.4	0.2		0.4	0.5	0.2	
Bleeding (%)	0.2	0.3	0.1		0.4	0.1	0.2		0.7	0.5	0.2	
Other (%)	0.4	0.8	0.4		0.5	0.7	0.4		0.0	0.2	0.4	

all 3 categories, pancreas graft thrombosis remained the major cause of technical failure, whereas the other factors accounted for only a small percentage of technical problems.

In SPK, the main risk factors for technical failure were donor age older than 30 years, increased preservation time over 12 hours, and the recipient being obese or on dialysis pretransplant. Centers with higher transplant volume showed a significantly lower relative risk for technical failure. The model could not confirm significant changes over time. Maintenance immunosuppression remained a risk factor for technical failure, which is most likely a sign that immunologic losses were falsely reported as technical losses.

In PAK, donor age older than 30 years and low center volume were the factors that significantly affected technical graft loss. Induction and maintenance therapy reached significance that again pointed to wrongly reported causes of graft loss. All other factors in the model did not reach significance.

In PTA, the transplant period reached significance with an increasing relative risk of technical failure over time. Recipient and donor age, as well as preservation time, did not show a statistically significant impact on technical failure owing to good donor selection. As in SPK and PAK, induction and maintenance therapy reached significance.

Immunologic Graft Loss

The immunologic graft loss for the SPK pancreas and kidney (**Fig. 4**A, B) significantly improved over time for the pancreas ($P = .0004$) but not for the kidney ($P = .45$). The improvement for the pancreas could be found between the outcomes of the periods of

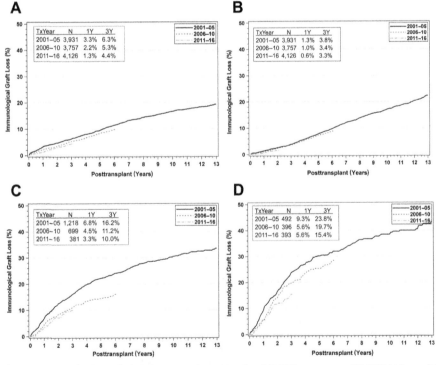

Fig. 4. Immunologic graft loss by transplant year for (A) SPK pancreas, (B) SPK kidney, (C) PAK, (D) PTA.

2001 to 2005 and 2011 to 2016. The immunologic loss was initially much lower for the SPK kidney but, over time, the differences between the 2 grafts shrunk. Of interest was the constantly ascending slope of the rate of kidney losses.

More impressive was the development in PAK (**Fig. 4C**). Here, a highly significant improvement in the reduction of immunologic loss was noted ($P<.0001$). The decrease in immunologic losses was between the periods of 2001 to 2005 and 2006 to 2010. No further progress could be found later on. In PAK, the initial slope of immunologic graft loss was steep but it slightly leveled off later on.

Immunologic pancreas graft loss remained a problem in PTA (see **Fig. 4C**). A significant reduction of the immunologic loss was found between the periods of 2001 to 2005 and 2011 to 2016. As in PAK, the slope was initially steep but then slightly decreased.

Table 7 shows the risk analysis for immunologic pancreas and pancreas-kidney graft loss in technically successful transplants. In all 3 categories, and in the SPK kidney, the relative risk of immunologic graft loss in recipients younger than the age of 30 years was significantly increased.

In SPK, black recipients and recipients receiving an organ from an older donor had a significantly higher relative risk of losing both of their grafts. Male recipients showed a significantly lower relative risk of losing their kidney but not their pancreas graft. For both organs, a treatment of an acute rejection episode during the first year posttransplant was a significant risk factor, more than doubling the risk of graft loss. Maintenance protocols were important for the pancreas but not for the kidney graft. HLA mismatching and center volume did not significantly affect immunologic loss in SPK. The decline in immunologic losses over time was significant for the pancreas but not for the kidney.

In PAK, a significantly increased risk in recipients with a panel reactive antibody (PRA) level greater than 20% and an HLA-A antigen mismatch could be found. Treatment of an acute rejection episode during the first year also increased the relative risk significantly. The overall use of induction therapy could lower the relative risk significantly compared with no induction therapy at all. The decline of immunologic loss over time was also significant in the multivariate model.

Male recipients showed a significantly lower relative risk for immunologic graft in PTA. Besides the increased risk in younger recipients only treatment of an acute rejection episode during the first year reached significance and more than doubling the relative risk of pancreas loss. The changes in immunologic graft loss were not significant over time.

Comparison of Recent Category Outcomes

Fig. 5 shows patient survival for the 3 transplant categories over the first 3 years for the years from 2011 to 2016. The outcome is not statistically significant between the 3 categories but, as expected, the highest patient survival rate could be observed in PTA and the lowest in PAK. **Fig. 6** shows the graft function of the pancreas and pancreas categories and the simultaneous kidney over the same transplant years. The best function could be seen in the SPK kidney; however, when the initial technical problems were eliminated, the SPK kidney and pancreas grafts were almost identical. The outcome of solitary transplants was equal to that of the SPK pancreas during the first 6 months but then dropped. PAK graft function improved over PTA graft function but the difference was not significant ($P = .67$). The differences in long-term graft function were mainly due to the differences in immunologic graft loss (**Fig. 7**). Although the difference between SPK kidney and pancreas was small, the immunologic graft loss of the solitary grafts was significantly higher. The pairwise comparison of the

Table 7
Risk analysis for immunologic pancreas and kidney graft loss for technically successful transplants performed from 2001 to 2005, 2006 to 2010, and 2011 to 2016

| | Pancreas | | SPK | | | | | |
| | | | Kidney | | PAK | | PTA | |
	RR (95% CI)	P	RR (95% CI)	P	RR (95% CI)	P	RR (95% CI)	P
Era								
2001–2005	1.00	.01	1.00	.48	1.00	.001	1.00	.29
2006–10	0.83 (0.68–1.00)		0.91 (0.74–1.15)		0.62 (0.46–0.83)		0.95 (0.68–1.33)	
2011–2016	0.71 (0.56–0.90)		0.85 (0.66–1.11)		0.58 (0.38–0.88)		0.73 (0.48–1.10)	
Recipient Age (y)								
18–29	1.62 (1.30–2.02)	<.0001	1.90 (1.51–2.38)	<.0001	1.63 (1.12–2.36)	<.0001	2.40 (1.74–3.31)	<.0001
30–44	1.00		1.00		1.00		1.00	
>45	0.61 (0.49–0.75)		0.58 (0.45–0.75)		0.64 (0.49–0.84)		0.58 (0.41–0.82)	
Recipient Gender								
Female	1.00	.25	1.00	<.0001	1.00	.16	1.00	.02
Male	0.91 (0.76–1.07)		0.69 (0.57–0.83)		0.85 (0.67–1.07)		0.71 (0.53–0.95)	
Recipient Race								
White	1.00	.0004	1.00	<.0001	1.00	.22	1.00	.84
Black	1.43 (1.17–1.75)		2.29 (1.86–2.82)		1.25 (0.86–1.81)		1.26 (0.58–2.73)	
Hispanic	0.78 (0.56–1.07)		1.21 (0.87–1.67)		0.99 (0.63–1.55)		1.16 (0.55–2.43)	
Other	1.30 (0.80–2.12)		1.67 (0.99–2.82)		—		—	
PRA								
<20%	1.00	.94	1.00	.22	1.00	.008	1.00	.96
≥20%	1.01 (0.76–1.35)		1.20 (0.89–1.62)		1.69 (1.15–2.49)		1.01 (0.66–1.56)	
Donor Age (y)								
<15	0.96 (0.72–1.29)	.002	0.97 (0.70–1.34)	.05	1.46 (1.04–2.04)	.06	1.11 (0.74–1.65)	.82
16–30	1.00		1.00		1.00		1.00	
31–45	1.37 (1.14–1.63)		1.27 (1.04–1.56)		1.23 (0.94–1.61)		0.96 (0.68–1.33)	

	HR (95% CI)	P	HR (95% CI)	P	HR (95% CI)	P	HR (95% CI)	P
HLA An MM								
0,1	1.00		1.00		1.00		1.00	
2	1.02 (0.87–1.21)	.79	1.07 (0.89–1.29)	.45	1.26 (1.06–1.49)	.003	0.92 (0.69–1.23)	.59
HLA B MM								
0,1	1.00		1.00		1.00		1.00	
2	0.89 (0.75–1.06)	.20	1.09 (0.88–1.34)	.44	1.43 (1.13–1.80)	.28	0.86 (0.67–1.10)	.25
HLA DR MM								
0,1	1.00		1.00		1.00		1.00	
2	1.13 (0.95–1.33)	.16	1.10 (0.91–1.32)	.35	1.14 (0.89–1.46)	.71	1.10 (0.83–1.46)	.49
Duct Management								
Bladder Drainage	1.00		1.00		1.00		1.00	
Eenteric Drainage	0.95 (0.73–1.24)	.70	0.59 (0.45–0.76)	<.0001	1.05 (0.83–1.32)	.74	0.84 (0.59–1.18)	.33
Induction								
None	1.00	.16	1.00	.07	1.00	.13	1.00	.93
NonDepl. AB	0.77 (0.58–1.03)		0.66 (0.47–0.92)		1.30 (0.87–1.95)		1.22 (0.61–2.45)	
Depl. Ab	0.93 (0.75–1.16)		0.91 (0.72–1.16)		0.92 (0.67–1.24)		1.03 (0.67–1.59)	
Both	0.63 (0.36–1.10)		0.73 (0.42–1.27)		0.71 (0.38–1.30)		1.13 (0.59–2.16)	
Maintenance Protocol								
TAC&MMF	0.86 (0.67–1.10)	.03	0.93 (0.71–1.21)	.86	1.07 (0.78–1.51)	.04	1.04 (0.72–1.52)	.12
TAC&MMF&Steroids	1.00		1.00		1.00		1.00	
SRL-Based	0.93 (0.70–1.23)		0.98 (0.72–1.33)		0.84 (0.58–1.22)		1.08 (0.72–1.63)	
Other	1.40 (1.08–1.83)		1.10 (0.80–1.53)		1.46 (1.08–1.98)		1.67 (1.09–2.55)	
Acute Rejection Treatment								
No	1.00	.0001	1.00	.0001	1.00	<.0001	1.00	<.0001
Yes	2.59 (2.15–3.10)		2.92 (2.38–3.55)		2.49 (1.92–3.23)		2.47 (1.83–3.33)	
Center Volume								
Low	1.00	.53	1.00	.67	1.00	.82	1.00	.29
Medium	1.17 (0.77–1.76)		0.84 (0.56–1.25)		0.86 (0.52–1.41)		0.56 (0.26–1.20)	
High	1.23 (0.84–1.81)		0.89 (0.61–1.29)		0.87 (0.54–1.38)		0.60 (0.30–1.17)	

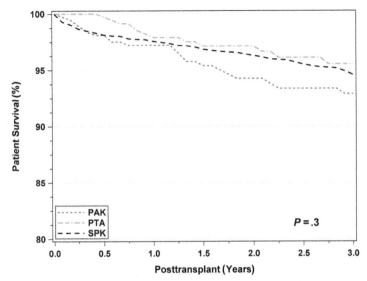

Fig. 5. Patient survival for primary deceased donor transplants performed between 2011 and 2016.

immunologic graft loss in all 3 categories was highly significant. The immunologic graft loss in PTA was significantly higher compared with the loss in PAK.

DISCUSSION

A plethora of literature exists that demonstrates the advantage of whole pancreas transplantation in comparison with other treatment options in patients with brittle diabetes and/or endstage renal disease.[2,3] Currently, it is the best short-term and

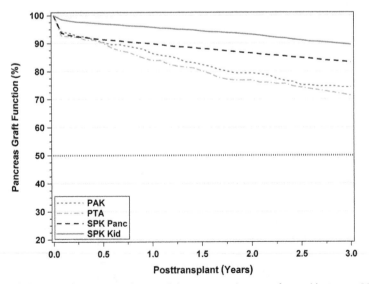

Fig. 6. Graft function for primary deceased donor transplants performed between 2011 and 2016. Kid, kidney; Panc, pancreas.

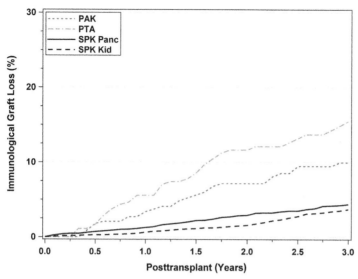

Fig. 7. Immunologic graft loss for primary deceased donor transplants performed between 2011 and 2016.

long-term treatment to achieve insulin-independence and good metabolic control, and may be help avoid, ameliorate, or even reverse secondary diabetic complications.[4–6] Regardless of this progress, the number of transplants declined significantly until 2015 and only in 2016, for the first time, was some recuperation of numbers noted. Of particular concern is the drop of PAK during this time period.[7,8] A PAK transplant offers the diabetic patient the opportunity to receive a living or deceased kidney to correct uremia and, subsequently, a solitary pancreas transplant. PAK had, on average, the oldest recipients and the mortality was the highest. The recipients had already undergone at least 1 transplant and represented, therefore, a population at high risk. Nevertheless, the outcome of PAK did not reach that of SPK but the gap is closing. PAK can be a life-preserving procedure because it avoids long-term dialysis and corrects the diabetes later on.[9] A kidney transplant alone would only correct the secondary diabetic complication of renal failure but not the underlying problem. A recurrence of diabetic nephropathy can be detected some years after posttransplant.[10] Despite the progress, many centers stopped performing PAK transplants and now only offer kidney transplant alone or SPK.

The number of PTA remained relatively stable over the analyzed time period. The outcome improved significantly in this population with severe brittle diabetes. Patient survival was the highest compared with the other categories. This shows that early correction of metabolic control with transplantation can be life-saving. Therefore, a solitary transplant should be considered early on before the patient develops end-stage renal disease.[11,12] There is still a reluctance to consider pancreas transplantation without the development of more severe diabetic secondary complications because many physicians still believe that exogenous insulin administration outweighs the surgical risk and the risk of long-term immunosuppression.

Most pancreas transplants were performed in combination with a kidney graft and here the outcomes improved significantly and the numbers increased in 2016 after a drastic decline.[13,14] When technical problems were excluded, SPK pancreas and kidney graft functions showed comparable outcome.

While the numbers were declining, the characteristics of recipients and donors were also changing. The median recipient age increased, most likely because of lower immunologic risk; however, with older age the likelihood of death could also increase. More patients with type 2 diabetes received a pancreas transplant and the number of black recipients increased. Black patients represented a larger proportion of type 2 than type 1 diabetics.[15] With the overall weight change in the US population, the weight at transplant also increased, which represented another technical risk factor.

The pancreas donor quality improved significantly with decreased age and more male donors, and trauma was more often reported as cause of death.[16] The pancreas preservation time dropped significantly with the decrease in transplant numbers.

Over the analyzed time period, a standardization of pancreas transplantation seemed to occur. Most transplant surgeons used enteric drainage and the use of the more physiologic portal drainage declined. Most recipients received induction therapy with depleting antibodies, and a maintenance protocol of tacrolimus with MMF. The use of steroid-free maintenance protocols increased between the periods from 2001 to 2005 and 2006 to 2010; however, from 2011 to 2016 the use of steroids increased again.

With the decline in transplants, the number of centers remained relatively stable but the center volume declined significantly. This had an effect on graft outcome[17,18] but not on patient survival. This will affect the education of future transplant surgeons. More and more centers perform only 1 to 2 pancreas transplants a year, and transplant fellows see fewer pancreas transplants.

With changes in recipient, donor, and transplant factors, an improvement in patient survival, graft function, and immunologic graft loss was noted. Patient survival at 3 years posttransplant reached greater than 93%, pancreas graft function in SPK was greater than 83% (SPK kidney >89%), and solitary pancreas graft was greater than 70%. These facts about pancreas transplantation should be brought out of the specialist's realm, informing physicians about those achievements so that they are better equipped to refer suitable patients for transplantation, and to manage, counsel, and support them when encountered within their own specialty.[19]

REFERENCES

1. Center for Disease Control and Prevention. National Diabetes Statistics Report, 2017. Atlanta (GA): Center for Disease Control and Prevention, U.S. Dept of Health and Human Services; 2017.
2. Bonner KP, Kudva YC, Stegall MD, et al. Should we be performing more pancreas transplants? Clin Transplant 2015;31:173–80.
3. Dean PG, Kukla A, Stegall MD, et al. Pancreas transplantation. BMJ 2017;357.
4. Dunn TB. Life after pancreas transplantation: reversal of diabetic lesions. Curr Opin Organ Transplant 2014;19(1):73–9.
5. Boggi U, Rosati CM, Marchetti P. Follow-up of secondary diabetic complications after pancreas transplantation. Curr Opin Organ Transplant 2013;18(1):102–10.
6. Lombardo C, Perrone VG, Amorese G, et al. Update on pancreatic transplantation on the management of diabetes. Minerva Med 2017;108(5):405–18.
7. Fridell JA, Mangus RS, Hollinger EF, et al. The case for pancreas after kidney transplantation. Clin Transplant 2009;23(4):447–53.
8. Kaufman DB. Pancreas-after-kidney transplantation: to have and not have not. Clin Transplant 2009;23(4):435–6.
9. Kleinclauss F, Fauda M, Sutherland DE, et al. Pancreas after living donor kidney transplants in diabetic patients: impact on long-term kidney graft function. Clin Transplant 2009;23(4):437–46.

10. Barbosa J, Steffes MW, Sutherland DE, et al. Effect of glycemic control on early diabetic renal lesions. A 5-year randomized controlled clinical trial of insulin-dependent diabetic kidney transplant recipients. JAMA 1994;272(8):600–6.
11. Niederhaus SV. Pancreas transplant alone. Curr Opin Organ Transpl 2015;20(1): 115–20.
12. Gruessner RW, Gruessner AC. Pancreas transplant alone: a procedure coming of age. Diabetes Care 2013;36(8):2440–7.
13. Stratta RJ, Fridell JA, Gruessner AC, et al. Pancreas transplantation: a decade of decline. Curr Opin Organ Transplant 2016;21(4):386–92.
14. Stratta RJ, Gruessner AC, Odorico JS, et al. Pancreas transplantation: an alarming crisis in confidence. Am J Transplant 2016;16(9):2556–62.
15. Gruessner AC, Laftavi MR, Pankewycz O, et al. Simultaneous pancreas and kidney transplantation-is it a treatment option for patients with type 2 diabetes mellitus? An analysis of the international pancreas transplant registry. Curr Diab Rep 2017;17(6):44.
16. Maglione M, Ploeg RJ, Friend PJ. Donor risk factors, retrieval technique, preservation and ischemia/reperfusion injury in pancreas transplantation. Curr Opin Organ Transplant 2013;18(1):83–8.
17. Alhamad T, Malone AF, Brennan DC, et al. Transplant center volume and the risk of pancreas allograft failure. Transplantation 2017;101(11):2757–64.
18. Kim Y, Dhar VK, Wima K, et al. The center volume-outcome effect in pancreas transplantation: a national analysis. J Surg Res 2017;213:25–31.
19. Dholakia S, Mittal S, Quiroga I, et al. Pancreas transplantation: past, present, future. Am J Med 2016;129(7):667–73.

Robotic Pancreas Transplantation

Mario Spaggiari, MD[a],*, Ivo G. Tzvetanov, MD[b], Caterina Di Bella, MD[c],
Jose Oberholzer, MD[d]

KEYWORDS

- Robotic transplant • Pancreas transplantation • Diabetes • Obesity
- Surgical-site infection

KEY POINTS

- Obesity is considered a relative contraindication to pancreas transplantation.
- The minimally invasive approach reduces wound-related complications and surgical-site infections.
- This approach offers an extended indication for pancreas transplantation to obese type 2 diabetic patients with suppressed C-peptide.

BACKGROUND AND INDICATIONS

Along with the increasing incidence of type 1 diabetes,[1] the prevalence of obesity in this population is escalating.[2] Outcomes after pancreas transplantation in select type 1 diabetic patients are excellent,[3] but can be burdened by significant complications that are more commonly observed in obese recipients.[4] Consequently, obesity is considered a relative contraindication to pancreas transplantation, because of an overall increase in surgical and wound-related complications, which increase risk of graft loss.[5–8] Moreover, the indication for pancreas transplantation has been extended to include selected, nonobese type 2 diabetic patients or obese diabetic patients with suppressed C-peptide. Among recipients of simultaneous pancreas-kidney transplants (SPK), the proportion of type 2 diabetic patients increased 4-fold from 1994 to 2010.[9]

Disclosure Statement: The authors have nothing to disclose.
[a] Department of Surgery, Division of Transplantation, University of Illinois at Chicago, 840 South Wood Street, Clinical Sciences Building, Suite 503, Chicago, IL 60612, USA; [b] Department of Surgery, Division of Transplantation, University of Illinois at Chicago, 840 South Wood Street, Clinical Sciences Building, Suite 520, Chicago, IL 60612, USA; [c] Department of Surgery, Division of Transplantation, University of Illinois at Chicago, 840 South Wood Street, Clinical Sciences Building, Suite 522, Chicago, IL 60612, USA; [d] Department of Surgery, Division of Transplantation, University of Virginia, Health System, Transplant Center, 1300 Jefferson Park Avenue, Fourth Floor, Charlottesville, VA 22903, USA
* Corresponding author.
E-mail address: mspaggia@uic.edu

Gastroenterol Clin N Am 47 (2018) 443–448
https://doi.org/10.1016/j.gtc.2018.01.010
0889-8553/18/© 2018 Elsevier Inc. All rights reserved.

As always, the dilemma persists in optimizing utility while ensuring equity access to organ transplantation. Lynch and colleagues[6] observed that although obese kidney transplantation recipients experienced surgical site infections and related graft and patient loss, those who did not present wound complications maintained comparable patient and graft outcomes as those with normal body mass index (BMI). Fridell and colleagues[10] found that the 1-year patient and graft survival was comparable between obese and nonobese pancreas recipients. More recently, Laurence and colleagues[4] reported that obese pancreas recipients with well-controlled cardiovascular risk have comparable survival outcomes but still have a significantly higher risk of wound-related complications and early rejection as compared with nonobese pancreas recipients. Therefore, organ transplantation in well-selected obese patients seems to be a worthy and reasonable pursuit; however, in this patient population, strategies that effectively reduce wound-related complications require further development to mitigate these increased risks. Minimally invasive approaches can reduce wound-related complications. With the availability of robotic assistance, more technically demanding procedures can be safely performed in a minimally invasive manner.

At the University of Illinois at Chicago, the authors performed the initial series of robotic-assisted pancreas transplantation in patients with type 1 and 2 diabetes, and they hypothesize that this novel approach could extend the acceptable BMI range.

SURGICAL TECHNIQUE

During the donor procurement, particular attention must be given to ligate all the small vascular tributaries to the pancreas in order to prevent bleeding at the time of reperfusion. Warm dissection of the entire organ should be favored for this purpose.

The benching of the transplant graft is performed as follows: the spleen is removed first; the root of the mesentery stump is oversewn with 4.0 Prolene; the proximal duodenal stump is oversewn with 4.0 Prolene. Then, the stump of the superior mesenteric artery and splenic artery are reconstructed with a "Y" iliac artery graft from the same donor. In order to minimize post-reperfusion bleeding, the organ is flushed with a solution of 1 L of University of Wisconsin Solution and methylene blue to address any visible leaking points.

Positioning of the patient and trocars placements are as illustrated in **Fig. 1**. In the case of SPK, the robotic cart has to be redocked after the pancreas transplant is completed, and symmetric contralateral ports for the robotic arms must be placed to the other side. Usually the pancreas goes to the left iliac fossa, whereas kidney goes to the right iliac fossa.

The patient is placed in a seated position with Yellofins stirrup devices and then tilted into steep Trendelenburg position. For insertion of the organs and hand assistance, a 7-cm supraumbilical midline incision is performed, and a GelPort is used. The rest of the trocars placement is as described in **Fig. 1**.

The authors have chosen to place the pancreas graft into the left iliac fossa with the head facing caudal for dorsal alignment of the portal vein with the left external iliac vein, and ventral alignment of the arterial Y-graft with the external iliac artery.

After mobilizing the descending colon, the left external iliac vessels are mobilized under appropriate hemostasis and lymphostasis. Bulldog vascular clamps are applied robotically during the anastomosis time. The implantation starts by performing the portal to iliac vein anastomosis in an end-to-side fashion with 5-0 expanded polytetrafluoroethylene suture. The arterial anastomosis between the Y-graft and the common iliac artery is performed in the same manner **(Fig. 2)**.

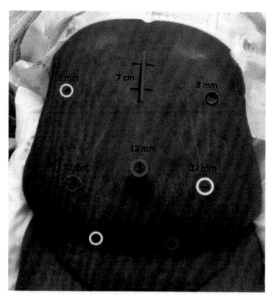

Fig. 1. Trocars position: 8-mm ports for the robotic arms; 12-mm ports for the laparoscopic assistance and robotic camera (*red*) and for the GelPort device (*red line*). ⬤: Pancreas transplant. ⬤: Kidney transplant.

The anastomosis between the donor duodenum and recipient ileum is performed with an EEA circular stapler (Covidien, Mansfield, MA, USA) by inserting the shaft through the GelPort to the fourth duodenum and the spike in a proximal ileum loop (>120 cm from the ileocecal valve). After firing the EEA, the end of the donor duodenum is closed using an Endo GIA (Ethicon Endo-Surgery, Cincinnati, OH, USA) (see **Fig. 2**).

In case the small bowel does not reach easily the graft duodenum, a bladder diversion can be performed. The duodeno-bladder drainage is performed by inserting an EEA circular stapler via the fourth portion of the duodenum. A small incision in the bladder is made to insert the headpiece of the EEA. The authors guide the spike of EEA to protrude from the anterior wall of the second portion of the duodenum. After firing the EEA, the end of the duodenum is closed using the Endo GIA.

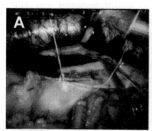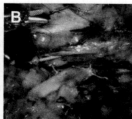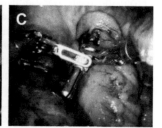

Fig. 2. (*A*) Portal to right external iliac vein anastomosis. (*B*) "Y" graft to external iliac artery completed anastomosis. (*C*) Enteric anastomosis between the second duodenum and the iliac loop: the robotic forceps engaged the spike of the EEA to the headpiece. The assistant at the table fires the stapler from the GelPort.

The technical aspects of the kidney transplant have been previously reported by the authors' group.[11,12]

The edited video of the operation is available if requested by the publisher.

WORLD EXPERIENCE IN ROBOTIC PANCREAS TRANSPLANTATION

From October 2015 to October 2016, 5 morbidly obese patients underwent robotic-assisted pancreas transplantation at the University of Illinois at Chicago. Four were men, and one was a woman. Type 1 diabetes was the underlying disease in 3 cases, and the remaining 2 presented with type 2 diabetes. Two recipients presented with class I obesity, 2 with class II obesity, and one with class III obesity. Preoperatively, the patients required on average 65 units of insulin per day. Three recipients underwent SPK; one patient had a pancreas after kidney transplantation, and one had a pancreas transplantation alone.

In the literature, there is only one series of 3 robotic pancreas transplant cases, reported by Boggi and colleagues.[13] In the experience of Boggi and colleagues, patients had normal BMI, whereas the authors clearly advocate the use of a minimally invasive technique to overcome the obesity-related surgical complications related to the access. Boggi and colleagues applied the vascular clamps manually through the GelPort, whereas the authors applied it robotically. Also, Boggi and colleagues performed the duodenal drainage manually through the GelPort, whereas the authors completed the anastomosis in a minimally invasive fashion with the EEA circular stapler.

COMMENTS

The rationale for performing pancreas transplantation in a minimally invasive fashion is to reduce the risk of access-related postoperative complications, which is more common in obese patients[4] and associated with inferior patient and graft survival following kidney transplantation.[6]

The recent literature about obesity and pancreas transplantation reports comparable outcomes between obese and nonobese recipients.[4,14] Laurence and colleagues[4] in a single-center analysis (368 patients divided by BMI, greater or lower than 30 kg/m^2) reported that the obese population (n = 60) had a higher incidence of wound complications and acute rejection. However, graft and patient survival was comparable between obese and normal weight recipients. Afaneh and colleagues[14] experienced similar results in a single-center study of 139 consecutive pancreas transplants that showed a significant association between higher BMI and perioperative morbidity, but no differences in terms of patient and graft outcome.

From the utility perspective in organ allocation, these recent findings are more encouraging than the results of older single-center studies and of a registry analysis that associated obesity with higher mortality risk and higher risk of graft loss.[15,16]

From the patient perspective, receiving a pancreas-kidney graft is associated with years of life gained, regardless of the BMI,[17] and is likely related to overall improved metabolic control with subsequent reduction in cardiovascular risk profile. The cardiovascular benefit is further supported by studies describing favorable changes such as carotid intima thickness.[18]

Intuitively, the best approach might be to have patients lose weight before transplantation, through either lifestyle changes or bariatric surgery. Medical weight loss has a very low success rate, and long-term results after bariatric surgery are not ideal either. Moreover, it has been reported that the postoperative mortality of bariatric surgery in patients with end-stage renal disease (ESRD; 3.5% at 30 days) is not negligible,[19] and one can reasonably presume that it is even higher in diabetic patients with ESRD.

Consequent to the assumption that type 2 diabetes is mainly due to insulin resistance and to a lesser degree the result of impaired insulin secretion, the utility of pancreas transplantation has been questioned. In reality, the pathogenesis of type 2 diabetes is more complex. The extent of β-cell mass loss impacts the severity of the disease and the type of response to the different treatments, including lifestyle changes and weight loss.[20] When β-cell mass loss reaches the point of no return, such as is often the case in patients with long-standing history of type 2 diabetes and ESRD, β-cell replacement therapy has been shown to restore normoglycemia.[21] There are ample data showing that outcomes after pancreas transplantation are comparable among type 1 and type 2 diabetic recipients.[21,22]

In conclusion, minimally invasive pancreas transplantation in obese patients is a novel strategy that could potentially provide better outcomes for selected insulin-dependent obese recipients.

REFERENCES

1. Patterson CC, Dahlquist GG, Gyurus E, et al. Incidence trends for childhood type 1 diabetes in Europe during 1989-2003 and predicted new cases 2005-20: a multicentre prospective registration study. Lancet 2009;373:2027–33.
2. Conway B, Miller RG, Costacou T, et al. Temporal patterns in overweight and obesity in type 1 diabetes. Diabet Med 2010;27:398–404.
3. Gruessner RW, Gruessner AC. Pancreas transplant alone: a procedure coming of age. Diabetes Care 2013;36:2440–7.
4. Laurence JM, Marquez MA, Bazerbachi F, et al. Optimizing pancreas transplantation outcomes in obese recipients. Transplantation 2015;99:1282–7.
5. Bedat B, Niclauss N, Jannot AS, et al. Impact of recipient body mass index on short-term and long-term survival of pancreatic grafts. Transplantation 2015;99: 94–9.
6. Lynch RJ, Ranney DN, Shijie C, et al. Obesity, surgical site infection, and outcome following renal transplantation. Ann Surg 2009;250:1014–20.
7. Everett JE, Wahoff DC, Statz C, et al. Characterization and impact of wound infection after pancreas transplantation. Arch Surg 1994;129:1310–6 [discussion: 1316–7].
8. Hanish SI, Petersen RP, Collins BH, et al. Obesity predicts increased overall complications following pancreas transplantation. Transplant Proc 2005;37:3564–6.
9. Gruessner AC. 2011 update on pancreas transplantation: comprehensive trend analysis of 25,000 cases followed up over the course of twenty-four years at the International Pancreas Transplant Registry (IPTR). Rev Diabet Stud 2011;8: 6–16.
10. Fridell JA, Mangus RS, Taber TE, et al. Growth of a nation part II: impact of recipient obesity on whole-organ pancreas transplantation. Clin Transplant 2011;25: E366–74.
11. Giulianotti P, Gorodner V, Sbrana F, et al. Robotic transabdominal kidney transplantation in a morbidly obese patient. Am J Transplant 2010;10:1478–82.
12. Oberholzer J, Giulianotti P, Danielson KK, et al. Minimally invasive robotic kidney transplantation for obese patients previously denied access to transplantation. Am J Transplant 2013;13:721–8.
13. Boggi U, Signori S, Vistoli F, et al. Laparoscopic robot-assisted pancreas transplantation: first world experience. Transplantation 2012;93:201–6.

14. Afaneh C, Rich B, Aull MJ, et al. Pancreas transplantation considering the spectrum of body mass indices. Clin Transplant 2011;25:E520–9.
15. Humar A, Ramcharan T, Kandaswamy R, et al. The impact of donor obesity on outcomes after cadaver pancreas transplants. Am J Transplant 2004;4:605–10.
16. Sampaio MS, Reddy PN, Kuo HT, et al. Obesity was associated with inferior outcomes in simultaneous pancreas kidney transplant. Transplantation 2010;89: 1117–25.
17. Wolfe RA, McCullough KP, Schaubel DE, et al. Calculating life years from transplant (LYFT): methods for kidney and kidney-pancreas candidates. Am J Transplant 2008;8:997–1011.
18. Larsen JL, Colling CW, Ratanasuwan T, et al. Pancreas transplantation improves vascular disease in patients with type 1 diabetes. Diabetes Care 2004;27: 1706–11.
19. Modanlou KA, Muthyala U, Xiao H, et al. Bariatric surgery among kidney transplant candidates and recipients: analysis of the United States renal data system and literature review. Transplantation 2009;87:1167–73.
20. Donath MY, Halban PA. Decreased beta-cell mass in diabetes: significance, mechanisms and therapeutic implications. Diabetologia 2004;47:581–9.
21. Wiseman AC, Gralla J. Simultaneous pancreas kidney transplant versus other kidney transplant options in patients with type 2 diabetes. Clin J Am Soc Nephrol 2012;7:656–64.
22. Sampaio MS, Kuo HT, Bunnapradist S. Outcomes of simultaneous pancreas-kidney transplantation in type 2 diabetic recipients. Clin J Am Soc Nephrol 2011;6:1198–206.

Moving?

Make sure your subscription moves with you!

To notify us of your new address, find your **Clinics Account Number** (located on your mailing label above your name), and contact customer service at:

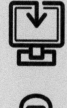

Email: journalscustomerservice-usa@elsevier.com

800-654-2452 (subscribers in the U.S. & Canada)
314-447-8871 (subscribers outside of the U.S. & Canada)

Fax number: 314-447-8029

Elsevier Health Sciences Division
Subscription Customer Service
3251 Riverport Lane
Maryland Heights, MO 63043

*To ensure uninterrupted delivery of your subscription, please notify us at least 4 weeks in advance of move.

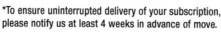
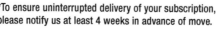

Printed and bound by CPI Group (UK) Ltd, Croydon, CR0 4YY

03/10/2024

01040392-0003